Bipolar Disorder in Youth

Bipolar Disorder in Youth

Presentation, Treatment, and Neurobiology

EDITED BY

Stephen M. Strakowski, MD

Senior Vice President
Strategy & Transformation, UC Health
Professor of Psychiatry & Behavioral Neuroscience
Psychology & BME, UC
University of Cincinnati College of Medicine, Cincinnati, OH

Melissa P. DelBello, MD, MS

Professor of Psychiatry and Pediatrics
Dr. Stanley and Mickey Kaplan Professor and Chair
Department of Psychiatry and Behavioral Neuroscience
University of Cincinnati College of Medicine, Cincinnati, OH

Caleb M. Adler, MD

Professor and Vice-Chair for Clinical Research
Department of Psychiatry and Behavioral Neuroscience
Co-Director, Division of Bipolar Disorders Research
University of Cincinnati College of Medicine, Cincinnati, OH

OXFORD
UNIVERSITY PRESS

OXFORD
UNIVERSITY PRESS

Oxford University Press is a department of the University of
Oxford. It furthers the University's objective of excellence in research,
scholarship, and education by publishing worldwide.

Oxford   New York
Auckland   Cape Town   Dar es Salaam   Hong Kong   Karachi
Kuala Lumpur   Madrid   Melbourne   Mexico City   Nairobi
New Delhi   Shanghai   Taipei   Toronto

With offices in
Argentina   Austria   Brazil   Chile   Czech Republic   France   Greece
Guatemala   Hungary   Italy   Japan   Poland   Portugal   Singapore
South Korea   Switzerland   Thailand   Turkey   Ukraine   Vietnam

Oxford is a registered trademark of Oxford University Press
in the UK and certain other countries.

Published in the United States of America by
Oxford University Press
198 Madison Avenue, New York, NY 10016

Library of Congress Cataloging-in-Publication Data

Bipolar disorder in youth : presentation, treatment, and neurobiology / edited by
Stephen M. Strakowski, Melissa P. DelBello, Caleb M. Adler.
 p. ; cm.
Includes bibliographical references.
ISBN 978–0–19–998535–7 (alk. paper)
 I. Strakowski, Stephen M., editor.   II. DelBello, Melissa P., editor.   III. Adler, Caleb M., editor.
[DNLM: 1. Bipolar Disorder—diagnosis.   2. Bipolar Disorder—therapy.   3. Adolescent.
4. Diagnosis, Differential.   5. Risk Factors.   WM 207]
RC516
616.89′5—dc23
2014019807

This material is not intended to be, and should not be considered, a substitute for medical or
other professional advice. Treatment for the conditions described in this material is highly
dependent on the individual circumstances. And, while this material is designed to offer accurate
information with respect to the subject matter covered and to be current as of the time it was
written, research and knowledge about medical and health issues is constantly evolving and dose
schedules for medications are being revised continually, with new side effects recognized and
accounted for regularly. Readers must therefore always check the product information and
clinical procedures with the most up-to-date published product information and data sheets
provided by the manufacturers and the most recent codes of conduct and safety regulation. The
publisher and the authors make no representations or warranties to readers, express or implied, as
to the accuracy or completeness of this material. Without limiting the foregoing, the publisher
and the authors make no representations or warranties as to the accuracy or efficacy of the drug dosages
mentioned in the material. The authors and the publisher do not accept, and expressly
disclaim, any responsibility for any liability, loss or risk that may be claimed or incurred as a
consequence of the use and/or application of any of the contents of this material.

9 8 7 6 5 4 3 2 1
Printed in the United States of America
on acid-free paper

Contents

SECTION 3.   Neurobiology of Bipolar Disorder
Section Editor: Stephen M. Strakowski

Contributors

Caleb M. Adler, MD
Department of Psychiatry & Behavioral
Neuroscience
University of Cincinnati College of
Medicine
Cincinnati, OH

Michael Berk, MD, PhD
Department of Psychiatry
Deakin University School of
Medicine
Geelong, Australia

Hilary P. Blumberg, MD
Department of Psychiatry
Yale University School of Medicine
New Haven, CT

Katherine E. Burdick, PhD
Departments of Psychiatry and
Neuroscience
Icahn School of Medicine at
Mount Sinai
New York, NY

Gabrielle A. Carlson, MD
Department of Psychiatry
Stony Brook University School of
Medicine
Stony Brook, NY

Kiki D. Chang, MD
Department of Psychiatry and Behavioral
Sciences
Stanford University School of Medicine
Stanford, CA

Alexandra Cottle
Center for Innovation in Pediatric
Practice
The Ohio State University
Columbus, OH

Anne Duffy, MD
Department of Psychiatry
Calgary University
Calgary, Alberta, Canada

Melissa P. DelBello, MD, MS
Department of Psychiatry & Behavioral
Neuroscience
University of Cincinnati College of
Medicine
Cincinnati, OH

Robert L. Findling, MD, MBA
Department of Psychiatry and
Behavioral Sciences
Johns Hopkins University, and
Vice President of Psychiatry Services and
Research
Kennedy Krieger Institute
Baltimore, MD

Barbara L. Gracious, MD
Center for Innovation in Pediatric
Practice
The Research Institute at Nationwide
Children's Hospital
The Ohio State University
Columbus, OH

Sathyan Gurumurthy, MD
Department of Psychiatry
The Ohio State University
Columbus, OH

Peirce Johnston, MD
Department of Psychiatry & Behavioral
Neuroscience
University of Cincinnati College of
Medicine
Cincinnati, OH

Gagan Joshi, MD
Department of Psychiatry
Massachusetts General Hospital
Boston, MA

Ellen Leibenluft, MD
Section on Bipolar Spectrum Disorders
Emotion and Development
National Institute of Mental Health
Bethesda, MD

Sarah M. Lytle, MD, MS
Division of Child and Adolescent
Psychiatry

University Hospitals Case Medical
Center
Cleveland, OH

Katie Mahon, PhD
Departments of Psychiatry and
Neuroscience
Icahn School of Medicine at
Mount Sinai
New York, NY

Anil K. Malhotra, MD
Department of Psychiatry Research
The Zucker Hillside Hospital
Glen Oaks, NY
and
The Feinstein Institute for Medical
Research
Manhasset, NY

Taylor M. McCabe, SN/STNA
Ohio Northern University
Ada, OH

Patrick D. McGorry, MD, PhD
Department of Psychiatry
Centre for Youth Mental Health
University of Melbourne
Melbourne, Australia

Robert K. McNamara, PhD
Department of Psychiatry and
Behavioral Neuroscience
University of Cincinnati College of
Medicine
Cincinnati, OH

David J. Miklowitz, PhD
Division of Child and Adolescent
Psychiatry
David Geffen School of Medicine at
UCLA
Los Angeles, CA

Sonal K. Moratschek, MD, MPH
Division of Child and Adolescent
Psychiatry
University Hospitals Case Medical
Center
Cleveland, OH

Alessandra M. Passarotti, PhD
Department of Psychiatry
University of Illinois at Chicago
Chicago, IL

Caroly Pataki, MD
Department of Psychiatry and
Biobehavioral Sciences
David Geffen School of Medicine
at UCLA
Los Angeles, CA

Luis Rodrigo Patino Duran, MD
Department of Psychiatry & Behavioral
Neuroscience
University of Cincinnati College of
Medicine
Cincinnati, OH

Mani N. Pavuluri, MD, PhD
Department of Psychiatry
University of Illinois at Chicago
Chicago, IL

Aswin Ratheesh, MD
Centre for Youth Mental Health
University of Melbourne
Melbourne, Australia

Jillian M. Russo, PsyD
Department of Psychiatry
Yale University School of
Medicine
New Haven, CT

Manpreet K. Singh, MD, MS
Department of Psychiatry and
Behavioral Sciences
Stanford University School of Medicine
Stanford, CA

Stephen M. Strakowski, MD
Department of Psychiatry & Behavioral
Neuroscience
University of Cincinnati College of
Medicine
Cincinnati, OH

Jeffrey R. Strawn, MD
Department of Psychiatry and Behavioral
Neuroscience
University of Cincinnati College of
Medicine
Cincinnati, OH

Kenneth E. Towbin, MD
Emotion and Development
Branch
National Institute of Mental
Health
U.S. Department of Health and Human
Services
Bethesda, MD

Timothy Wilens, MD
Department of Psychiatry
Massachusetts General Hospital
Harvard Medical School
Boston, MA

Sonja M. C. de Zwarte, MS
Department of Psychiatry
Yale University School of Medicine
New Haven, CT

Prologue

R.J., a 10-year-old boy with a bilineal family history of bipolar disorder, came with his parents to our offices. He tearfully cried, "My mood swings are critical—I need help!" Within minutes, he jumped on the exam room chairs and sang. He could not stop moving or climbing so that the energy level in the exam room was high, affecting everyone present. He growled "like a lion" to show us that he was "very scary." His labile affect ranged from euphoria and elation to sadness and irritability. He spoke so rapidly that he was difficult to interrupt. R.J. reported he could not fall asleep at night because his thoughts went too fast, and he "never" feels tired. He and his parents described that this behavior had been ongoing for several weeks, but it intensified after he started taking an antidepressant that he was prescribed during a recent hospitalization for suicidal and homicidal ideation, extreme irritability, and anger outbursts. It was difficult to comprehend how R.J, his parents, and his teachers were managing these "critical" mood swings and the associated disruptive behaviors.

Two weeks following his initial presentation, R.J. and his parents returned for follow-up. After discontinuing the antidepressant and starting a mood-stabilizing medication, R.J. declared that his moods were "still critical, but not as much" and according to his parents, R.J. was beginning to function well at home and at school. During the next month, he steadily improved to the point of being "like the old R.J."

Bipolar Disorder in Youth: A Decade of Progress

Although once thought to be relatively uncommon compared with adult-onset bipolar disorder, it is now widely accepted that bipolar disorder also occurs in youth and is a serious mental health disorder with significant morbidity and mortality.[1] Youth with bipolar disorder exhibit impaired relationships with family and peers and dysfunction at home and school.[2] Indeed, recent studies suggest that healthy social-, emotional-, and neuro-developmental processes are interrupted or delayed when the onset of bipolar disorder occurs during childhood or adolescence.

The evaluation and treatment of bipolar disorder in children and adolescents have been surrounded by considerable controversy, in part because the clinical manifestations of bipolar disorder in youth are distinct from those of adults.[3] Furthermore, the field has been challenged with underdiagnosing, overdiagnosing, and misdiagnosing bipolar disorder in children and adolescents.[4] Nonetheless, during the past decade, significant advances have been made toward better understanding the phenomenology, neurobiol-ogy, outcome, and treatment of childhood and adolescent bipolar disorder, leading to improvements in the assessment and identification of this population.[5] Earlier recogni-tion of symptoms accelerates treatment initiation, thereby improving outcome for these youth. Furthermore, researchers have identified prodromal clinical features and risk and resilience factors for childhood and adolescent bipolar disorder, leading to preliminary studies of early interventions.[6–9]

Investigators have also made considerable progress toward establishing evidence-based interventions for mania in children and adolescents.[10] However, first-line treatments (e.g., second-generation antipsychotics) are frequently associated with side effects, including significant metabolic concerns, which adversely impact adherence and outcome.[11] Therefore, alternative treatment strategies for symptom management and to improve the tolerability of existing medications are needed.

The consequences of having the onset of bipolar disorder during important stages of neurodevelopment are likely to have lifelong implications compared to having the onset of bipolar disorder during adulthood, after a majority of neuro-development has occurred. Novel neuroimaging methods have clarified the neural circuitry of pediatric bipolar disorder, which in part, is distinct from that of adult bipolar disorder. However, methodological limitations persist in studies of neural markers of illness onset, progression, and treatment response, which include the diagnostic heterogeneity of most samples of children and adolescents with bipolar disorder.[12] Throughout this book, then, novel approaches that may accelerate iden-tification of neural markers and personalized medicine for bipolar disorder in youth are considered.

This book highlights the substantial progress that has been made in understanding and treating bipolar disorder in children and adolescents. Although significant advance-ments have also occurred in identifying prodromal manifestations of bipolar disorder in youth, the next era of research will need to clarify risk and resilience factors that con-tribute to the onset and progression of bipolar disorder in order to develop targeted pre-vention and early intervention and improve the outcome for youth with and at risk for developing bipolar disorder.[13–15]

Organization of the Book

The chapters of this book provide a comprehensive review of recent diagnostic, treatment, and neurobiological research and controversies in the field of bipolar disorder in youth. Important topics of investigation are examined, including differences in clinical presentation between adults and youth, underlying genetic and neural abnormalities, and state-of-the-art treatment strategies. Other areas of interest are considered, including how to assess and treat youth at risk for bipolar disorder, and whether clinical differences between adults and youth are the result of developmental differences in symptom manifestation, distinct underlying genetic and neurophysiological abnormalities, or the same illness occurring at very different developmentally vulnerable periods.

The book is organized into three main sections. The first section focuses on the phenomenology and diagnosis of children and adolescents with and at high risk for developing bipolar disorder. In the first chapter of this section, Duffy describes prodromal presentations and early symptom manifestations that predate the onset of bipolar disorder in children and adolescents, particularly those who have clinical and familial risk factors. Next, Carlson and Pataki discuss the clinical characteristics, comorbidities, and diagnostic dilemmas associated with bipolar disorder in children and adolescents, while addressing the controversies that surround the diagnosis. In the third chapter of this section, Towbin and Leibenluft review the differential diagnosis for bipolar disorder as well as the evolving role and impact of the newest version of the *Diagnostic and Statistical Manual of Mental Disorders* (DSM), DSM-5,[16] on diagnosing bipolar disorder in youth. Comorbidity is the rule, rather than the exception for youth with bipolar disorder. Specifically, behavioral (e.g., ADHD, conduct disorder), anxiety, and substance use disorders commonly co-occur in these children and adolescents.[17] Furthermore, bipolar youth with co-occurring disorders are more challenging to diagnose, have a poorer outcome, and are more difficult to treat than those without psychiatric comorbidities.[18] In Chapter 5, Joshi and Wilens discuss practical strategies for evaluating, diagnosing, and treating bipolar disorder in youth with co-occurring psychiatric disorders.

Family and twin studies consistently reveal that bipolar disorder is a familial illness, suggesting that genetics represent a strong risk factor.[19] However, there are also environmental risk and resilience factors that contribute to the onset of bipolar disorder.[13] Therefore, the last two chapters of this section provide a comprehensive update regarding genetic and environmental risk factors. First, Mahon, Burdick, and Malhotra explore the genetics of childhood and adolescent bipolar disorder. Results of genetics investigations are inconsistent, in part, due to the phenotypic heterogeneity of the disorder. The authors provide suggestions on how to manage these obstacles so that the field advances more rapidly. In the last chapter of this section, McNamara and Strawn review nongenetic risk and resilience factors associated with the onset and prevention, respectively, of bipolar disorder. Improvements in identifying children and adolescents at genetic and environmental risk for bipolar disorder will ultimately lead to the development of targeted early intervention and prevention strategies. In summary, the first section of the book provides an in-depth review of the phenomenology, clinical characteristics, and risk factors that contribute to the development of bipolar disorder in children and adolescents. With this knowledge, young people will receive more accurate and efficient assessments and treatments for bipolar disorder.

The second section of the book focuses on treatment. The ultimate goal of intervention is to develop primary and secondary prevention strategies for bipolar disorder. Although risk, resilience, and biological markers have been identified, the specificity and sensitivity of each of these to predict the onset of bipolar disorder in at-risk youth remain unknown. In a provocative chapter, Ratheesh, Berk, and McGorry provide a thoughtful appraisal of the risks and benefits of current evidence-based early interventions. Additionally, the authors describe the ethical hurdles to developing more rational treatment strategies for children and adolescents with early symptoms and signs of bipolar disorder.

During the same period of time when there has been an epidemic of pediatric bipolar disorder diagnoses and a dramatic increase in the number of second-generation antipsychotic prescriptions,[20–21] there has been an explosion of controlled studies that provide evidence-based guidance for treating bipolar youth.[10] During the past decade, there have been more than a dozen double-blind placebo-controlled studies examining treatments for manic children and adolescents. However, data to support treatments for depression associated with bipolar disorder and maintenance interventions are lacking. Lytle, Moratschek, and Findling review evidence-based pharmacologic treatments for the different illness phases.

Psychotherapeutic interventions have considerably fewer side effects than pharmacological treatments. Moreover, data are rapidly expanding to support the efficacy of several specific psychotherapies for childhood and adolescent bipolar disorders. In Chapter 10, Miklowitz describes the role of psychotherapy in treating bipolar youth and their families and reviews evidence to support different types of therapies, including psychoeducational, cognitive, and family modalities. Finally, in the last chapter of the treatment section, Gracious, Gurumurthy, Cottle, and McCabe examine the growing evidence to support alternative and complementary treatments for youth with and at risk for bipolar disorder and suggest future directions to advance this field.

During the past decade evidence-based research has shifted the debate from whether bipolar disorder in children and adolescents exists to how to best use neuroimaging to determine the neural underpinning of pediatric bipolar disorder. The third and final section of the book highlights the neurodevelopment of bipolar disorder in youth. In the first chapter of this section, Russo, de Zwarte, and Blumberg describe normal and abnormal neurodevelopmental processes in at-risk youth in the context of prodromal manifestations of the illness. Bipolar disorder is a progressive illness, and therefore, some neurobiological alterations are present at illness onset and some develop over time. In Chapter 13, Pavuluri describes the neural circuits associated with the symptoms of bipolar disorder and the neuro-progressive changes following the onset of bipolar disorder, with particular attention to prefrontal-amygdala connectivity. Additionally, the neural basis of bipolar disorder in youth are explored in the context of the National Institute of Mental Health's Research Domain Criteria (RDoC),[22] which is a novel approach for classifying psychopathology based on dimensions of behavior and neurobiological measures rather than the more classic categorical criteria sets (e.g., *DSM*). As expected, neurocognitive impairments are associated with neural alterations in youth with and at risk for bipolar disorder. In Chapter 14, Passarotti provides a synopsis of the neurocognitive deficits commonly exhibited by bipolar youth, particularly in the domains of emotion processing, working memory, cognitive flexibility, executive functions, and attention. These deficits may persist during euthymic periods, worsen with illness onset and progression, and are associated with poor outcomes.[23] They also reflect the underlying functional neuroanatomic abnormalities observed with imaging. Finally, in the last chapter of this section, Singh and Chang examine the neural effects of psychotropic medications in youth with and at risk for bipolar disorder and consider the progress, challenges, and limitations of using neuroimaging to identify biomarkers of treatment effects and response. Applying innovative neuroimaging techniques to predict medication response and establishing targeted treatment strategies for a specific individual with bipolar disorder will help guide us into the area personalized medicine. In the final chapter of the book, Patino Duran and colleagues reflect on the major research findings in the field and offer suggestions for future investigations.

The incorporation of *DSM-5*, RDoC, and personalized medicine into clinical practices and research studies will force the field of pediatric bipolar disorder to undergo a paradigm shift so that dimensional levels of behaviors and symptoms are considered and defined by neurobiological characteristics. This approach will lead to better characterization of risk and resilience factors, so that children and adolescents with and at risk for bipolar disorder have better outcomes.

In conclusion, the information provided in this book will guide clinicians, researchers, parents, and other individuals involved in the care of children and adolescents with and at risk for developing bipolar disorder to provide state-of-the-art assessments and interventions for these youth. Despite the past decade of substantial growth in evidence-based strategies for these youth, gaps in how to identify those at highest risk for developing the illness and provide optimal treatments for children and adolescents with and at risk for bipolar disorder remain.

Melissa P. DelBello, MD
Caleb M. Adler, MD
Stephen M. Strakowski, MD

References

1. Chang K. Adult bipolar disorder is continuous with pediatric bipolar disorder. *Can J Psychiatry* 2007;52:418–25.

2. DelBello MP, Hanseman D, Adler CM, Fleck DE, Strakowski SM. Twelve-month outcome of adolescents with bipolar disorder following first hospitalization for a manic or mixed episode. *Am J Psychiatry.* 2007;164:582–90.

3. Geller B, Luby J. Child and adolescent bipolar disorder: a review of the past 10 years. *J Am Acad Child Adolesc Psychiatry.* 1997; 36:1168–176.

4. Carlson GA, Klein DN. How to understand divergent views on bipolar disorder in youth. *Annu Rev Clin Psychol.* 2014;10:529–51.

5. DeFilippis M, Wagner KD. Bipolar disorder in adolescence. *Adolesc Med State Art Rev.* 2013;24:433–45.

6. Duffy A. The early natural history of bipolar disorder: what we have learned from longitudinal high-risk research. *Can J Psychiat.* 2010;55:477–85.

7. Berk M, Hallam KT, McGorry PD. The potential utility of a staging model as a course specifier: a bipolar disorder perspective. *J Affect Disord.* 2007;100:279–81.

8. Miklowitz DJ, Chang KD. Prevention of bipolar disorder in at-risk children: theoretical assumptions and empirical foundations. *Dev Psychopathol.* 2008;20:881–97.

9. McNamara RK, Strawn JR, Chang KD, DelBello MP. Interventions for youth at high risk for bipolar disorder and schizophrenia. *Child Adolesc Psychiatr Clin N Am.* 2012; 21:739–51.

10. Correll CU, Sheridan EM, DelBello MP. Antipsychotic and mood stabilizer efficacy and tolerability in pediatric and adult patients with bipolar I mania: a comparative analysis of acute, randomized, placebo-controlled trials. *Bipolar Disord.* 2010;12:116–41.

11. DeHert M, Dobbelaere M, Sheridan EM, Cohen D, Correll CU. Metabolic and endocrine adverse effects of second-generation antipsychotics in children and adolescents: a systematic review of randomized, placebo controlled trials and guidelines for clinical practice. *Eur Psychiatry.* 2011;26:144–58.

12. Schneider MR, DelBello MP, McNamara RK, Strakowski SM, Adler CM. Neuroprogression in bipolar disorder. *Bipolar Disord.* 2012;14:356–74.

13. McNamara RK, Nandagopal JJ, Strakowski SM, DelBello MP. Preventative strategies for early-onset bipolar disorder: towards a clinical staging model. *CNS Drugs.* 2010;24:983–96.

14. Ketter TA, Wang PW. Predictors of treatment response in bipolar disorders: evidence from clinical and brain imaging studies. *J Clin Psychiatry.* 2002;63(Suppl. 3):21–5.

15. Duffy A, Horrocks J, Doucette S, Keown-Stoneman C, McCloskey S, Grof P. The developmental trajectory of bipolar disorder *BJP.* 2014;204:122–8.

16. American Psychiatric Association. *Diagnostic and Statistical Manual of Mental Disorders.* 5th ed. Arlington, VA: American Psychiatric Publishing; 2013.

17. Joshi G, Wilens T. Comorbidity in pediatric bipolar disorder. *Child Adolesc Psychiatr Clin N Am.* 2000;18:291–319, vii–viii.

18. Birmaher B, Axelson D, Goldstein B, et al. Four-year longitudinal course of children and adolescents with bipolar spectrum disorders: the Course and Outcome of Bipolar Youth (COBY) study. *Am J Psychiatry.* 2009;166:795–804.

19. Mick E, Faraone SV. Family and genetic association studies of bipolar disorder in children. *Child Adolesc Psychiatr Clin N Am.* 2009;18:441–53.

20. Olfson M, Blanco C, Wang S, Laje G, Correll CU. National trends in the mental health care of children, adolescents, and adults by office-based physicians. *JAMA Psychiatry.* 2014;71:81–90.

21. Zito JM, Burcu M, Ibe A, Safer DJ, Magder LS. Antipsychotic use by medicaid-insured youths: impact of eligibility and psychiatric diagnosis across a decade. *Psychiatr Serv.* 2013;64:223–9.

22. Insel T, Cuthbert B, Garvey M, et al. Research domain criteria (RDoC): toward a new classification framework for research on mental disorders. *Am J Psychiatry.* 2010;167, 748–51.

23. Joseph MF, Frazier TW, Youngstrom EA, Soares, JC A quantitative and qualitative review of neurocognitive performance in pediatric bipolar disorder. *J Child Adolesc Psychopharmacol.* 2008;18: 595–605.

Phenomenology and Diagnosis

Section Editor: Caleb M. Adler

Progression of Bipolar Disorder in Youth

Defining the Early Clinical Stages in the Development of Bipolar Disorder

Anne Duffy

Overview and Context

The course of established recurrent mood disorders, including melancholia and bipolar disorder, has been described since antiquity. Our current diagnostic classification system of mood disorders remains anchored in 19th-century descriptions of adult patients admitted to asylums and organized into a unitary construct by Kraepelin in order to differentiate recurrent mood disorders from chronic progressive psychotic illnesses. Ironically, more recent modifications to the diagnostic criteria have broadened the mood diagnostic categories to include psychotic spectrum illnesses, thus blurring the distinction between mood and psychotic disorders in terms of illness course and treatment response. What has not changed is the fact that diagnostic approaches in psychiatry remain focused on describing end-stage illness syndromes, rather than on mapping the early natural history in the development of these brain diseases. Furthermore, our diagnostic approach does not take into consideration other predictive factors, such as the nature of the clinical course (episodic, partial remitting, deteriorating) or the family history (what illnesses manifest in other family members), which would help to identify and differentiate between emerging psychiatric disorders earlier. This approach is problematic given that symptoms alone are nonspecific and cross diagnostic boundaries, syndromes do not correlate well with treatment response or prognosis, and there are no reliable biomarkers or pathophysiological correlates to help validate diagnoses as yet. With increased convergent information suggesting that earlier effective treatment may be neuroprotective[1] and associated with better outcomes,[2] there is increasing urgency to describe the early natural history in the development of major psychiatric disorders. Therefore, this chapter will focus on key findings demonstrating that bipolar disorder is often preceded by risk syndromes, in some cases years prior to the defining index hypomanic/manic/mixed episode. These observations underscore the need to incorporate the natural history of psychiatric diseases in our diagnostic approach and add support for the importance of the early identification and intervention effort under way in psychiatry.

Natural History of Bipolar Disorder—What We Knew

Clinical descriptions consistent with manic and melancholic states can be traced to the ancient Greek and Roman times. The circular nature of manic depressive episodes and the close relationship between them were also noted in writings of 17th-century clinical researchers, including Thomas Willis (1622–1675).[3] As part of the French psychiatric movement in the early 1800s, alternating states of manic excitement and melancholic inhibition with remitted intervals in the same patient were described most notably by Esquirol (1838), Falret (1851), and Baillarger (1854). The concept of a unified illness with alternating manic and depressive states was not well accepted until Kraepelin's proposal to unify recurrent (periodic or cyclic) disorders under one category, putting melancholia (unipolar depression) and manic depressive insanity (bipolar disorder), with and without psychotic features, together. His reasoning was based on longitudinal observations of patients in psychiatric hospitals and predicated on the assumption of a shared pathological process that was heritable.[4] Interestingly, Kraepelin recognized that mood was not the main diagnostic criterion, but rather part of an excited or inhibited broader syndrome. He later elaborated on the distinction between acquired (intoxication, brain injury, paresis due to tertiary syphilis) and constitutional disorders (periodic, degenerative states, neuroses).

Kraepelin left an import legacy to psychiatry practice and research. First, rather than focusing on enumerating nonspecific symptoms, he approached psychiatric diagnosis from the perspective of identifying and differentiating brain diseases. This strategy led him to study the onset, evolution, and outcome of psychiatric disease trajectories in order to work out which presentations likely shared underlying pathophysiological factors and which represented different processes. Furthermore, he described the complexity of the acute syndromes, which included not only a mood component but also psychotic features, neurocognitive deficits, and activity changes.[3] Kraepelin also emphasized the fundamental core differences in clinical course between the periodic mood disorders and the progressive deteriorating psychotic disorders. Consistent with this speculation of a shared pathophysiology between recurrent melancholia and bipolar disorder are findings from family studies showing the cosegregation of these two diseases,[5] their shared response to lithium prophylaxis,[6] and overlapping biomarkers, including HPA axis dysregulation.[7,8]

In a recent comprehensive review and reanalysis of modern follow-up studies of adults patients with bipolar disorder, Angst and Sellaro[9] made conclusions that largely confirm key observations made by Kraepelin over 125 years earlier.[10] Specifically, diagnosable manic or hypomanic episodes typically have an early-adulthood onset, the course remains typically recurrent, and the bulk of evidence suggests that there is no progressive shortening of cycle lengths once recurrence risk is taken into account (time from the end of one acute episode to the onset of the next). The median episode lengths and proportion of activated to depressed syndromes appear quite stable over the course of illness in both men and women, with the latter having more depressive episodes comparatively. The median episode length in individuals with bipolar disorder in clinical settings is estimated at 3–6 months, with rapid cycling only seen in a minority as a transient feature rather than a course trait. It was estimated that individuals with a diagnosis of bipolar disorder spend 2 months per year in an episode of one polarity or another.

Collectively, these observations do not support the current popular view that bipolar disorder is a neuroprogressive illness in the majority of patients, nor are they consistent with a kindling model proposed by Post.[11] In fact, prospective longitudinal data from a large well-characterized cohort reported by the IGSLi group demonstrate that patients with a highly recurrent untreated illness course continue to show a good response and remission stability throughout a 20-year observation period.[12]

However, as pointed out by Grof[6,13,14] and others,[15] the current concept of bipolar disorder has broadened and includes disorders that previously would have been conceptualized as psychotic spectrum illnesses. This broadening of the bipolar concept has undoubtedly contributed to the findings of an overlap in biomarkers between schizophrenic and bipolar populations;[16] observations of more chronic, less episodic illness course; lower response rates to lithium prophylaxis with rebound upon discontinuation; and increased response rates to atypical antipsychotics.[6] The inclusion of lithium nonresponsive patients in studies has undoubtedly also contributed to the reconceptualization of bipolar disorder as a neuroprogressive (deteriorating) illness.[17,18] In a typical Canadian tertiary care mood disorders program, it was recently estimated that only 30% of bipolar patients met the predictive profile of a classical episodic lithium responsive subtype.[19] Response to lithium prophylaxis following a highly recurrent natural course of illness is one way to identify a classical, more homogeneous subtype of bipolar disorder well suited to biological studies and likely representing the form of illness Kraepelin described.[20]

Evolution of Bipolar and Related Mood Disorders—What We Now Know

As is the case with most medical diseases, we are increasingly aware that major psychiatric disorders evolve from reliable antecedent risk syndromes or early clinical stages to end-stage, full-threshold disorders.[21] The Dunedin Longitudinal Birth Cohort study demonstrated that most psychiatric disorders in adults have their origins in childhood and adolescence, but that the early risk syndromes may be quite different in nature (phenotypically) to that of the end-stage illness (heterotypic continuity).[22] The idea of using clinical staging models to describe the early natural history of psychiatric diseases was championed by McGorry and systematically studied in regard to the developmental trajectory into schizophrenia.[23,24] Essentially the related studies showed the benefits of early identification, intervention, and specialty follow-up 3–5 years after an index psychotic episode (youth-specific secondary prevention), as well as the benefits of identifying an "ultra-high-risk" group (prodromal signs and symptoms) and providing low-intensity interventions (with high benefit-to-risk ratio) to prevent progression to index psychotic episode.[25]

Attention has been more recently focused on describing the early natural history of bipolar disorder and identifying risk syndromes representing the early clinical stages, as well as prodromal states heralding the imminent onset of bipolar-related mood episodes. Given the very high heritability of bipolar disorder,[26] studying the offspring of well-characterized affected parents is an important strategy to map the natural history of illness development, identify risk and resiliency factors, and characterize biological markers associated with illness onset and progression. There are several international longitudinal high-risk studies that have provided important complementary findings and insights into the early natural history of bipolar disorder (as reviewed by Duffy et al.[27,28]). Taken together, despite different methods and variance in the high-risk families, studies have shown that bipolar disorder most often debuts as a major depressive episode in adolescence or early adulthood.[29] This finding is very important because, unlike schizophrenia, the index episode of illness is not phenotypically the same as the index diagnostic episode—that is, the first major mood episode is most often depressive, not hypomanic/manic/mixed. This observation from high-risk longitudinal studies is consistent with findings from retrospective studies of bipolar patients,[30] family studies of bipolar probands (in which recurrent depressive disorders are considered a part of the phenotype segregating in families[5,31]), and prospective studies of depressed adolescents who "convert" to bipolar disorder.[32] The implication is that a valid staging model for bipolar disorders cannot simply be extrapolated from the ultra-high-risk prodromal criteria studied in psychotic disorders. That is, prodromal criteria to mania are much further down the clinical course in bipolar disorder than are prodromal criteria to psychosis in schizophrenia.

Puberty has been long recognized to mark a high-risk developmental period for the onset or progression of psychiatric disorders, including mood disorders.[33] In high-risk offspring of bipolar parents, puberty is associated with the onset of clinically significant mood psychopathology. Specifically, offspring appear more likely to break down under stress with clinically significant depressive symptoms (adjustment disorders) that previously they would have managed and adequately coped.[27,34] Furthermore, recent and consistent reports have demonstrated that earlier childhood presentations of anxiety and sleep disorders confer a greater risk of subsequent depressive and bipolar mood disorders in high-risk offspring.[35,36] These observations resonate with the long-standing reports of circadian rhythm disturbances as central features predicting the onset and recurrence of mood episodes.[37–40]

Taking these observations into account, Duffy et al. recently proposed a clinical staging model describing the development of bipolar disorder from stage 0 (clinically well, but at confirmed familial risk) to stage 4 (full threshold diagnosable bipolar illness).[21] Subsequent analyses using multistate models[41] showed that children at confirmed genetic risk of developing bipolar disorder tend to move through the proposed clinical staging sequence in a forward progressive manner (see Fig. 1.1) without skipping stages; however, they may enter the model at any stage (not all manifest stage 1 for example). Furthermore, there are differences in the breadth of the stages differentiating those at risk for classical recurrent mood disorders (lithium responsive) and those on a more psychotic-mood trajectory (lithium nonresponsive). This model provides a refined developmentally sensitive phenotype that should advance both early diagnosis and intervention clinical practice, as well as research directed at identifying biomarkers of stage progression and characterizing genetically sensitive causal pathways. Furthermore, staging also makes it possible to separate the primary disease process from secondary complications and burden of illness effects at a clinical and a psychobiological level. This separation is extremely important because most research to date in bipolar disorder has been in adults with established illness, which confounds effects of the disease with those of its consequences. For example, in high-risk offspring the emergence of diagnosable substance use disorders converges with the age of onset of the first major mood (depressive) episode,[42] and depending on the severity, duration, and drug of choice, it likely alters the pathophysiology, clinical course, and treatment response of the underlying primary disease process.

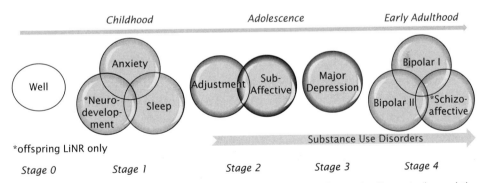

FIGURE 1.1 A clinical staging model affords the opportunity to refine early diagnosis (beyond the *DSM*); it is an organizing framework for neurobiological research and enables the recognition of critical periods for effective intervention. The longitudinal prospective study of high-risk individuals is extremely important for investigating and mapping biomarkers and pathways to the clinical phenotype.

What is interesting about findings from longitudinal studies across different high-risk groups is the degree of overlap in reported antecedent risk syndromes. For example, childhood anxiety and sleep disorders have been described as predictive antecedent syndromes in those at risk of developing primary psychotic, mood, and substance use disorders. However, it is the nature of the family history and the clinical course that gives these nonspecific early presentations a specific predictive meaning.[2] At the same time, there are certain early risk syndromes that are differentially present. Specifically, as described by Murray et al.[43] there are important and reliable dissimilarities in the early developmental history of children who go on to develop bipolar disorder compared to those who develop schizophrenia. Namely, the latter have evidence of increased pre- and perinatal complications and other early environmental influences (urban, winter/spring birth), childhood antecedents that include motor, cognitive, and language impairment not seen in children at risk for or who develop bipolar disorder.[44,45] Although there is evidence of some shared genetic factors between schizophrenia and bipolar disorder, these diseases are characterized by clearly very different developmental trajectories. While cross-sectional assessment may initially be confusing in determining what specific illness trajectory a given symptomatic youth may be on, the combination of developmental trajectory, course of illness, family history and other risk factors should clarify the clinical picture far beyond that of the *Diagnostic and Statistical Manual of Mental Disorders* (*DSM*) or the *International Classification of Diseases* (*ICD*) approach.

Implications for Clinical and Research Practice in Bipolar Disorder

Psychiatry has had a curious developmental trajectory in its own right—influenced by politics and strongly held beliefs, and straying at times from the evidence base. Happily, there appears to be a growing recognition that among the exploding diagnoses of mental health (or illness) conditions, there are primary prototypical disorders that represent brain diseases. These diseases have strong, but complex, genetic origins that manifest through childhood and adolescence, developing into full-threshold recognizable clinical syndromes in adulthood. Up until recently, unlike other areas of medicine, psychiatry has focused its efforts clinically and in research on established (end-stage) illnesses. As argued by McGorry[23] and others,[46] clinical staging represents an important heuristic concept that can advance early recognition and intervention efforts. As recently articulated by Scott et al.[47] clinical staging (1) is a validated approach in general medicine; (2) places a person on a continuum of disorder allowing for stage-specific and individualized treatment; (3) is based on the assumption that earlier stage treatments have a more favorable benefit-to-risk ratio and are associated with a better response likelihood and prognosis; (4) provides stage appropriate intervention that should change the progression of disease and the distribution of disease over clinical stages over time; and finally (5) guides research into associated stage-specific biomarkers that should lead to further refinement and validation of the clinical staging model.

On the other hand, clinical staging needs to be taken in the context of those at identifiable risk and not in unselected general population samples, in order to balance the risk of overlabeling with the clear benefits of early detection in known high-risk populations. That is, we need to reliably differentiate normative and transient experiences in adolescents from reliable signs and syndromes representing early-stage phenotypes or risk syndromes. Limiting clinical staging to those at confirmed genetic risk and/or help seeking should accomplish this goal. It is also important to factor in predictive influences that can lend important meaning to the clinical stages in order to determine as early as reliably possible different illness trajectories that might clinically overlap, but that originate from different underlying pathophysiological origins and respond differentially to treatment interventions.

Some argue that most cases of bipolar disorder in clinical practice are "sporadic" and not informed by family history. However, this argument is likely a result of: (1) phenocopies (clinical presentations that initially look like bipolar disorder, but are not); (2) a lack of rigorous history taking and not following individuals long enough to meet extended family members; and (3) not taking the full phenotypic spectrum into consideration (in relatives of a bipolar proband, cyclothymia, bipolar not otherwise specified, or bipolar I/II, recurrent major depression and suicide are part of the phenotypic spectrum). Based on heritability estimates of approximately 85%, it would be the exception rather than the rule to not find a positive family history to inform diagnosis in the case of a patient with a primary recurrent mood disorder.

Staging models of bipolar disorder proposed by others largely derive from clinical and research experience with those at ultra-high risk of developing schizophrenia[48,49] and focus on the prodrome of the index manic episode.[50] When you consider the full clinical trajectory of bipolar disorder in high-risk youth, this focus seems skewed too far toward end-stage illness and ignores a substantial proportion of morbidity mostly related to the depressive polarity of the illness. Major depressive episodes in high-risk youth are associated with suicidality[51] and with substance use disorders,[42] as well as school dropout and psychological processes that are associated with illness progression.[52] This approach of focusing on the prodrome to index psychotic episode (or mania), while fitting a model of schizophrenia, does not seem adequate or well suited for a clinical staging and early intervention approach for bipolar disorder.

In summary, we are at an exciting crossroads in psychiatry. On the one hand, there is increasing recognition of the importance of mapping the trajectory into major mood and psychotic illnesses to identify early clinical stages that would support early identification and intervention. We also have a better idea of how to study gene-by-environment interactions and complex genetically sensitive pathways into psychiatric disorders. On the other hand, there is a popular movement toward studying overlapping nonspecific symptoms and syndromes out of the important context of familial risk and developmental longitudinal course. If we persist with a clinical staging model focusing on carefully longitudinally studied well-characterized high-risk cohorts in an integrative way, we should be able to make major advances in identifying associated biological markers and early intervention targets. This direction would be the next step, as envisioned by Kraepelin all those years ago. Let's hope that we continue to learn from the history of medicine, to remind us of what we know and direct us to what we need to know and how best to get there.

Author Disclosure

Dr. Duffy has no conflicts to disclose. She is funded by the Canadian Institute of Health Research.

References

1. Hajek T, Cullis J, Novak T, et al. Brain structural signature of familial predisposition for bipolar disorder: replicable evidence for involvement of the right inferior frontal gyrus. *Biol Psychiatry.* 2013;73(2):144–52.
2. Duffy A, Carlson GA. How does a developmental perspective inform us about the early natural history of bipolar disorder? *J Can Acad Child Adolesc Psychiatry.* 2013;22(1):6–12.
3. Trede KSP, Baethge C, Gerhard A, Maggini C, Baldessarini RJ. Manic-depressive illness: evolution in Kraepelin's textbook, 1883–1926. *Harvard Rev Psychiatry.* 2005(May/June):155–78.
4. Kendler KS. Kraepelin and the differential diagnosis of dementia praecox and manic-depressive insanity. *Compr Psychiatry.* 1986;27(6):549–58.
5. Rice J, Reich T, Andreasen NC, et al. The familial transmission of bipolar illness. *Arch Gen Psychiatry.* 1987;44(5):441–7.
6. Grof P, Muller-Oerlinghausen B. A critical appraisal of lithium's efficacy and effectiveness: the last 60 years. *Bipolar Disord.* 2009;11(suppl 2):10–9.
7. Carroll BJ, Feinberg M, Greden JF, et al. A specific laboratory test for the diagnosis of melancholia. Standardization, validation, and clinical utility. *Arch Gen Psychiatry.* 1981;38(1):15–22.
8. Duffy A, Lewitzka U, Doucette S, Andreazza A, Grof P. Biological indicators of illness risk in offspring of bipolar parents: targeting the hypothalamic-pituitary-adrenal axis and immune system. *Early Interv Psychiatry.* 2012;6(2):128–37.
9. Angst J, Sellaro R. Historical perspectives and natural history of bipolar disorder. *Biol Psychiatry.* 2000;48(6):445–57.
10. Angst J GA. Diagnosis and course of affective psychoses: was Kraepelin right? *Eur Arch Psychiatry Clin Neurosci.* 2008;258(suppl 2):107–10.
11. Post RM. Transduction of psychosocial stress into the neurobiology of recurrent affective disorder. *Am J Psychiatry.* 1992;149(8):999–1010.
12. Berghofer A. Lithium and suicide. *BMJ.* 2013;347:f4449.
13. Grof P. Sixty years of lithium responders. *Neuropsychobiology.* 2010;62(1):8–16.
14. Grof P, Alda M, Ahrens B. Clinical course of affective disorders: were Emil Kraepelin and Jules Angst wrong? *Psychopathology.* 1995;28 Suppl 1:73–80.
15. Alda M. The phenotypic spectra of bipolar disorder. *Neuropsychopharmacology.* 2004;14:94–9.
16. Gershon ES, Alliey-Rodriguez N, Liu CY. After GWAS: searching for genetic risk for schizophrenia and bipolar disorder. *Am J Psychiatry.* 2011;168(3):253–6.
17. Berk M, Conus P, Kapczinski F, et al. From neuroprogression to neuroprotection: implications for clinical care. *Med J Aust.* 2010;193(4 suppl):S36–40.

18. Berk M, Kapczinski F, Andreazza AC, et al. Pathways underlying neuroprogression in bipolar disorder: focus on inflammation, oxidative stress and neurotrophic factors. *Neurosci Biobehav Rev.* 2011;35(3):804–17.

19. Garnham J, Munro A, Slaney C, et al. Prophylactic treatment response in bipolar disorder: results of a naturalistic observation study. *J Affect Disord.* 2007;104(1–3):185–90.

20. Grof P, Duffy A, Alda M, Hajek T. Lithium response across generations. *Acta Psychiatr Scand.* 2009;120(5):378–85.

21. Duffy A, Alda M, Hajek T, Sherry SB, Grof P. Early stages in the development of bipolar disorder. *J Affect Disord.* 2010;121(1–2):127–35.

22. Kim-Cohen J, Caspi A, Moffitt TE, Harrington H, Milne BJ, Poulton R. Prior juvenile diagnoses in adults with mental disorder: developmental follow-back of a prospective-longitudinal cohort. *Arch Gen Psychiatry.* 2003;60(7):709–17.

23. McGorry PD, Nelson B, Goldstone S, Yung AR. Clinical staging: a heuristic and practical strategy for new research and better health and social outcomes for psychotic and related mood disorders. *Can J Psychiatry.* 2010;55(8):486–97.

24. McGorry PD, Purcell R, Hickie IB, Yung AR, Pantelis C, Jackson HJ. Clinical staging: a heuristic model for psychiatry and youth mental health. *Med J Aust.* 2007;187(7 Suppl):S40–2.

25. McGorry PD, Nelson B, Amminger GP, et al. Intervention in individuals at ultra high risk for psychosis: a review and future directions. *J Clin Psychiatry.* 2009;70(9):1206–12.

26. Bienvenu OJ, Davydow DS, Kendler KS. Psychiatric "diseases" versus behavioral disorders and degree of genetic influence. *Psychol Med.* 2011;41(1):33–40.

27. Duffy A. The early natural history of bipolar disorder: what we have learned from longitudinal high-risk research. *Can J Psychiat.* 2010;55(8):477–85.

28. Duffy A, Doucette S, Lewitzka U, Alda M, Hajek T, Grof P. Findings from bipolar offspring studies: methodology matters. *Early Interv Psychiatry.* 2011;5(3):181–91.

29. Hillegers MH, Reichart CG, Wals M, Verhulst FC, Ormel J, Nolen WA. Five-year prospective outcome of psychopathology in the adolescent offspring of bipolar parents. *Bipolar Disord.* 2005;7(4):344–50.

30. Angst J, Gerber-Werder R, Zuberbuhler HU, Gamma A. Is bipolar I disorder heterogeneous? *Eur Arch Psychiatry Clin Neurosci.* 2004;254:82–91.

31. Winokur G, Tsuang MT, Crowe RR. The Iowa 500: affective disorder in relatives of manic and depressed patients. *Am J Psychiatry.* 1982;139(2):209–12.

32. Strober M, Carlson G. Predictors of bipolar illness in adolescents with major depression: a follow-up investigation. *Adolesc Psychiatry.* 1982;10:299–319.

33. Silberg J, Pickles A, Rutter M, et al. The influence of genetic factors and life stress on depression among adolescent girls. *Arch Gen Psychiatry.* 1999;56(3):225–32.

34. Shaw JA, Egeland JA, Endicott J, Allen CR, Hostetter AM. A 10-year prospective study of prodromal patterns for bipolar disorder among Amish youth. *J Am Acad Child Adolesc Psychiatry.* 2005;44:1104–11.

35. Duffy A, Horrocks J, Doucette S, Keown-Stoneman C, McCloskey S, Grof P. Childhood anxiety: an early predictor of mood disorders in offspring of bipolar parents. *J Affect Disord.* 2013;150(2):363–9.

36. Nurnberger JI J, McInnis M, Reich W, et al. A high-risk study of bipolar disorder. Childhood clinical phenotypes as precursors of major mood disorders. *Arch Gen Psychiatry.* 2011;68(10):1012–20.

37. Bauer M, Glenn T, Grof P, et al. Comparison of sleep/wake parameters for self-monitoring bipolar disorder. *J Affect Disord.* 2009;116(3):170–5.

38. Grof E, Grof P, Brown GM, Arato M, Lane J. Investigations of melatonin secretion in man. *Prog Neuro-Psychopharmacol Biol Psychiatry.* 1985;9(5–6):609–12.

39. Deshauer D, Grof E, Alda M, Grof P. Patterns of DST positivity in remitted affective disorders. *Biol Psychiatry.* 1999;45(8):1023–9.

40. Deshauer D, Duffy A, Meaney M, Sharma S, Grof P. Salivary cortisol secretion in remitted bipolar patients and offspring of bipolar parents. *Bipolar Disord.* 2006;8(4):345–9.

41. Duffy A, Horrocks J, Doucette S, Keown-Stoneman C, McCloskey S, Grof P. The developmental trajectory of bipolar disorders. *Br J Psychiatry.* 2014;204(2):122–8.

42. Duffy A, Horrocks J, Milin R, Doucette S, Persson G, Grof P. Adolescent substance use disorder during the early stages of bipolar disorder: a prospective high-risk study. *J Affect Disord.* 2012;142(1–3):57–64.

43. Murray RM, Sham P, Van Os J, Zanelli J, Cannon M, McDonald C. A developmental model for similarities and dissimilarities between schizophrenia and bipolar disorder. *Schizophrenia Res.* 2004;71(2–3):405–16.

44. Cannon M, Caspi A, Moffitt TE, et al. Evidence for early-childhood, pan-developmental impairment specific to schizophreniform disorder: results from a longitudinal birth cohort. *Arch Gen Psychiatry.* 2002;59(5):449–56.

45. MacCabe JH, Murray RM. Intellectual functioning in schizophrenia: a marker of neurodevelopmental damage? *J Intellectual Disabil Res.* 2004;48(Pt 6):519–23.

46. Hickie IB, Scott J, McGorry PD. Clinical staging for mental disorders: a new development in diagnostic practice in mental health. *Med J Aust.* 2013;198(9):461–2.

47. Scott J, Leboyer M, Hickie I, et al. Clinical staging in psychiatry: a cross-cutting model of diagnosis with heuristic and practical value. *Br J Psychiatry.* 2013;202(4):243–5.

48. Berk M, Hallam KT, McGorry PD. The potential utility of a staging model as a course specifier: a bipolar disorder perspective. *J Affect Disord.* 2007;100(1–3):279–81.

49. Reinares M, Colom F, Rosa AR, et al. The impact of staging bipolar disorder on treatment outcome of family psychoeducation. *J Affect Disord.* 2010;123(1–3):81–6.

50. Conus P, Ward J, Hallam KT, et al. The proximal prodrome to first episode mania—a new target for early intervention. *Bipolar Disord.* 2008;10(5):555–65.

51. Lewitzka U, Doucette S, Seemuller F, Grof P, Duffy AC. Biological indicators of suicide risk in youth with mood disorders: what do we know so far? *Curr Psychiatry Rep.* 2012;14(6):705–12.

52. Knowles R, Tai S, Christensen I, Bentall R. Coping with depression and vulnerability to mania: a factor analytic study of the Nolen-Hoeksema (1991) Response Styles Questionnaire. *Br J Clin Psychol.* 2005;44(Pt 1):99–112.

Presentation of Mania/Bipolar I in Youth

Comparison With Adults

Gabrielle A. Carlson and Caroly Pataki

Evolution of the Bipolar Controversy

Much of the controversy around the diagnosis of bipolar disorder in youth addresses whether its clinical picture, and especially mania, presents differently across the life span.[1] It has been difficult to resolve this issue due to a combination of philosophical and methodological factors.[2] Carlson and Klein have noted that divergent viewpoints regarding the phenomenology of type I bipolar disorder in youth have led clinicians and researchers to use different interpretations of the *Diagnostic and Statistical Manual of Mental Disorders* (*DSM*) criteria to diagnose bipolar disorder, within and across age groups.[3] This state of affairs has evolved for a number of reasons.

Changes in the conceptualizations of attention-deficit/hyperactivity disorder (ADHD) and oppositional behavior led to the elimination of the "mood" component of low frustration tolerance, variability, and mood lability from the criteria when the *DSM-III* evolved ADHD from the *DSM-II* concept of hyperkinetic reaction of childhood.[4,5] Mood symptoms were included in the text only as secondary symptoms and were thus not included in subsequent structured and semistructured interviews developed to study ADHD. The only condition in which hyperactivity, impulsivity, distractibility, and irritable mood co-occur as primary criteria is mania.

Changes in the conceptualization of mania and bipolar disorder also have impacted the way in which manic and mixed episodes are diagnosed. The *DSM* from the third edition to the fourth edition (text revision) defined mania primarily by symptoms—that is, expansive, irritable, or elevated mood with associated symptoms/behaviors, without an associated daily time frame.[6] Thus, an individual who endorsed sufficient symptoms could be diagnosed with a manic episode regardless of the daily extent of a given symptom or the degree to which individual symptoms overlapped; this deficiency was remedied in DSM-5.[7] These ambiguities led to differing interpretations of how persistent manic symptoms needed to be over the course of a day for diagnostic purposes. This ambiguity, coupled with a lack of clarity around the "irritability" element of mania and the imprecise definition of "episode," may have made it difficult to distinguish a hyperactive, distractible, impulsive, emotionally labile, overly reactive, and irritable child with ADHD from a child with mania. In addition, because irritability has been retained as a depression criterion in recent versions of the DSM only for children and adolescents, bipolar youths may be more likely to be diagnosed with a mixed episode than are adults.[8] The duration requirement of at least a week for the "distinct period" in mania was also eliminated, allowing a distinct period to last only minutes to hours, further confusing mood lability with a manic episode. Finally, no offset was described to delineate a manic episode; focusing on symptoms without a comprehensive longitudinal history that includes defined episodes makes it difficult to distinguish a child with emotionally reactive ADHD from one with mania.

Differences in structured and semistructured diagnostic interviews used for youths and adults may influence diagnostic differences between age groups as well. Conditions that are typically thought to begin in childhood have developmental qualifiers; for example, ADHD criteria note that hyperactivity is "maladaptive and inconsistent with developmental level." However, no developmental qualifiers for mania or mood regulation are used, in part because such parameters have not been adequately researched.[9] This lack of developmental perspective may skew diagnoses, with younger subjects more apt to be diagnosed with ADHD than mania.

There are also potential informant issues in diagnosing bipolar disorder in younger individuals.[10] While some symptoms are readily observable, more internal symptoms, including hallucinations, racing thoughts, and even euphoria may be less amenable to outside observation.[9] Further, there is also the problem of ascertaining whether mania is lasting "most of the day, every day" in children who spend much of their day away from home. Unfortunately, teacher information is rarely solicited in studies of children with bipolar disorder, and even when obtained, teacher information has often been discounted on the grounds that teachers may not be qualified to identify mania.[10] While this may be true, in situations where parents describe symptoms of both mania and ADHD, while teachers observe no behavior problems at all, there is a clear diagnostic question.[11] This is not a question of misidentifying manic symptoms; this is a question of whether manic symptoms are occurring most of the day, every day.

In addition, structured and semistructured interviews geared to diagnosing bipolar disorder often make no attempt to collect a *history* systematically,[12] and they are inconsistent in how they operationalize the DSM criteria and manic symptoms.[13,14] The Washington University version of the Schedule for Affective Disorders and Schizophrenia for children (WASH U K-SADS), for example, elicits information as to the current episode, including dates of onset and offset for each symptom, from both the parent and child.[15] The dates on which point these symptoms overlap are used to define the presence of an episode. Strictly speaking, however, this methodology is not entirely consistent with the *DSM*, which assumes that symptoms should onset and offset contemporaneously over the course of mania or depression.

The handling of comorbid symptoms also varies with clinicians and researchers. Some investigators "double-count" symptoms across all disorders to which they might apply. For instance, if distractibility is present, it is counted as a symptom of both ADHD and mania. Investigators who double-count symptoms believe that it is not possible to know which condition is accounting for the psychopathology; therefore, they include the item in diagnosing multiple disorders. Other investigators take a more conservative approach, requiring manic symptoms to be over and above symptoms of comorbid conditions—or requiring that the "comorbid" symptoms represent an intensification of the original symptomatology. Not surprisingly, the former approach yields higher rates of ADHD comorbidity, and it may potentially yield a population of youthful bipolar patients that differs from adult populations. Finally, in some studies clinicians do not conduct the interview, though the investigators provide many checks and balances to overcome this potential issue.[16]

Outpatient versus inpatient status and the age range of the samples (and thus mean age) also vary enough between studies to make interpretation difficult. The result of these ambiguities and inconsistencies between studies is to make it quite difficult to truly address the question of how the phenomenology of bipolar disorder differs across the age range.

CASE EXAMPLE 1 Prepubertal Mania and Attention-Deficit/Hyperactivity Disorder

Seth, age 10, has been described in detail elsewhere.[17] Referred by both school and his mother for explosive outbursts when he felt thwarted, insulted, or provoked, he needed to be seen for an emergency consultation. At the time of his initial assessment, he appeared agitated, with rapid, pressured, and off-topic speech. He "did not remember" his property-destroying outbursts, neither what he did nor why they occurred. His problems were not acute. He had been a mildly language-delayed, hyperactive, dangerously impulsive toddler with sleep problems. Seth had witnessed his father beating his mother, and his mother often fled the house, usually taking the children. In his Head Start program, Seth began to throw "megawatt fits." After receiving a diagnosis of ADHD, Seth was started on methylphenidate, which seemed to make his behavior worse, and by age 5 a diagnosis of bipolar disorder was made based on his extreme rages. Subsequently, he was treated unsuccessfully with risperidone, aripiprazole, divalproex, oxcarbazepine, and topiramate. He had been psychiatrically hospitalized and was taking 25 mg of atomoxetine, 0.1 mg of clonidine, and 25 mg of lamotrigine nightly at the time.

Seth was admitted to the hospital at this time, and his medications were discontinued. His Young Mania Rating Scale (YMRS) score based on nurse observations was similar to the score of 16 based on parent observations.[18] He did not seem to understand consequences for his behaviors and was behind academically. Although he could not shed any light on his mood symptoms, Seth's language impairment, co-occurring anxiety, and ADHD symptoms were obvious. He was treated with mixed amphetamine salts, which reduced but did not eliminate his distractibility, impulsivity, and excessive talking.

Seth improved initially but for reasons not clear, he then appeared to get worse. He started writing poems to his teacher, became unaccountably silly, became more disruptive at bedtime, and responded explosively to any kind of limit. His weekly nurse-YMRS score increased to 38, indicating increased irritability and energy (despite decreased sleep), elevated mood, rapid and pressured speech, grandiosity, and erotic and hypersexual behavior. These behaviors continued despite discontinuing stimulant medication. Both his mother and outside teacher, witnessing these events, indicated he had had such "spells" before. They usually lasted several days but could persist up to a week.

Lithium carbonate was started but needed to be supplemented with risperidone (0.5 mg twice a day). Mixed amphetamine salts were started again, which improved his concentration; repeat IQ testing revealed a 16-point increase, mostly due to improvements in the areas of working memory and processing speed. Nevertheless, it was felt that Seth needed ongoing structure, special education, and close medication monitoring, so he was discharged to a day treatment program. Final diagnoses included bipolar disorder, most recent episode manic; ADHD, combined type; oppositional defiant disorder; specific learning disorder: reading and math; and language disorder not otherwise specified.

Family history was significant for his mother's postpartum depression, and her mother was said to have been manic-depressive. Biological father had numerous learning disabilities and a history of substance abuse.

Seth was admitted to the hospital again 2 years later when he had an explosive outburst, threatening to hurt his elderly grandmother. On that admission, however, there were no symptoms of mania, and it became apparent quickly that his mother had pushed the panic button, fearing that he was developing a manic episode. He was discharged shortly thereafter and ultimately moved out of state.

Seth presented many of the issues that complicate the identification and treatment of bipolar I disorder in children. It may be difficult to distinguish a specific mood episode from a backdrop of ADHD, low frustration tolerance with oppositionality, anxiety, and agitation. His psychosocial situation was tumultuous, and had we not actually witnessed the manic episode, and captured it with the YMRS score of 38, it may well have gone unrecognized. On the other hand, he had periods of time when he became aggressive but was not manic.

The effect of different interpretations of the *DSM* criteria in making the diagnosis of mania impacts age-related comparisons of bipolar disorder, type I prevalence.[19]

Conservatively diagnosed bipolar disorder, type I rates are lower in community studies of youths compared with adults. This differs from rates in studies using more liberal definitions of bipolar disorder, type I, which yield rates of bipolar disorder in youths that are the same as those observed in adults. Rates of co-occurring ADHD are similarly lower in studies using more conservative interpretations of the criteria for bipolar disorder, type I in children and adolescents. Rates of both bipolar disorder, type I and of ADHD are also lower in the offspring of bipolar disorder probands, and outcomes more closely approximate that of adults in studies using more conservative criteria for bipolar disorder.

However, even disregarding differing definitions of mania, there appears to be a developmental relationship between ADHD and bipolar disorder, with higher rates in youth with an earlier onset (Table 2.1).[20-29] Faraone and colleagues reported the rate of comorbid ADHD in youth with bipolar disorder to be 93% in children, 88% in teens with a childhood onset, and 59% in teens with adolescent-onset mania.[21] The Course and Outcome of Bipolar Youth study (COBY) similarly reported rates of ADHD in their subjects with bipolar spectrum disorders to vary by age as follows: Comorbid ADHD was present in 71.7% in children less than 12 years of age, 69.3% of teens with childhood onset of a bipolar spectrum disorder, but only 31.1% of adolescents with an adolescent-onset bipolar disorder.[22] In Masi and colleagues' study of bipolar disorder in Italy, rates of ADHD in mania are about half of what is seen in the United States (37.8%), though the average age of the children studied is older than US samples (12.3 years).[23] His teenage subjects, however, are approximately the same age as samples studied in the United States (14–16 years), and ADHD rates are nonetheless lower.[23,29] Comparatively low rates of ADHD are seen in several studies of bipolar teenagers outside of the United States (Table 2.2). In adults with bipolar disorder, rates of ADHD/childhood externalizing disorders are also low, generally reported to be 10%–20%.[30-33]

Oppositional defiant (ODD)/conduct disorder (CD) rates also appear to be more common in younger people diagnosed with bipolar disorder (Table 2.1) than in teens, and they are more common in teens than in adults. Carlson and colleagues used a secondary analysis of the epidemiologic catchment area (ECA) data to demonstrate that in the sample of 132 adults who met criteria for mania, rates of CD significantly differed between bipolar subjects under age 30 (32.6%) than those over that age (16.3%).[34] The general prevalence rate of CD among young adult respondents was 7.75%. Rates of CD were especially high in those young bipolar patients with substance use problems, 52%, versus 14.8% of those without substance abuse. This high rate of substance abuse comorbidity in young bipolar patients may have implications for rates in adults with mania.

Manic Symptom Differ Between Children, Adolescents, and Adults With Bipolar Disorder

Several studies have compared rates and severity of manic symptoms between children and teens with bipolar disorder, type I using structured/semistructured interview data. Geller and colleagues, for example, examined prepubertal versus postpubertal youth.[15]

TABLE 2.1 Comparison of Child, Adolescent, and Adult Clinical Features and Outcome

	Findling et al. (2001)[24]	Masi et al. (2006)[23]	Faraone et al. (1997)[21]	Geller et al. (2002)[15] (2008)[27] (child)	Birmaher et al. (2009)[22] (child)	Birmaher et al. (2009)[22] (teen)	Carlson and Strober (1978)[25]	Jairam et al. (2004)[26]	Srinath et al. (1998)[28]	Faraone et al. (1997)[21]	Findling et al. (2001)[24]	Masi et al. (2006)[23] (2007)[29]
n	56	80	68	115	244		54	25	30	17	34	56
Interview	KSADS	KSADS	KSADS-E	WASH U KSADS	KSADS PL		SADS	DICA-R MAGIC	ISCA	KSADS-E	KSADS	KSADS
DSM version	DSM-IV	DSM-IV	DSM-IIIR	DSM-IV	DSM-IV		DSM-IIIR	DSM-IIR and DSM-IV	DSMIIIR	DSMIIIR	DSM IV	DSM IV
Age (baseline), years	8.5 (1.9)	12.3 (2.9)	7.9 (2.6)	11.1	13.2 (3.0)		16	14.1 (1.40)	13.9	15.8 (2.0)	14.5 (1.7)	15.2 (1.8)
Age onset, years	5.0 (2.6)	7.7 (2.1)	4.6 (3.0)	8.3 (3.7)	9.3 (4.1)		n/a	13.7 (1.7)	13.8	14.6 (1.5)	9.5 (4.4)	13.0 (1.4)
% male	75	67.5	78	77	52.6		48	60	50	65	64.7	48.2
% hospitalized at intake	25	38.7	None	None	~16%		100	80	100	none	41.2	?38.7
% ADHD	75	37.8	93	93.9	71.7	31.1	14.8	4	0	59	61.8	8.9
% ODD	N/A	35.9	91	81.7	43.4	31.1		28		71	n/a	10.7
% CD	N/A			19.1	6.4	15.6	11.1	4	7		n/a	
% psychosis	17.9	42.2a	31	[73]	41.4% for BP-I—rates lower for BP-II and BP-NOS		28	60	63	35	14.7	66.7a
% substance	0	n/a	0	35.2	0	23.3	9.3	0	0	35	17.6	n/a

ADHD, attention-deficit/hyperactivity disorder; BP, bipolar; CD, conduct disorder; DICA-R, Diagnostic interview for children and adolescents-revised; ISCA, interview schedule for children and adolescents; ODD, oppositional defiant disorder; KSADS PL, K-SADS Present and Lifetime.

Birmaher and coauthors in the COBY sample, and Faraone and coinvestigators, also each reported on samples of youth divided into those with childhood-onset bipolar disorder, teens with childhood-onset bipolar disorder, and teens with adolescent-onset bipolar disorder.[21,22] Neither Geller and colleagues nor Faraone and colleagues found a significant difference in rates of specific manic symptoms, with the exception of irritability and elevated energy, which were higher in younger patients.[15,21] Masi and colleagues reported that elation and episodicity occurred in teens, but chronic elation and irritability were more common in younger patients.[23,29] On the other hand, the COBY study found that adolescents with adolescent-onset mania had more severe symptoms than children, for most manic symptoms.[22] Elation, grandiosity, decreased need for sleep, accelerated speech, racing thoughts, goal-directed hyperactivity, delusions, and increased productivity were all more severe in teens. Only mood lability was more severe in children, and there were no differences between the two age groups in severity of irritability, flight of ideas, hallucinations, or hypersexuality.

Three studies used a rating scale to examine differences in manic symptoms. Demeter and colleagues found no age effects using the K-SADS Mania Rating Scale (KMRS), a severity measure of manic symptoms.[35,36] In contrast, Torpor and colleagues conducted a factor analysis on the KMRS for the COBY sample, finding both similarities and differences in various factors by age.[37] For children with childhood onset of symptoms, two factors emerged, "activated/pleasure seeking" and "labile/disorganized." One former factor was also present for adolescents with childhood onset of symptoms. The "activated/pleasure seeking" factor also emerged in adolescents with adolescent onset of symptoms, along with a new factor called "disorganized/psychotic." The teen sample reported by Demeter and colleagues, however, showed KMRS scores across all measures that were similar to Birmaher's COBY childhood-onset sample;[35] the reason for this discrepancy is not clear.

Safer and coauthors examined baseline YMRS data from several treatment studies;[38] they found that preadolescents had significantly higher irritability and motor activity scores on the YMRS than adolescents, who had higher aggression and irritability scores than adults. Adults with mania, however, scored comparatively higher on the grandiosity and sexual interest items. Comparative studies of adolescent and adult mania are considerably more similar in methodology. Ten relevant studies are included in Table 2.2.[39-48] Almost all of these studies compare phenomenology by age of onset rather than age at index (first manic of mixed) episode. While the definition of "young" or "early onset" may vary from adolescent (ages 12–18 years) to include patients under 40 years of age, "adult" onset either starts at the end of the early-onset age range or allows a gap between early and later onset, so there is a clearer demarcation between groups. All but two studies use patients hospitalized for mania, so there is at least some control for severity.[41,45] In addition, investigators can observe or have immediate access to information about mania rather than relying on retrospective recall. That said, age of onset is mostly retrospective—though in some cases of first episode or first hospitalization for mania, age of onset is relatively close to age at index.

TABLE 2.2 Early- and Late-Onset Sample Descriptions

Study	Definition of Early Versus Late	How Assessed	Findings for Early-Onset Patients Compared to Older Onset
McGlashan et al.[39] Inpatient-Chestnut Lodge 1950–1975 N = 66	Age at first symptoms ≤19 years; ≥20 years	*DSM-III* Chart abstract; follow-up study	Higher rate of prior hospitalization Higher rate of psychosis Higher rate of psychotic assaultiveness More likely schizoaffective More trouble with the law
Carlson et al.[40] County-wide sample of first hospitalized patients for psychosis 1989–1995 N = 53	Age met criteria Early onset: ≤20 years Later onset: ≥30 years	*DSM-IV* SCID SAPS BPRS Consensus child psychopathology	Teen mean AAO: 17.7 ± 1.6 AAI: 18.3 ± 1.7 Adult mean AAO: 38.3 ± 8.9 AAI: 39.4 ± 8.2 More conduct disorder More behavior problems More substance abuse at onset Worse school performance More paranoia; grandiosity More mixed episodes Higher BPRS rating
Schurhoff et al.[41] Inpatients—Paris, Fr. N = 97	Age met criteria for episode Early onset: ≤age 18 years Late onset: ≥40 years	*DSM-IV* DIGS	Teen mean AAO: 15.5 ± 1.9 AAI: 33.6 ± 11.9 Adult mean AAO: 48.5 ± 7 AAI: 60.2 ± 9.2 More mixed episodes More psychosis More panic disorder Poorer lithium response
Schultze et al.[42] Inpatients in Germany N = 90	Age criteria met for major mood episode Early onset: up to age 20 years Late onset: >35 years	*DSM-IV* SCID OPCRIT	Current age: EO: 35 ± 13; LO: 54 ± 10 More delusions More hallucinations
Kennedy et al.[43] All cases of first-episode mania from 1965 to 1999 presenting for service; Camberwell, London N = 246	Age at which treatment was sought for mania Early onset: <40 years Late onset: >40 years	Case record review using Operational Checklist for psychotic disorders (OPCRIT)	Higher rates of acute onset Violence at intake More irritability More reckless behavior More psychotic symptoms Less euphoria Less sociability
Suominen et al.[44] Inpatients and outpatients from Helskinki programs N = 191	Age onset of *DSM-IV* criteria Early onset: <age 18 years Late onset: age 18–51 years	*DSM-IV* SCID Beck Depression Inventory Beck Anxiety Inventory Scale for Suicidal Ideation	Teen mean AAO: 14.2 ± 3.4 AAI: 30.5 ± 11.6 Adult mean AAO: 27.8 ± 8.8 AAI: 40.8 ± 11.1 Female gender Rapid cycling Lifetime psychotic symptoms Index episode mixed Suicidal ideation Lifetime comorbidity

(continued)

TABLE 2.2 Continued

Study	Definition of Early Versus Late	How Assessed	Findings for Early-Onset Patients Compared to Older Onset
Hamshere et al.[45] Sample acquired by advertisements in UK N = 1,225	Age of impairment from mood symptoms Early onset: 6–22 years Middle onset: 25–37 years Late onset: 40–73 years	All available notes Schedule for Assessment in Psychiatry (SCAN) Narratives reviewed by two investigators Bipolar Affective Disorder Scale (BARS)	18.7 (3.7) Higher rates of rapid cycling More manic and depressive episodes More psychosis
Sax et al.[46] First hospitalization for affective psychosis— Univ. of Cincinnati N = 88	Age at index hospitalization Early onset: <18 years Typical onset: 20–25 years Late onset: >35 years	DSM-IIIR SCID SAPS HAM D YMRS	More suicidality More agitation Greater energy More abnormal thought content Less insomnia Fewer somatic symptoms
McElroy et al.[47] hospitalization for treatment of acute mania—Univ. of Cincinnati N = 128	Onset of first mood episode meeting DSM-IIIR criteria Hosp. age Teen 12–18 years; adult 19–45 years	DSM-IIIR SCID SAPS YMRS HAM-D	Teen mean AAO: 12 + 2 AAI: 15 + 2 Adult mean AAO: 22 + 6 AAI: 28 + 6 Lower rates of psychosis Less thought disorder Less substance abuse disorder More mixed episodes
Patel et al.[48] First psychiatric admit— Univ. of Cincinnati Hosp. N = 161	Age onset of criteria <age 18 years >20 years, typical onset	DSM-IV WASH U KSADS SCID YMRS HAM-D SAPS	Teen mean AAO: 13.2 + 3.3 AAI: 17.2 + 5.1 Adult mean AAO: 24.2 + 3.5 AAI: 26.1 + 5.1 Onset episode more likely mixed Index episode more likely mixed; less likely psychotic Rates of substance and alcohol abuse were lower

AAI, age at index episode; AAO, age at onset; BPRS, brief psychiatric rating scale; DIGS, diagnostic interview for genetic studies; EO, early onset; HAD-D, hamilton depression rating scale; LO, late onset ; SAPS, scale for the assessment of positive symptoms; SCID, structured clinical interview for DSM.

Three studies were chart reviews using systematic data abstraction systems.[39,42,43] The rest used structured/semistructured interviews, usually the Structured Clinical Interview for *DSM-III-R* or *DSM-IV*.[40,41,44–48] Investigators focused on different aspects of phenomenology. However, almost all studies addressed rates of psychosis, or different aspects of psychosis (e.g., hallucinations, delusions, thought disorder), and almost all described the type of onset episode or index episode (i.e., manic, mixed, or depressed). Other features highlighted sometimes were aggression/behavior problems, anxiety, suicidality, and substance abuse.

With the exception of the samples from the Cincinnati group, who used similar assessment procedures with slightly different samples,[46–48] most studies report higher rates of psychosis in adolescent-onset patients than in the comparison group.[39–45] The fact that psychosis is reported in both adolescent-onset patients and in early-onset patients who are older at the time of interview suggests that a possible early-onset phenotypic variation is occurring, rather than that the psychotic symptoms associated with mania are more common in adolescents experiencing mania.

Studies in which episode type was defined invariably reported mixed episodes and rapid cycling occurring more often in the younger onset samples.[40,41,44,47,48] Perhaps not surprisingly, behavior disorder problems (e.g., aggression, trouble with the law, conduct disorder, behavior problems) were also the domain of early-onset patients.[39,40,43] Elevated rates of substance abuse were less consistent; again, they were reported less commonly in the early-onset patients studied by the Cincinnati group,[46–48] and more commonly in youths observed by other investigators.

In summary, compared to later onset patients, bipolar patients with early onset have more complicated manic episodes, with increased rates of psychosis, comorbidity with behavior problems, anxiety, depression, and possibly substance abuse. It is not clear whether it is the episode itself that is more complicated or the fact that affective symptoms are superimposed on underlying comorbid problems. Conversely, "typical" or later onset patients had more classic-appearing mania with possibly a more clearly defined demarcation from premorbid, normal behavior.

CASE EXAMPLE 2 Bipolar Disorder, Type I in Early Adolescence

Duncan, a 12-½-year-old pubertal seventh grader, was referred for an outpatient evaluation after what was felt to be an acute reaction to OROS methylphenidate. At that time, Duncan was frankly psychotic, delusional, and nearly incoherent. Unlike Seth, who had demonstrated behavior problems his whole life, Duncan had been a good student until approximately 6 months prior to the evaluation request. He had been on the football and wrestling teams at school, and he has been described by teachers as a "great," "enthusiastic," "respectful," "kind" child.

Approximately 6 months prior to his hospitalization, Duncan underwent a dramatic personality change. Initially, he was more conscientious and harder working in school than he had been in earlier grades. Parents were pleased at how much energy he was devoting to his studies. He was talkative (though that was not a new symptom) and very upbeat. However, to their chagrin, he became increasingly disinhibited and defiant, acting in outlandish ways in school, his behavior escalating to the point that his school suggested that he get "tested" psychiatrically. Examples of Duncan's disrespectful comments to teachers included, "You old piece of shit, you should die or retire." Besides being insulting, he repeatedly asked teachers and classmates for candy, swearing at them when they refused. He asked a classmate whether he had masturbated before and on one occasion blurted out: "Suck my dick!" Previously a kind youth, he became a bully. He approached a peer, grabbed his lunch, and threw it in a mud puddle saying, "It was in my way," and then reportedly looked up with a nasty grin. When the principal took him to task for his transgressions, he said that he was part of a "bigger plan" and "wouldn't be punished." According to his parents, these behaviors were very out of character for Duncan.

Duncan was evaluated at the time by a child psychiatrist, who elicited long-standing symptoms of somewhat poor focus and disorganization, diagnosed ADHD, and prescribed a low dose of OROS methylphenidate. Over the next several months there was behavioral improvement. However, Duncan suddenly became "itchy," and extremely anxious, short of breath, and dizzy. He experienced intrusive thoughts of Miley Cyrus with drugs and needles. He said he felt "100% smart and 100% protective," and he felt like people were watching and following him. Medication was discontinued, but it took 2 weeks before Duncan's unusual thoughts abated.

Duncan then became increasingly depressed, quiet, and clingy, following his parents around the house. He ultimately got through this depression, but then started to get hyperactive, provocative, and "bad" again. OROS methylphenidate was restarted. Several says later, Duncan became so slowed down he was almost catatonic. He failed final exams miserably. He was sent home from school because he was "practically a zombie," in the school psychologist's words. Concerned that Duncan's mental state had nothing to do with stimulant response, the school psychologist referred him for psychiatric consultation.

When seen in consultation a few days later, Duncan looked very subdued. When asked why he was so sad, he launched into a completely unrelated monologue. Duncan's thoughts were so slow he could only complete the first page of a five-page rating scale. He endorsed many ADHD symptoms and admitted that he often lost his temper and was argumentative. He denied general worry, separation anxiety, depression, or mania. In response to being questioned about his psychotic symptoms, Duncan responded, "Whenever I heard something, it was just like echoing. I don't know." He said he thought he smelled chemicals.

Duncan was given a series of cognitive tasks at which he performed very poorly. He could not remember or summarize a short paragraph read to him. Given a series of facts to recall, he remembered only one. Duncan was unable to draw inferences. For instance, the sentence "Mary and Susie play with each other every day after school. Each night, before they go to bed, they argue and fight. How do Mary and Susie know each other?" The answer is that they are sisters. Duncan first said, "They don't know each other." After the paragraph was read to him again, he responded, "They know each other." He later added: "They play with each other after school." Duncan was unable to draw a correct inference from any single sentence. Finally, when given a picture story book where it was necessary to look at pictures to tell the story, Duncan could not do it because, he said, "You can't read a book unless there are words in it."

There was a family history of alcoholism, his mother had received electroconvulsive therapy for a severe postpartum depression, and his grandmother had been psychiatrically hospitalized with a "nervous breakdown," the details of which were unknown.

Duncan was experiencing a clear change from his prior functioning. It does sound like he had had ADHD symptoms before his episodes, but, unlike Seth's symptoms, they were not serious enough to warrant treatment. The doctor evaluating him started stimulants, thinking that Duncan had deteriorated in middle school the way children with untreated ADHD often do. However, this was not the case with Duncan—his grades had actually improved.

The acronym HIPERS provides an easy way to remember manic symptoms and to explain Duncan's psychopathology: *H* (hyperactivity) *I* (irritability) *P* (psychosis-grandiosity) *E* (elated/expansive mood) *R* (rapid speech and racing thoughts) *S* (sleep-does not need or want any). Applied to Duncan, we see hyperactivity (goal directed and pleasure oriented) in his money and sweets seeking. The fact that he had actually worked more effectively for some months before his behavior deteriorated may have been hypomania that was prodromal to the subsequent manic episode. His nasty, defiant behavior, kicking a child's lunch into the mud because it was "in his way" is a manifestation of irritability. What Duncan told his principal about having a "plan" that exempts him from consequences was clearly grandiose. His "100% smart and 100% protective" and "like people were watching and following" him were both grandiose and paranoid symptoms. He had what may be olfactory hallucinations, too. Descriptions of Duncan when he is doing nasty things to people sounds clearly elated. He grinned and got pleasure out of inflicting pain—something that did not characterize this child's typical personality. Duncan was also described as talking too much and sometimes did not make sense. The only manic symptom that could not be documented was a reduced need for sleep.

Duncan had become quite obnoxious. Had his behaviors not been such a change from who he had been only a few months earlier, he would have been considered oppositional defiant or even conduct disordered. The bullying, pestering people for sweets, and worrying about a pop star's drug problems were, in fact, his "pathoplastic" (i.e., unique to Duncan) manifestations of manic symptoms. What was especially striking about Duncan was the level of psychomotor retardation that accompanied what appeared to be depressive symptoms. Psychomotor retardation is rare in depressed children and is commonly seen in adults with bipolar depression.[49] In Duncan's case, he appeared to have days at a time when, in addition to being slowed physically and cognitively, he felt depressed and anxious. The crying outbursts, morbid preoccupations, and many aches and pains were also a part of his depressive episodes. They had nothing to do with stimulant administration, occurring several months after stimulants started at a low dose. He became manic again and following that experienced a psychomotor-retarded depression, which caused him to be sent home from school. It was not surprising that he failed his final exams. His mental status during the psychiatric evaluation was of a child who could not think and whose conversation was thought disordered. Again, it is his history that clarified the behaviors, not just the behaviors themselves.

Duncan's episodes appeared to follow one another without much, if any, euthymia between them. He appeared to have a "rapid cycling pattern," and within some of his episodes, a case could be made that symptoms were mixed. Psychotic symptoms were vague and not sustained. Even his paranoia was not especially intense.

Adolescent Mania and Substance Abuse

The differential diagnosis of mania and ADHD is not usually as complicated in teens and young adults as in prepubertal children. That is probably because the hyperactivity and impulsivity of ADHD has been attenuated by adolescence, and it is therefore easier to distinguish the increased energy and hyperactivity seen in new-onset mania from the background of chronic ADHD symptoms. However, substance abuse adds its own age-dependent complication, especially since substance abuse occurs more often in teens with ADHD[50] and, as noted earlier, oppositional defiant and conduct disorder.[34] The following case has been followed for two decades as part of the Suffolk County Mental Health Project, a county-wide study of 15-year-olds to 60-year-olds hospitalized for a first episode of psychosis between 1989 and 1995.[51-52] In this study, patient information was collected from hospitals, schools, parent/spouse/friend coinformants, and from the subjects themselves using the Structured Clinical Interview for *DSM-IV* and other systematic assessments.[53] Subjects were seen at baseline; at 6, 24, and 48 months; and at 10 and 20 years, with telephone information obtained in between visits. Consensus diagnoses were made by a team of psychiatrists, and they included an interviewer who was blind to prior diagnoses.

CASE EXAMPLE 3 Bipolar Disorder in a Young Adult With a Comorbid Substance Use Disorder

Mason was a college freshman who was expelled from school when, in a fit of rage, he threw his roommate's TV out of the window. He was taken to a psychiatric emergency room, where he presented with "extreme argumentativeness and grandiose delusions." He himself denied having any problems outside of being a "hyperactive insomniac." Although he had a history of attention problems and hyperactivity in public school, he denied that it caused any impairment. His mother, on the other hand, said that his grades suffered in high school, he had low self-esteem, and that he was always sensitive to criticism. His real problems started at age 16, with the development of polysubstance abuse, including daily marijuana use, cocaine use several times a month, drinking up to twelve cans of beer several times a week, and experimenting with hallucinogens. In fact, a week prior to the emergency room visit, Mason took LSD; shortly thereafter he thought that he could be a famous actor and get on TV to tell the viewers what was wrong with the world. He was expansive, had pressured speech and racing thoughts, was very energetic, and was not sleeping.

Mason was hospitalized and treated with lithium carbonate and haloperidol. It took a month for his manic symptoms to remit. Several months later, he developed a depressive episode with a full complement of depressive symptoms. He refused to take lithium, saying he did not like how he felt on it. He was treated first with a tricyclic antidepressant and then with fluoxetine. Neither antidepressant precipitated another manic episode. He continued daily marijuana use and occasional LSD use. Over the next year, Mason's mood was stable, but he entered a drug rehabilitation program. The rehabilitation program appeared to be successful in decreasing his substance abuse. Over the next 4 years, he had mood fluctuations with a prominence of depressive symptoms and an occasional full depressive episode. He was treated with antidepressants only.

At a 10-year follow-up, it was determined that Mason had not met criteria for any affective or psychotic episodes over the 4- to 10-year interval, though he still sometimes had subthreshold cyclothymia. These mood changes lasted hours and usually abated with exercise and rest. He got drunk several weekends each month at parties and had one DUI, but he was not alcohol dependent. He smoked marijuana a few times per year and occasionally used cocaine and ecstasy, but he did not meet abuse criteria for any illicit drugs. There did not appear to be a relationship between drug use and any mood fluctuations. He had returned to college, obtained a degree, and was gainfully employed in the film industry; he did not have grandiose ideas of changing the world, and he functioned well socially. Interestingly, he had not been prescribed psychotropic medication for the prior 6 years and was in psychotherapy three times per week.

Over the next 10 years, Mason continued to do well. He was successful in his work and socially. He still drank frequently but did not meet abuse or dependence criteria. He still dabbled in illicit drugs and stumbled upon mixed amphetamine salts given to him by a friend. He found that amphetamine salts helped his focus enormously, and he used it when he had to get a project to completion quickly. He experienced one threshold depressive episode that lasted 3 months and remitted without treatment.

Was there a relationship between Mason's substance abuse and development of bipolar disorder? It is obviously impossible to say. He had been abusing drugs for 2 years before the onset of his first mood episode. Why and whether the LSD used prior to the onset of his first manic episode was a biological precipitant is unknown. It did appear, however, that his moods were more unstable while he continued to abuse drugs heavily, and they seemed to subside after his stint in rehab, even though he never gave up drug use completely. We have observed the relationship between mood improvement and decreased substance abuse in the Suffolk County Mental Health Project sample.[51]

Although much has been written about antidepressants precipitating mania in patients with bipolar I disorder,[54,55] Mason took antidepressants on a number of occasions without mania; his mood stabilized, by and large, without medication at all.

Mason's ADHD had posed more difficulty for him in school than he wanted to admit, at least according to his mother, who was an informant during the first years of the follow-up study. He would not accept treatment for it. However, when he stumbled onto the efficacy of stimulant medication, he self-medicated seemingly appropriately. That is, stimulants were never drugs of abuse for Mason.

Finally, there is an interesting relationship between the pathoplastic and pathologic aspects of Mason's symptoms. His grandiose delusions when first ill revolved around becoming a famous TV personality who would change the world. It may not be a coincidence that he ended up working in the creative end of the film industry.

Psychosis in Bipolar Disorder

While ADHD and externalizing disorders pose the most difficult differential diagnosis challenge in prepubertal children, psychosis and its differential diagnosis becomes a problem in adolescence and young adulthood that is usually not an issue in children—though reports of non-mood-related hallucinations that might be falsely attributed to a mood disorder are not rare in community samples of children.[56] As noted in Table 2.1, with the exception of data from Geller and Findling, psychosis rates are always lower in children than in teens.[15,24] The significance of psychotic symptoms, however, remains poorly understood.

The following young woman, who also was part of the Suffolk County Mental Health Project, illustrates someone whose psychopathology exemplifies this point. With the exception of the baseline research diagnosis, there was no consensus over follow-up as to whether she had bipolar disorder type I or schizoaffective disorder, bipolar type. This problem rarely, if ever, arises with prepubertal mania.

CASE EXAMPLE 4 Bipolar Disorder in a Young Adult With Psychosis

Felicia was 21-years-old when first hospitalized. She had an uncomplicated childhood, was friendly and social, and was in honors programs throughout high school. She was attending an Ivy League college and was home on Christmas break when her family noted that she was uncharacteristically irritable and critical of her parents. She showed no interest in church attendance, though church had been an important part of her life. She appeared depressed and complained that she had no friends and that no one liked her. She did not mail Christmas cards or buy Christmas presents. She withdrew from her family, had trouble sleeping, and complained of difficulty studying for exams. She began drinking more heavily. She returned to college and developed a belief that others were talking about her and that her roommate was sending her hints and messages by leaving slippers on her dresser or putting a cup on the windowsill. Felicia became suicidal, at which point her parents were asked to take her home. She was taken to a psychiatrist who hospitalized her, at which point she consented to be a part of the study. Her baseline research diagnosis based on this presentation was major depressive disorder with mood incongruent psychotic features.

During the latter part of her hospitalization, Felicia became agitated, talkative, expansive, and self-confident. She picked constant fights with her parents. She was observed to be manic, treated with lithium carbonate, and discharged after improving enough to return to college and graduate. Subsequently, however, the jobs she took did not seem commensurate with her previous level of function. She worked as a sales clerk and bartender. She subsequently became very focused on religion, noting that "developing a relationship with God helped me find peace."

Four years after the initial depressive episode, Felicia developed a period of "confusion" during which she was hyperreligious, had racing thoughts, grandiosity, trouble concentrating, and excessive talking. She denied this was a manic episode, however, and felt it had nothing to do with having discontinued her medication, based on a message she saw in the Bible. She was brought to a psychiatry emergency room, where she was hospitalized with confusion and auditory hallucinations that included Satan's talking to her. Lithium and antipsychotic medications were restarted, and her acute psychosis subsided. However, she was tangential and circumstantial in her conversations, and she remained overly preoccupied with religion and God. She did not resume the level of social contacts she had experienced in the past. Nevertheless, she was able to return to school and obtain a nursing degree.

At the 10-year follow-up, Felicia had been psychiatrically hospitalized numerous times with paranoid and/or religious delusions, auditory hallucinations (sometimes with multiple voices), hyperreligiosity, and with speech described as pressured and circumstantial at times; or with a poverty of speech, thought blocking, and psychomotor retardation at other times. Between episodes, she believed that people were talking about her or taking special notice of her. Although Felicia was working full time, she did not have much of a social life. She did maintain a relationship with her family, though that too was occasionally strained.

Over the following 10 years, Felicia was somewhat more adherent to medication, though she did sometimes discontinue her medications, invariably ending up in the hospital—usually with manic symptoms of irritability, agitation, expansiveness, grandiosity, and bizarre, racing thoughts of things patently untrue (e.g., the Mafia was after her, she was sexually abused by a relative with whom there is no evidence she even spent time alone). Her employer has been tolerant of her psychiatric issues, and she has been able to keep her job. There have been no serious relationships, and she reports that she does not have much time to engage in recreational activities.

There were two sources of diagnostic controversy. The first was whether her chronic referential thinking (between episodes) constituted psychosis. The second was whether what appeared to be social and academic decline represented negative symptoms. Felicia had always been involved in her church, though not unusually so when she still lived at home. It is relevant that this interest became one of the foci of her delusions, another case of the pathoplastic nature of personality or interest on subsequent psychotic symptoms. She had been an academic achiever who was socially connected. This changed after her first episode of psychosis, and although Felicia has functioned fairly well at least occupationally and particularly on medication, she has shown evidence of significant change in her personality and has never returned to her premorbid level of function.

Whether Felicia has a "schizoaffective" disorder or bipolar disorder with a relatively poor outcome may be a matter of interpretation. In prepubertal children, however, patients who are given the diagnosis of bipolar disorder rarely present with this clinical picture. In part, this may be because most are not old enough to have established a stable, premorbid level of function. In addition, the nature of standardized interview instruments does not allow investigators to deconstruct a child's stories. The question of psychosis involves distinguishing between true psychosis and nonspecific odd beliefs and transitory hallucinations that are not uncommon in children, may be developmental, and often do not meet criteria for any specific disorder.[57]

Conclusions

This chapter has outlined several issues that make the comparison of bipolar symptomatology between children, adolescents, and adults potentially quite difficult. Studying bipolar disorder requires the use of standardized assessments. However, the most commonly used instruments were not designed to obtain qualitative information. Furthermore, they were patterned after *DSM* criteria that were not meant to be all-inclusive. The interviews themselves were developed to be comprehensive and to allow interviewers to obtain enough information to decide whether a symptom is present or absent, or at best to rate a symptom as mild, moderate, or severe. Including age-appropriate or pathoplastic information in clinical studies requires a good interview and a way of comparing the information obtained across individuals. Qualitative changes in symptomatology with age are rarely recorded systematically and thus are not available for study.

In addition, to qualify for a bipolar diagnosis, a child, adolescent, or adult by definition has to meet diagnostic criteria, so it may not be surprising that interview studies show more similarities than differences between age groups.[35] Where there are differences in phenomenology, they may be at least, in part, developmental (e.g., higher rates of ADHD and behavior disorders in younger patients).[20] Even increased rates of comorbid substance abuse might reflect developmental issues, since substance abuse occurs more often in the context of ADHD and conduct disorder.[34] Further, distinguishing manic symptoms from the backdrop of other psychopathology is not always easy. In children, confusion with ADHD is common; in teens and young adults, comorbid substance abuse is particularly common; and in adults, bipolar disorder is often confused with depression and anxiety.[58,59]

The reason for long-standing observations of higher rates of psychosis in patients with teenage and young adult onset remains poorly understood, as do differences in the nature of the psychosis observed and the significance of psychosis in mood disorders.[59,60] We have suggested that it is the presence of psychosis that has frequently led to confusion with schizophrenia in these patients. [25,60]

Summary

Age-related comparisons of bipolar disorder have been severely complicated by the lack of diagnostic homogeneity across age groups and instruments.[2] Furthermore, many comparisons of bipolar disorder classify individuals by age of onset, while symptoms are measured later in the course of illness—a patient classified as having had illness onset at 18 years old might be studied at the age of 30. Other concerns include age-related differences in comorbidity; research criteria used to delineate samples restrict the range of symptomatology so the bulk of group variability will encompass nondiagnostic symptoms. This phenomenon may exaggerate some differences, potentially giving misleading findings around variation in rates of comorbid ADHD, behavior disorders, and mixed episodes. Other comorbid symptoms and diagnoses also appear to be more prominent in younger patients with bipolar disorder, including psychosis and substance abuse. Symptom expression, however, is unique to each patient—the so-called pathoplastic effects. These are likely to vary with age, but they are typically not recorded, leaving a substantial hole in our ability to truly compare the pathology of bipolar disorder in children, adolescents, and adults with the disorder.

Author Disclosure

Drs. Carlson and Pataki have no conflicts to disclose. Dr. Carlson receives research funding from GSK, BMS/Otuska, Pfizer, Merck/Schering Plough, and the National Institute of Mental Health.

References

1. Harrington R, Myatt T. Is preadolescent mania the same condition as adult mania? A British perspective. *Biol Psychiatry.* 2003;53:961–9.
2. Kowatch RA, Youngstrom EA, Danielyan A, Findling RL. Review and meta-analysis of the phenomenology and clinical characteristics of mania in children and adolescents. *Bipolar Disord.* 2005;7:483–96.
3. Carlson GA, Klein DN. How to understand divergent views on bipolar disorder in youth. *Annu Rev Clin Psychol.* 2014;10:529–51.
4. American Psychiatric Association. *Diagnostic and Statistical Manual of Mental Disorders.* 3rd ed. Washington, DC: American Psychiatric Association; 1980.

5. American Psychiatric Association. *Diagnostic and Statistical Manual of Mental Disorders*. 2nd ed. Washington, DC: American Psychiatric Association; 1968.

6. American Psychiatric Association. *Diagnostic and Statistical Manual of Mental Disorders*. 4th ed. Text rev. Washington, DC: American Psychiatric Association; 2000.

7. American Psychiatric Association. *Diagnostic and Statistical Manual of Mental Disorders*. 5th ed. Washington, DC: American Psychiatric Association; 2013.

8. American Psychiatric Association. *Diagnostic and Statistical Manual of Mental Disorders*. 3rd ed. Rev. Washington, DC: American Psychiatric Association; 1987.

9. Carlson GA, Meyer SE. Phenomenology and diagnosis of bipolar disorder in children, adolescents, and adults: complexities and developmental issues. *Dev Psychopathol*. 2006;18:939–69.

10. Youngstrom EA, Findling RL, Calabrese JR. Who are the comorbid adolescents? Agreement between psychiatric diagnosis, parent, teacher, and youth report. *J Abnorm Child Psychol*. 2003;31:231–45.

11. Carlson GA, Blader JC. Diagnostic implications of informant disagreement of manic symptoms. *J Child Adolesc Psychopharmacol*. 2011;5:399–405.

12. Andreasen NC. DSM and the death of phenomenology in America: an example of unintended consequences. *Schizophr Bull*. 2007;33:108–12.

13. Carlson GA. Will the child with mania please stand up? *Br J Psychiatry*. 2011;198:171–2.

14. Galanter CA, Hundt SR, Goyal P, Le J, Fisher PW. Variability among research diagnostic interview instruments in the application of DSM-IV-TR criteria for pediatric bipolar disorder. *J Am Acad Child Adolesc Psychiatry*. 2012;51:605–21.

15. Geller B, Zimerman B, Williams M, Delbello MP, Frazier J, Beringer L. Phenomenology of prepubertal and early adolescent bipolar disorder: examples of elated mood, grandiose behaviors, decreased need for sleep, racing thoughts and hypersexuality. *J Child Adolesc Psychopharmacol*. 2002;12:3–9.

16. Wozniak J, Monuteaux M, Richards J, Lail KE, Faraone SV, Biederman J. Convergence between structured diagnostic interviews and clinical assessment on the diagnosis of pediatric-onset mania. *Biol Psychiatry*. 2003;53:938–44

17. Carlson GA. Treating the childhood bipolar controversy: a tale of two children. *Am J Psychiatry*. 2009;166:18–24.

18. Young RC, Biggs JT, Ziegler VE, Meyer DA. A rating scale for mania: reliability, validity and sensitivity. *Br J Psychiatry*. 1978;133:429–35.

19. American Psychiatric Association. *Diagnostic and Statistical Manual of Mental Disorders*. 4th ed. Washington, DC.: American Psychiatric Association; 1994.

20. Pataki C, Carlson GA. The comorbidity of ADHD and bipolar disorder: any less confusion? *Curr Psychiatry Rep*. 2013;15:372.

21. Faraone SV, Biederman J, Mennin D, Wozniak J, Spencer T. Attention-deficit hyperactivity disorder with bipolar disorder: a familial subtype? *J Am Acad Child Adolesc Psychiatry*. 1997;36:1378–87.

22. Birmaher B, Axelson D, Strober M, et al. Comparison of manic and depressive symptoms between children and adolescents with bipolar spectrum disorders. *Bipolar Disord*. 2009;11:52–62.

23. Masi G, Perugi G, Toni C, et al. Attention-deficit hyperactivity disorder—bipolar comorbidity in children and adolescents. *Bipolar Disord*. 2006;8:373–81.

24. Findling, RL, Gracious BL, McNamara NK, Youngstrom EA, Demeter CA. Rapid, continuous cyucling and psychiatric co-morbidity in pediatric bipolar I disorder. *Bipolar Disord*. 2001;3:202–10.

25. Carlson GA, Strober M. Manic-depressive illness in early adolescence. A study of clinical and diagnostic characteristics in six cases. *J Am Acad Child Psychiatry*. 1978;17:138–53.

26. Jairam R, Srinath S, Girimaji SC, Seshadrei SP. A prospective 4–5 year follow-up of juvenile onset bipolar disorder. *Bipolar Disord*. 2004;5:386–294.

27. Geller B, Tillman R, Bolhofner K, Zimerman B. Child bipolar I disorder: prospective continuity with adult bipolar I disorder; characteristics of second and third episodes; predictors of 8-year outcome. *Arch Gen Psychiatry*. 2008;65:1125–33.

28. Srinath S, Janardhan RYC, Girmaji SR, Seshadri SP, Subbakrishna DK. A prospective study of bipolar disorder in children and adolescents from India. *Acta Psychiatr Scand*. 1998;6:437–42.

29. Masi J, Perugi G, Millepiedi S, et al. Clinical implications of DSM-IV subtyping of bipolar disorders in referred chidlren and adolescents. *Am Acad Child Adolesc Psychiatry*. 2007;46:1299–306.

30. Bernardi S, Cortese S, Solanto M, Hollander E, Pallanti S. Bipolar disorder and comorbid attention deficit hyperactivity disorder. A distinct clinical phenotype? Clinical characteristics and temperamental traits. *World J Biol Psychiatry.* 2010;11:656–66.

31. Carlson GA, Bromet EJ, Sievers S. Phenomenology and outcome of subjects with early—and adult-onset psychotic mania. *Am J Psychiatry.* 2000;157:213–9.

32. Perlis RH, Miyahara S, Marangell LB, Wisniewski SR, Ostacher M. STEP-BD Investigators. Long-term implications of early onset in bipolar disorder: data from the first 1000 participants in the systematic treatment enhancement program for bipolar disorder (STEP-BD). *Biol Psychiatry.* 2004;55:875–8.

33. Sachs GS, Baldassano CF, Truman CJ. Comorbidity of attention deficit hyperactivity disorder with early and late bipolar disorder. *Am J Psychiatry.* 2000;157:466–8.

34. Carlson GA, Bromet EJ, Jandorf L. Conduct disorder and mania: what does it mean in adults? *J Affect Disord.* 1998;48:199–205.

35. Demeter CA, Youngstrom EA, Carlson GA, et al. Age differences in the phenomenology of pediatric bipolar disorder. *J Affect Disord.* 2013;147(1–3):295–303.

36. Axelson D, Birmaher BJ, Brent D, et al. A preliminary study of the Kiddie Schedule for Affective Disorders and Schizophrenia for School-Age Children mania rating scale for children and adolescents. *J Child Adolesc Psychopharmacol.* 2003;13(4):463–70.

37. Topor DR, Swenson L, Hunt JI, et al. Manic symptoms in youth with bipolar disorder: factor analysis by age of symptom onset and current age. *J Affect Disord.* 2013;145:409–12.

38. Safer DJ, Magno Zito J, Safer AM. Age-grouped differences in bipolar mania. *Compr Psychiatry.* 2012;53:1110–7.

39. McGlashan TH. Adolescent versus adult onset of mania. *Am J Psychiatry.* 1988;145:221–3.

40. Carlson GA, Bromet EJ, Sievers S. Phenomenology and outcome of subjects with early—and adult-onset psychotic mania. *Am J Psychiatry.* 2000;157:213–9.

41. Schürhoff F, Bellivier F, Jouvent R, et al. Early and late onset bipolar disorders: two different forms of manic-depressive illness? *J Affect Disord.* 2000;58:215–21.

42. Schulze TG, Müller DJ, Krauss H, et al. Further evidence for age of onset being an indicator for severity in bipolar disorder. *J Affect Disord.* 2002;68(2–3):343–5.

43. Kennedy N, Boydell J, Kalidindi S, et al. Gender differences in incidence and age at onset of mania and bipolar disorder over a 35-year period in Camberwell, England. *Am J Psychiatry.* 2005;162(2):257–62.

44. Suominen K, Mantere O, Valtonen H, et al. Early age at onset of bipolar disorder is associated with more severe clinical features but delayed treatment seeking. *Bipolar Disord.* 2007;9:698–705.

45. Hamshere ML, Gordon-Smith K, Forty L, et al. Age-at-onset in bipolar-I disorder: mixture analysis of 1369 cases identifies three distinct clinical sub-groups. *J Affect Disord.* 2009;116(1–2):23–9.

46. Sax KW, Strakowski SM, Keck PE Jr, et al. Comparison of patients with early-, typical-, and late-onset affective psychosis. *Am J Psychiatry.* 1997;154(9):1299–301.

47. McElroy SL, Strakowski SM, West SA, Keck PE Jr, McConville BJ. Phenomenology of adolescent and adult mania in hospitalized patients with bipolar disorder. *Am J Psychiatry.* 1997;154(1):44–9.

48. Patel NC, Delbello MP, Keck PE Jr, Strakowski SM. Phenomenology associated with age at onset in patients with bipolar disorder at their first psychiatric hospitalization. *Bipolar Disord.* 2006;8(1):91–4.

49. Mitchell PB, Frankland A, Hadzi-Pavlovic D, et al. Comparison of depressive episodes in bipolar disorder and in major depressive disorder within bipolar disorder pedigrees. *Br J Psychiatry.* 2011;199:303–9.

50. Wilens TE. The nature of the relationship betweenattention-deficit/hyperactivity disorder and substance use. *J Clin Psychiatry.* 2007;68(Suppl 11):4–8.

51. Bromet EJ, Schwartz JE, Fennig S, et al. The epidemiology of psychosis: the Suffolk County Mental Health Project. *Schizophr Bull.* 1992;18:243–55.

52. Carlson GA, Kotov R, Chang SW. Ruggero C, Bromet EJ. Early determinants of four-year clinical outcomes in bipolar disorder with psychosis. *Bipolar Disord.* 2012;14:19–30.

53. Spitzer RL, Williams JBW, Gibbon M, First MB, Endicott J, Klein DF *User's Guide for the Structured Clinical Interview for DSM Disorder III-R*. Washington, DC: American Psychiatric Press; 1990.

54. Carlson GA, Finch SJ, Fochtmann LJ, et al. Antidepressant-associated switches from depression to mania in severe bipolar disorder. *Bipolar Disord*. 2007;9:851–9.

55. Ghaemi SN, Hsu DJ, Soldani F, Goodwin FK. Antidepressants in bipolar disorder: the case for caution. *Bipolar Disord*. 2003;5:421–33.

56. Carlson GA. Affective disorders and psychosis in youth. *Child Adolesc Psychiatr Clin N Am*. 2013;22:569–80.

57. Frazier JA, Carlson GA. Diagnostically homeless and needing appropriate placement. *J Child Adolesc Psychopharmacol*. 2005;15:337–42.

58. Angst J, Azorin JM, Bowden CL, et al. Prevalence and characteristics of undiagnosed bipolar disorder in inpatients with a major depressive episode: the BRIDGE study. *Arch Gen Psychiatry*. 2011;68:791–8.

59. Ballenger JC, Reur VI, Post, RM. The "atypical" clinical picture of adolescent mania. *Am J Psychiatry*. 1982;139:602–6.

60. Joyce PR. Age of onset in bipolar affective disorder and misdiagnosis as schizophrenia. *Psychol Med*. 1984;13:145–9.

Differential Diagnosis of Bipolar Disorder in Children and Youth

Kenneth E. Towbin and Ellen Leibenluft

Background and Overview

The differential diagnosis of pediatric bipolar disorder has been a topic of intense interest in the child psychiatry literature for the past two decades. Historically, bipolar disorder has been viewed as an illness characterized by episodes of mania or hypomania, as well as depression. As detailed later in this chapter, the defining features of an episode are the occurrence of a distinct change in mood from the patient's baseline, accompanied by the onset or clear worsening of associated cognitive and behavioral symptoms. Controversy arose in the late 1990s when researchers in child psychiatry suggested that the presentation of bipolar disorder in youth was fundamentally different from the episodic phenotype seen in adults because bipolar disorder in youth was instead characterized by severe nonepisodic irritability[1,2] or by extremely brief episodes (i.e., only hours long) whose symptoms could not be differentiated from those of comorbid illnesses, such as attention-deficit/hyperactivity disorder (ADHD).[3,4] Concurrent with this proposed reformulation of the diagnostic criteria for bipolar disorder presenting in youth, there was a significant rise in the rate at which the diagnosis of bipolar disorder was being assigned to American youth in both outpatient[5] and inpatient[6] settings.

Data suggest that the prevalence of nonepisodic irritability in children is higher than that of strictly diagnosed, episodic bipolar disorder.[7,8] Therefore, while the reasons for the rise in the rate of the pediatric bipolar disorder diagnosis is not known, one plausible explanation is that clinicians were tending increasingly to assign the diagnosis of bipolar disorder to youth with nonepisodic irritability. However, this diagnostic practice runs counter to data indicating that nonepisodic severe irritability should *not* be viewed as a phenotype of bipolar disorder. Specifically, longitudinal studies demonstrate that youth with irritability are at increased risk for unipolar depressive and anxiety disorders in adulthood, rather than for the onset of manic episodes.[9] Therefore, in the guidance provided later in this chapter, we emphasize the importance of identifying distinct episodes of mania or hypomania when determining whether a child or adolescent should be viewed as having bipolar disorder.

We begin the chapter by describing the criteria for bipolar disorder in *DSM-5*,[10] including a discussion of how these criteria differ from those in *DSM-IV-TR*.[11] We focus in particular on challenges that arise when clinicians apply these criteria to youth. We then discuss the differential diagnosis of major depressive disorder versus bipolar disorder, and of disruptive mood dysregulation disorder (DMDD) versus bipolar disorder; DMDD is a new diagnosis in *DSM-5*[10] designed to capture children with severe, nonepisodic irritability. Finally, although psychosis and irritability may arise in depressive or manic episodes, clinicians must be mindful that they also appear in other childhood psychopathologies. Thus, we conclude with sections discussing the diagnostic features of psychosis and irritability in bipolar disorder.

DSM-5 Bipolar Disorder

DSM-5[10] bipolar disorder has three subtypes, bipolar disorder type 1 (BP-1), bipolar disorder type 2 (BP-2), and other specified bipolar and related disorder (OSBP). Some clinicians use "bipolar disorder" interchangeably with "bipolar spectrum" to denote all three subtypes, while others use "bipolar disorder" to refer to only to BP-1 and BP-2. Of note, the criteria for each of the diagnoses in the bipolar disorder section of *DSM-5*[10] do not differentiate children or adolescents from adults. However, while the *DSM-5*[10] criteria do not differ developmentally, many developmental issues arise when applying the criteria, as described subsequently.

Bipolar I Disorder: The Manic Episode

The sine qua non for the diagnosis of BP-1 is a history of at least one manic episode. In the criteria for a manic episode, the A section requires a change in mood and activity from baseline, whereas the B section specifies associated symptoms. When the A criteria arise and continue for at least a week and are accompanied by significant worsening, or the first appearance, of B symptoms, this defines a manic episode. When diagnosing a manic episode in youth, it is particularly important to be mindful that the A and B symptoms of a manic episode must be temporally linked in this way.

Manic Episode "A" Criteria

The A criteria emphasize the pivotal feature of a manic episode: a distinct change in mood from baseline that is characterized by elevated/expansive mood or irritability, *and* is accompanied by increased energy and/or goal-directed behavior. All of these symptoms must be distinctly different from that person's usual baseline functioning, and they must be apparent most of the day most days for at least 1 week.

Compared to adults, it is more challenging to judge whether a child, particularly a younger child, is displaying elevated/expansive mood. Exaggerated positive emotional responses and expansive ideas can be normative for young children, especially when the child is excited by exceptionally positive events (e.g., visiting a theme park or anticipating birthday gifts and celebrations). Similarly, it is common for immature children (e.g., children who are developmentally approximately 3–7 years old, irrespective of their chronological age) to exhibit exuberant responses. When clinicians compare the excessive emotional responses of an immature child to those of children who are developmentally normative, they may misinterpret a child's immaturity as symptoms of elevated or irritable mood. Thus, while it is important to assess any clinical symptom with respect to a child's developmental age, rather than to his or her chronological age, this principle is particularly important when assessing elevated mood.

It is also helpful to bear in mind that an episode is defined by a change in mood that departs from *that person's* typical (baseline) mood state. For example, when deciding whether a person's mood is elevated, the clinician should compare the child's behaviors and statements to *what is typical for that child under similar circumstances*, rather than to the behavior of other children of the same age. In addition, a gauge of maturity for children is their ability to control their emotional responses to conform to the demands of their environment. Thus, when assessing a child who is exhibiting dysregulated behavior, it is essential to ascertain whether that behavior is distinctly different from baseline, or whether that child frequently exhibits such behavior.

DSM-5[10] differs from *DSM-IV-TR*[11] in that the *DSM-5* A criteria are not solely about mood. That is, the *DSM-5*[10] A criteria require a distinct period of "persistently increased goal-directed activity or energy" that must co-occur with the abnormally elevated, expansive or irritable mood. In this way, a change in mood *and* a change in goal-directed activity or energy frame the episode. The additional requirement of abnormally increased energy to the *DSM-5*[10] A criteria presents a somewhat narrower concept of a manic episode than *DSM-IV-TR*. For children and adolescents, particularly those who are immature or have ADHD with hyperactivity, the critical question to consider when assessing a possible manic episode is whether the child's activity or energy during the putative episode clearly exceeds his or her hyperkinetic baseline. In this way, the clinician can avoid inappropriately "double counting" increased energy toward both mania and ADHD.

In both *DSM-IV-TR*[11] and *DSM-5*[10] the duration of a manic episode is at least 7 days, and a hypomanic episode at least 4 days. However, compared to *DSM-IV-TR*, *DSM-5* imparts a clearer concept of an episode by specifying the *extent* of the change in mood. In *DSM-IV-TR*, the criteria required "persistently elevated, expansive or irritable mood lasting at least 1 week." However, this terminology was ambiguous regarding exactly how persistent the abnormal mood must be during that week to meet the threshold. *DSM-5*[10] establishes that, in a manic episode, the individual must display altered mood and energy "most of the day, nearly every day." The latter terminology mirrors that in the mood criteria for a major depressive episode—that is, sadness or anhedonia most of the day, nearly every day.

The inclusion of the modifying phrase "most of the day, nearly every day" in the criterion is particularly helpful when weighing whether irritability is a symptom of a manic episode in a developmentally immature child. Commonly, children who have developmental disorders or are highly impulsive have brief outbursts of irritability, sometimes multiple times per day. However, these outbursts are an incomplete picture of the child's mood throughout the day. The concept of "most of the day" directs the clinician's focus to the child's mood when he or she is not in the midst of an outburst, rather than focusing exclusively on mood during brief outbursts. The criterion specifies that the child should display irritability throughout the day, not exclusively when confronted with frustration or disappointment. In addition, when assessing any child, including (but not limited to) children who are immature or have developmental disorders, it is important to once again remember that the definition of a manic episode requires a change relative to that child's usual functioning. Thus, when deciding whether impulsive outbursts are indicative of a manic episode, the clinician must consider whether they are distinctly different from the child's usual behavior or a continuation of a characteristic pattern for that child; only the former would support the diagnosis of a manic episode.

As with irritability, when deciding whether the elevated mood of a child with a developmental delay or disorder exceeds the threshold for a manic episode, the clinician should remember that the abnormal mood must be "present most of the day nearly every day." A developmentally immature or highly impulsive child may display elevated mood in response to hearing of plans for exciting, pleasing activities, or when engaging in such activities. Generally, these responses do not last most of a day, and they are typical for how that child responds in these contexts. Thus, the response is not sufficiently long-lasting to qualify for mania, and it also does not signify a departure from that child's usual functioning. Of course, when a child's response to *unusual* circumstances includes changes in mood and activity from his or her baseline, such changes also should not be viewed as symptoms of a manic episode merely because they differ from the child's day-to-day behavior.

Manic Episode "B" Criteria

The B criteria include symptoms that are associated with a manic episode; many of them are less specific than the A criteria. Two concepts can be helpful when assessing B criteria. The first concept is that of a manic episode as a "bundle" of symptoms. That is, the "A" and "B" criteria must have their onset (or, in the case of the B criteria, either have their onset or worsen—see later) at the same time. *DSM-5*[10] establishes this principle clearly by noting that the B criteria must be present during the time that the "A" criteria are met, that is, "during the period of the mood disturbance and increased energy or activity."

The second concept concerns the fact that five of the seven B criteria (distractibility, agitation, pressured speech, flight of ideas, and racing thoughts) are not specific to manic episodes but instead are criteria or associated features of multiple other disorders. However, as with the A criteria, the B symptoms must "represent a noticeable change from usual behavior" if they are to "count" toward a manic episode. Therefore, when children with other disorders are assessed for a manic episode, extra care must be taken to determine not only whether a B criterion symptom meets a clinical threshold but also whether it was present prior to the onset of the A criteria symptoms and, if so, whether it worsened during the time that the A criteria are present. A common example involves assessing distractibility in a child with ADHD and a possible manic episode. In this instance, it is important for the clinician to assess whether the child's distractibility worsened markedly at the same time that he or she was exhibiting abnormal mood and activity. Such distinct worsening would be required for the distractibility to be considered a symptom of mania.

Among the B criterion symptoms, grandiosity and inflated self-esteem are particularly difficult to assess in children and adolescents because one feature of immaturity is inaccurate perception of one's skills and abilities. In developmentally immature children (e.g., preschoolers, those with intellectual disability) this feature is readily observed and unremarkable. Similarly, there is good evidence that adolescents often miscalculate their abilities, in that they may have excessively high regard for their skills or hold unrealistic ideas about their capacities.[12,13] The challenge for the child psychiatrist evaluating an immature individual is discerning when these inaccurate self-assessments exceed the threshold for grandiosity or inflated self-esteem of a manic episode. In addition, it is again helpful to remember that, for the symptoms of grandiosity and inflated self-esteem to be indicative of a manic episode, they must be *significantly* more pronounced than that individual's usual, everyday functioning. In addition, it is important to assess not only the child's grandiose cognitions but also how they affect the individual's behavior. Thus, when a child exhibits behaviors during an episode that are unusual for him and stem from having an uncharacteristically high opinion of himself, this supports the diagnosis of a manic episode. For example, an adolescent who makes disparaging remarks about his teacher (e.g., saying to his parents at home, "I can teach the class better than he can") may be offering an opinion that is consonant with his typical level of high self-admiration. However, when a student who typically is well mannered and appropriate in the classroom thinks he can do a better job than the teacher *and* creates a disturbance in his attempts to take over the classroom, this clinical presentation is more consistent with inflated self-esteem.

Similar considerations arise with regard to the Criteria B symptom "lack of regard for potentially painful consequences." Developmentally immature children assess their abilities inaccurately and, congruent with this, are limited in their ability to predict the consequences of their actions. Since they cannot grasp the range of possibilities or predict accurately how others will respond, they cannot use these predictions to modulate their behavior appropriately. Thus, what may appear to be a lack of regard for potentially painful consequences may instead be an inability to predict that the consequences of a given action may be painful. Moreover, as noted earlier for both the A criteria and the other B symptoms, the assessment of "lack of regard for potentially painful consequences" requires consideration of whether the child's cognitions and behavior represent a distinct change from baseline. Finally, it is important to consider whether the child takes actions that reflect his lack of consideration for the consequences. Merely voicing ideas about wishes or fantasies without engaging in behaviors based on these thoughts would not be sufficient to meet this criterion. However, the 8-year-old who is typically hesitant and considerate, but now thinks that he is keeping the neighborhood safe from intruders by donning camouflage clothing, gripping a hunting knife, and staying out late while creeping from one neighbor's yard to another's, has not considered the consequences of alarming his neighbors or being injured.

B-criteria symptoms such as distractibility, talkativeness, racing thoughts, flight of ideas, and involvement in activities that have a high risk of painful consequences are also symptoms of other childhood disorders. This lack of specificity of symptoms can be confusing for clinicians who are asked to determine the presence of a manic episode in children with preexisting, comorbid disorders that are also characterized by these symptoms. In contrast, true grandiosity, decreased need for sleep, and increased goal-directed behavior are relatively specific to a *DSM-5*[10] manic episode. Deciding whether the less specific symptoms are part of a manic episode turns on whether they appear exclusively, or significantly worsen, during the period when the A criteria are met. *DSM-5*[10] makes this clear when it emphasizes that B criteria represent a "noticeable change from the child's usual behavior" and "are present to a significant degree." Particular care is needed when making the diagnosis of a manic episode in children with developmental disorders or conditions that entail rapid changes in mood, irritability, or impulsivity. Since such symptoms are widespread in ADHD, conduct disorder, oppositional defiant disorder, generalized anxiety disorder, autism spectrum disorder, and posttraumatic stress disorder (PTSD), making the diagnosis of a manic episode when these disorders also are present requires particular care. It is crucial to define clearly the time frame of the manic episode and to exclude any B-criteria symptoms during the episode that are not clearly worse than at baseline.

Impairment, Psychosis, and Hospitalization

The diagnosis of mania is made when the child meets both symptom and impairment criteria. Impairment from mania is indicated by severely compromised functioning, the emergence of psychosis, and/or hospitalization. For children and youth with BP-I, compromised functioning arises when symptoms of the mood disorder produce a marked decline in performance at school, in interactions with peers, and/or in relationships at home. Established routines of hygiene, nutrition, and care of personal belongings or pets are likely to be disrupted. Once again, a crucial consideration is whether the child's excessive activity, irritability, or elevated mood is the source of this deterioration. For example, a child who, as a result of severe ADHD, typically shows significant limitations in his ability to care for his belongings, independently manage his personal hygiene, and maintain friendships may be markedly impaired. However, when these impairments characterize his baseline functioning, they cannot be considered to be part of a putative manic episode. They should be viewed indicative of mania only when there is a substantial decline in abilities that occurs concurrently with the appearance of the A and B criteria symptoms of a manic episode.

Several important features of psychosis in children are relevant to the diagnosis of bipolar disorder. First, clinicians must be mindful of child development when assessing psychosis. Immature children (e.g., those who are very young or have intellectual or language-based learning disabilities) may describe their experiences in concrete ways that can be misinterpreted as the presence of hallucinations. For example, a child reported a "voice" telling him to "do bad things" when asked to describe these experiences says, "It's like on TV with a devil on one shoulder and an angel or the other side." On further exploration with the child it became clear that he was describing his inner moral conflict, not actually experiencing hallucinations. Self-report or parents' speculations about what their child may be experiencing have limited reliability for making a determination about the presence of visual or auditory hallucinations in a young child. However, parental report about behavior (e.g., the child's comments and nonverbal actions) that accompany self-reported hallucinations can corroborate the child's report. Also, psychosis is typically accompanied by very significant impairment. Reports of psychosis without concomitant evidence of impairment at school and/or with peers should receive particular scrutiny. In addition, odd ways of perceiving or thinking that are present at baseline should not be viewed as symptoms of either mania or psychotic depression.

Of course, psychosis may appear in other disorders and is not specific to bipolar disorder. Being familiar with the differential diagnosis of psychosis is particularly important in a child with a comorbid anxiety disorder (such as PTSD, panic disorder, or separation anxiety disorder), sleep disorders, developmental disorders, or epilepsy. For example, a child with separation anxiety who has auditory hallucinations in response to circumstances that force him to be apart from his parents does not carry the same prognosis as a child who experiences hallucinations without any precedent or threat. In addition, when a youth's first psychosis is of very recent onset (e.g., days to weeks ago), it can be exceptionally difficult to distinguish between a manic episode and incipient schizophrenia. Generally, both the course of the illness over an extended period (e.g., 6 months) and a detailed review of premorbid functioning are necessary to tease out the pattern and associated features. Only then can the clinician determine the likelihood of an episodic or persistent psychotic disorder.

The hospitalization criterion can be problematic when making the diagnosis of a manic episode in children or youth. Several features should be considered. First, in many places in the United States, inpatient pediatric psychiatric care is unavailable. The child's impairment during an episode may well exceed the threshold of dangerousness that would warrant hospitalization, but inpatient treatment is simply not an option. Thus, level of impairment may be a more reliable measure. A further complication is that the threshold for hospitalization differs regionally. Beyond symptom severity, the decision to hospitalize a child can be influenced heavily by the setting where the child is evaluated, the time of day, availability of outpatient services, insurance resources, and the parents' distress or mental state when the child is brought to the emergency room.[14] Importantly, if a hospitalization occurs, it supports the diagnosis of a manic episode only if inpatient care resulted from a distinct episode characterized by the A- and B-criteria symptoms that were described previously. For example, if a child with a history of chronic irritability is hospitalized because she exhibits aggressive or threatening behavior, this hospitalization in itself does not attest to her having BP-1 because a manic *episode* is not defined solely by the occurrence of hospitalization or aggression. Both hospitalization and aggression can occur for a variety of reasons, and more clinical information is needed to decide whether the hospitalization is the result of a manic episode.

Preschoolers

The rapid developmental transitions and relatively wide range in normative behavior characteristic of the preschool age group make diagnosing a manic episode particularly challenging for children who are this age. Preschoolers' marked sensitivity to environmental context and the fact that developmental lags or disabilities may be present, but not yet identified, further complicate the diagnostic process. The literature contains a number of case reports of preschool bipolar disorder[15,16] but, in many instances, distinct episodes are not described, and the clinical picture is more one of chronic severe irritability and mood lability, with some waxing and waning of symptoms. Empirical investigations[17,18] have been undertaken to address the challenges of identifying bipolar disorder in early childhood.

Of note, the AACAP practice parameters for the assessment of children with bipolar disorder[19] recommend caution when applying the diagnosis of bipolar disorder to preschool children, noting that the validity of the diagnosis in young children has yet to be established. Further, these practice parameters note that, while the assignment of a bipolar disorder diagnosis is often a prelude to the initiation of aggressive pharmacotherapy, it is essential to consider carefully developmental, environmental, and social factors that might contribute to the child's symptoms and that should be addressed by treatment.

Bipolar II Disorder: The Hypomanic Episode

Distinguishing whether a child has had a hypomanic or a manic episode is necessary in order to differentiate BP-II versus BP-I illness. *DSM-5*[10] lays out two features that differentiate a manic episode from a hypomanic one: duration and impairment. In contrast to a manic episode, in which the duration is at least 1 week, a hypomanic episode lasts at least 4 consecutive days.

When a hypomanic episode lasts a week or more, this criterion may cause the diagnostician some confusion. To decide whether a mood episode that lasts a week or more is hypomanic or manic, the clinician must explore how much impairment occurred during this time. The impairment of a hypomanic episode is less than "marked" but is "associated with an unequivocal change in functioning that is uncharacteristic of the individual when not symptomatic," while that of a manic episode must be "severe," as discussed previously.

Thus, the differences between a hypomanic and manic episode are ones of degree. The same A and B criteria must be met. Both manic and hypomanic episodes show mood changes that are "unequivocal," "uncharacteristic" of that child at his or her baseline, noticeable to those around the child, *and* observable in a variety of settings. Also the pervasiveness of the mood (A-criteria) symptoms during the requisite time period is the same for hypomanic and manic episodes, that is, "most of the day, most days." Thus, determining whether a child had a hypomanic or manic episode requires the clinician to look closely at changes in the child's functioning and the resulting impairment.

Whereas *DSM-5*[10] does not require a history of a major depressive disorder in order to meet criteria for BP-I illness, the diagnosis of BP-II requires a history of both a hypomanic episode plus a separate time when the child met full criteria for a major depressive episode. If a person has only had a hypomanic episode without having ever displayed a major depressive episode, the appropriate diagnosis would be "other specified bipolar and related disorder" (see later).

Clinical Approach to Assessing Mania and Hypomania

As described earlier, ascertaining whether a child meets criteria for a manic or hypomanic episode requires both a longitudinal (historical) perspective and a firm grasp of the concept of a mood episode. The longitudinal perspective encompasses the child's functioning prior to the mood episode (i.e., the premorbid baseline), the child's functioning during the episode, and his or her functioning after (or between) episodes. It is essential to take a detailed and careful history in order to understand how the mood episode unfolded, in terms of the onset, severity, and duration of symptoms, as well as the resulting impairment. A longitudinal view also dictates that information solely based on one point in time is insufficient to make the diagnosis.

Given that a mood episode is based on a period of time during which the child's mood and functioning are clearly and noticeably different from that child's baseline, the clinical approach should be geared to gather information about mood and behavior at two pivotal times: during the proposed episode and at baseline. Behaviors during the proposed episode then can be compared to the baseline of that child's typical mood and day-to-day adaptive functioning. For example, a parent may provide a clinical history consisting of a detailed list of behaviors and events that she sees as symptoms of her child's "mania." The parent indicates her hope that, if the clinician can grasp how aggressive and destructive the child has been, the diagnosis will be clear. In this example, while the parent's concern about the child's behaviors is understandable, the clinician would still need to learn considerably more about the child in order to make a diagnosis. That is, determining whether the child had a manic episode would require the clinician to discern the child's baseline functioning in mood, sleep, agitation, distractibility, thinking, speech, and so on. Once a clear picture of the child's baseline mood and function has been acquired, the clinician can then compare this picture to these same features during the proposed episode.

Thus, in keeping with the fact that the pivotal feature of a mood episode is the emergence of a "distinct period," the interview should begin with defining two time periods (i.e., the baseline and the time of the proposed mood episode) for the interviewer, the parent, and the child. Starting with this distinction will frame the discussion so that everyone can compare the child's functioning at these two time points. In order to describe how the child's behavior was uncharacteristic for him or her during the putative manic episode, both parent and child need to orient their observations to the same time period that is thought to encompass the possible episode, and to compare these observations to the child's baseline.

Having established both the time period of the possible manic episode and a time period that could serve as a representative baseline, the clinician must then obtain information from the both the child and the parent about the specific mood and behavioral changes characteristic of a manic episode. This information includes both objective data (e.g., sleep time, activity level, behaviors associated with irritable or elated mood) and subjective data (e.g., subjective mood, racing thoughts, inflated self-esteem). Of course, obtaining consistent data from both informants and from subjective and objective sources enhances the reliability of the clinical picture. Generally, in order to obtain the highest quality information, it is best to interview the child and parent separately. The clinician may find that, for some criteria, the child's reports are more informative but, for others, it may be the parent's. Speaking with each alone allows them to give their views without concern about interruption or about the other's response. When there are disparate reports, and the parent and child are able to cooperate in providing information, the clinician can reconcile disparities by bringing the parent and child together and having them collaborate to clarify the picture. When they cannot collaborate, then it falls to the clinician to use his or her best judgment to decide which reporter's views on a particular symptom are more reliable.

Along this same line, the criteria indicate that the disturbance is "noticeable to others" (hypomania) and/or causes severe impairment (mania). To establish this criterion, it is incumbent on the clinician to learn whether teachers, coaches, activity leaders, friends, or neighbors made comments to the child or the parent about the child's functioning during the time of the proposed episode. Reports from health care providers who saw the child during this time also are very valuable. For example, when hearing reports from home consistent with a child suffering from a severely impairing manic episode, the clinician would expect to have some corroboration suggesting that, during this time, the child had problems performing in class, adhering to rules at school, and relating to peers, and that the child's therapist observed a change in the child's behavior. In short, it is important that these different informants report that the child's behaviors are significantly different from his or her usual ones.

Frequently, the clinical picture is ambiguous and leaves too much room for doubt about a specific diagnosis. While the primary concern should always be for the safety of the person and those around him or her, there are circumstances when deferring the diagnosis, monitoring the child, and obtaining more information before initiating treatment is the most sensible approach. Once the clinician, parents, and child are attuned to the mood and behavioral features of a manic episode, they can make prospective observations that will assist the clinician in making an accurate diagnosis. Also, when parents or the child believe that an episode is developing, they can be seen for an office visit that will allow the clinician to observe symptoms directly, learn about the child's subjective state, and compare for himself or herself the child's baseline status versus the episodic symptoms. Importantly, seeing a person at baseline and again during a proposed episode also facilitates the diagnostic process by minimizing recall bias that can affect parent and child reports.

Other Specified Bipolar Disorder

Other specified bipolar and related (OSBR) disorder is a category of conditions that are closely related to BP-I and BP-II disorder but do not meet criteria for either. Specifically, the diagnosis applies to clinical conditions in which there is a period (or periods) that resemble manic or hypomanic episodes, during which there is clear impairment, and they are noticeable to those around the child, but full criteria for BP-I or BP-II are not fulfilled. A careful reading of the description makes clear that the pivotal feature of an episode—that is, a time in which the symptoms are distinctly different from the child's usual functioning—is a core feature of OSBR, just as it is for BP-I and BP-II.

DSM-5[10] offers several examples that illustrate the application of this diagnosis. The first is "short duration hypomanic episodes" in those who have a lifetime history of a major depressive episode that occurred at different times than the hypomanic state, and in whom the hypomanic state lasted for less than 4 days. The second example, a converse of the first, concerns individuals with a lifetime history of at least one major depressive episode and of hypomanic events that are long enough to meet *DSM-5*[10] criteria, but that fall one or two symptoms short of the required number of "B" criteria. Once again, the episode of major depression must have occurred at a separate time from the "nearly hypomanic" episode. Compared to individuals who have only a major depressive episode, those with impairing episodes of hypomania that last no more than 2 or 3 days, or that are one or two symptoms shy of meeting full criteria, may be more likely to evolve into BP-II and may therefore benefit from different treatment.

In child and adolescent psychiatry, this OSBR diagnosis is particularly relevant for children described as bipolar disorder-not otherwise specified (BD NOS) in *DSM-IV*, and in particular those children with BD NOS as defined by the Course and Outcome of Bipolar Youth (COBY) study.[20] While other pediatric bipolar investigators have examined children diagnosed with BD NOS (see Table 1 in Reference 21), the COBY study included the most clearly defined, thoroughly characterized, and prospectively studied cohort with BD NOS. In the COBY study, children who displayed a total of four lifetime days of episodic hypomanic symptoms that were clearly different from their baseline function, but insufficient in duration and/or number to meet criteria for hypomania, were given the diagnosis of BD NOS.[20] Specifically, in COBY, the diagnosis of BD NOS was given to children presenting no more than one symptom short of the full criteria for hypomania. Of note, the definition of "a day" was a total of 240 minutes over a 24-hour period; the days or minutes need not be continuous. However, more recently several COBY investigators have suggested that, to increase the clinical utility of the criteria, a "day" that counts toward the diagnosis should include symptoms that are apparent "most of that day," and at least one period of hypomanic or manic symptoms should be at least 2 days long.[22]

As mentioned earlier, a third example of an OSBR disorder is individuals who meet criteria for a hypomanic episode yet have never had an episode of major depression and thus do not fulfill criteria for BP-II. Many clinicians would consider such people to have a high risk for developing BP-II or BP-I. Thus, providing this diagnostic category can facilitate research and assist with justifying treatment interventions that might reduce morbidity or prevent the development of "full-fledged" bipolar disorder.

The last example of OSBR in the *DSM-5*[10] takes note of people who experience impairment from episodic hypomanic symptoms and episodic depressive symptoms but have never experienced an episode of hypomania or major depression that would meet full criteria for the diagnosis. In children and youth, this OSBR designation is described as applying to individuals who, for less than a year, have been persistently in a subthreshold mood, more days than not, without a period of more than 2 months without mood symptoms. Because this is a vaguely defined group that has received virtually no attention in the literature, this diagnosis should be assigned only after the clinician has ascertained that there is no more appropriate diagnosis.

Cyclothymic disorder describes a clinical picture that closely resembles this latter OSBR group in that the child has experienced only subthreshold "near-episodes." Such a subthreshold mood state must be present most days, and the child must not have experienced more than 2 months without mood symptoms. However, in contrast to the OSBR example in the preceding paragraph, for children and youth the duration of cyclothymic disorder must be more than 12 months.

Clinicians considering the diagnosis of cyclothymic disorder face significant challenges. The text implies that the diagnosis may be appropriate for individuals who are "regarded as temperamental, moody, unpredictable. . . but there are no specific criteria for this. One does not know how many mood symptoms constitute a subthreshold episode or 'moodiness.'" The criteria do not rely on a distinct difference that the clinician might use to distinguish between mood symptoms and that child's baseline functioning, as discussed for manic or hypomanic episodes earlier. It may be especially challenging when assessing children and youth who display intense responses to situational stressors such as a suboptimal educational setting, strife at home, or loss of a stable residence. The vagueness of these criteria, coupled with the limited clinical research about the course or treatment of children with cyclothymia, makes the criteria difficult to apply.[23]

Major Depression Versus Bipolar Disorder

Two crucial questions confront the clinician who sees a child with a first-ever episode of major depression. First, is the clinical condition solely major depression, or is this presentation the leading edge of a bipolar disorder that is first manifest as an episode of major depression? Second, how can one differentiate major depression, particularly an agitated depression, from an irritable manic or mixed episode in children?

There is ample reason to want to differentiate an episode of depression due to bipolar disorder from one that is a manifestation of unipolar major depressive disorder. The treatment of bipolar depression requires different pharmacological approaches than does major depression.[24,25] Also, compared to people with unipolar depression, those with bipolar depression are less likely to recover, and their recovery is likely to take longer.[26] In addition, the risk of recurrence for bipolar depression is much greater than for unipolar depression, and bipolar depression carries an increased risk for suicide, substance abuse, and severe morbidity.[26–28]

In children and adolescents presenting with a first episode of major depression, the literature gives inconsistent rates for the risk of ultimately developing bipolar disorder (i.e., mania or hypomania). Inconsistencies in the literature can be explained by differences in methods, such as the diagnostic criteria and whether cohorts are ascertained from inpatient or outpatient populations. For prepubertal children with depression, the risk for later developing mania (bipolar disorder) is quite unclear. For children, the risk of subsequent bipolar disorder has been reported from 0%[29] to no difference in rate from a control cohorts of children with psychiatric disorders without depression[30] to "a significantly increased" rate compared to healthy children.[31]

Compared to prepubertal children with major depression, adolescents with major depression appear to have a greater risk of later bipolar disorder. Longitudinal clinical studies report risks of subsequent bipolar disorder ranging from 6%[31] to 9%[32] to 19% (Rao et al., 1995).[33] While one must acknowledge the limitations of studies relying on retrospective recall, 50% of adults with BP-1 report that their first mood episode was major depression during childhood or youth.[34,35] Thus, although there appears to be a relatively higher risk for subsequent bipolar disorder among individuals who have their first depressive episode in adolescence, quantifying that risk has proven elusive.

Psychosis during depression is the most consistently cited clinical feature that appears to be associated with a high risk for subsequent bipolar disorder. Children with bipolar disorder appear to display psychosis during major depression more frequently than children with unipolar major depression. For example, children and youth with a first major depressive episode that includes psychosis carry a risk of 13%–28% for developing bipolar disorder later.[36,37] Therefore, youth with psychotic depression, including those who have no prior hypomanic/manic episode, should be monitored closely for emergence of bipolar disorder. Similarly, it is important to inquire about family history because, in children with major depressive disorder (MDD), a history of bipolar disorder in a first-degree relative is associated with increased risk for eventual bipolar disorder. Strober and Carlson[38] reported a 5-fold greater risk (50% vs. 10%) of subsequent BP-1 among children with MDD plus a first-degree relative with bipolar disorder, compared to children with MDD without any family history for bipolar disorder.

In predicting bipolar disorder in a child with MDD, additional features that have been suggested are the presence of subthreshold symptoms of mania during depression. A body of work[39,40] suggests that, among youth with major depression and subthreshold hypomanic symptoms (i.e., elevated mood lasting 4 days, but only two B-criteria symptoms, or irritable mood with only three B-criteria symptoms that were not noticeable to others) carried a 5-fold greater risk for later development of BP-1 or BP-2 compared to those with "pure" major depression.[40]

Since irritability may be prominent in youth who have agitated major depression or a manic or mixed episode, it is useful to review what clinicians should consider in deciding which among these diagnoses is more likely. The task is made more difficult because criteria for a depressive episode, including "insomnia," "agitation," and "diminished ability to concentrate," can bear a superficial resemblance to "decreased need for sleep," "psychomotor agitation," and "distractibility," respectively, that are criteria for manic/hypomanic episodes. Thoughtful data gathering and being mindful of the differences among these clinical presentations may help resolve the confusion.

First, it is critical that the practitioner assess the entire clinical picture. Despite the fact that the child's irritability is often his or her most impairing symptom, and therefore may be of greatest concern for the parent, the clinician should look beyond the irritability alone and gather systematic information about other associated clinical features. For example, manic/hypomanic episodes are generally characterized by a mixture of irritable and elevated mood, whereas in depression irritability usually coincides with sad mood or anhedonia. Several large studies have found that, among children with bipolar disorder, reports based on their most severe manic/hypomanic episode revealed that the great majority had experienced episodes characterized by both elevated mood *and* irritability; only 10% had "irritable-only" episodes of mania/hypomania.[41,42] The fraction of those who displayed irritable-only manic episodes exclusively during their lifetime was smaller yet. Thus, when deciding whether irritability is a symptom of a depressive or manic/hypomanic episode, it can be helpful to inquire about the presence of elevated mood, inflated self-esteem, and/or grandiosity at some times during the episode, and about whether there is a past (lifetime) history of episodes with elevated mood. Of course, it also is necessary to seek information about changes in sleep, weight/appetite, goal-directed activity, energy, self-esteem, thoughts of death, and so on. In some cases, as noted earlier, only longitudinal follow-up or seeing the child at the height of an episode will resolve remaining doubts.

"Insomnia" (a symptom of major depressive disorder) may be confused with a "decreased need for sleep" (a symptom of hypomania and mania) because both are characterized by abnormally decreased sleep duration. However, individuals with insomnia awaken with difficulty in the morning and feel fatigued or foggy for all or part of the day. In contrast, children with decreased need for sleep awaken earlier than usual, do not feel fatigued, and feel no need to restore sleep during the day. The subjective reports typically given by children who experience decreased need for sleep during hypomanic/manic episodes are that they did not detect any ill effects from the 2 or more hours less sleep they have been getting each night.

The agitation of a depressive episode may have different clinical features than that of a manic/hypomanic one. The psychomotor agitation of depressive disorders typically is repetitive, aimless restlessness such as rubbing, hand wringing, or pacing. Agitation during manic/hypomanic episodes typically accompanies increased goal-directed behavior and is characterized by excessive energy or rapid, frenzied motion while attempting to carry out tasks or projects. Rapid talking, gesticulating, pacing, and accessory movement while doing tasks that demand concentration contribute to this frantic picture.

The descriptions offered for the "loss of concentration" that arises during a depressive episode could be read as much the same as the "distractibility" of a manic/hypomanic one. However, once again, the contexts of these two symptoms give them a different character. Loss of concentration during depression is typically experienced as feeling too slowed down to focus or keep things in memory, having intrusive negative thoughts that interrupt one's focus, or not being able to marshal the motivation to carry out the task. This contrasts with the distractibility of manic/hypomanic episodes, which is experienced as the loss of a "mental filter" that would permit one to concentrate. Patients describe that, during a manic/hypomanic episode, they are constantly being bombarded by thoughts and ideas that appear and disappear quickly, so that they are unable to think clearly.

Thus, clinicians should remember that a first-ever mood episode that meets criteria for a major depressive episode could eventually develop into one of three diagnostic endpoints. That is, an episode of major depression could be a single (lifetime) episode of depression, the first of a series of depressive episodes of *recurrent* major depression, or the initial manifestation of bipolar disorder that has yet to show a manic/hypomanic episode. Being mindful of these three outcomes is relevant for the treatment one chooses, what one monitors during treatment, and the psychoeducational work with the child and family.[43,44]

Disruptive Mood Dysregulation Disorder Versus Bipolar Disorder

Irritability is a common symptom and may be the most common reason parents give for bringing their children to psychiatric attention.[45] While children with episodic irritability, by definition, should be assessed carefully for major depression and bipolar disorder, there are children who show *chronic* and severe irritability lasting a year or longer.

Prior to *DSM-5*[10] there was no satisfactory diagnostic location for this syndromal presentation.[46] That is, while these children typically meet criteria for oppositional defiant disorder (ODD), ODD also encompasses children with relatively mild impairment, or impairment only at home, as well as children with oppositional features only without irritability. The absence of a suitable diagnosis undermined attempts to investigate, treat, or obtain services for children impaired by this serious condition. Data accumulating in the early 2000s suggested that a sharp rise in the rate of bipolar disorder diagnoses in children might have resulted, in part, from assigning bipolar disorder to chronically irritable children who did not have episodes of hypomania or mania.

Research over the last decade suggested that the syndrome of chronic irritability could be reliably diagnosed in children and, when such children were compared to those with bipolar disorder, their outcome was likely to be different. Specifically, the data suggested that children with chronic irritability had a substantial risk of developing depression or anxiety disorders in adulthood,[7,47,48] but they did not have an increased risk of developing bipolar disorder. Moreover, rates of bipolar disorder among first-degree relatives of children with chronic irritability were much lower than among relatives of children with bipolar disorder.[49] Furthermore, there was evidence for fundamental neurobiological differences between bipolar disorder and the phenotype of chronic irritability,[50-52] although there were also shared features.[53,54] As a result, *DSM-5*[10] defined a new diagnosis, disruptive mood dysregulation disorder (DMDD). The decision to create this new diagnosis was based on accumulating data indicating important differences in the course, family history, and neurobiological measures of children and youth who display a syndrome of chronic irritability compared to those with bipolar disorder.

DSM-5[10] DMDD criteria hinge on two primary components: chronically irritable mood and a routine display of angry outbursts. The criteria specify that the syndrome of chronically irritable mood must be severely impairing in at least one setting (home, school, peers) and at least mildly impairing in another. Irritability should be present "most of the day most days" for at least a year, without any period of 3 months or more when it is quiescent, and the outbursts should occur at least three times per week throughout this time. When there is chronic irritability with frequent angry outbursts, impairment, and it appears before age 10, this presentation is DMDD.

When differentiating bipolar disorder from DMDD, the first rule for the clinician to recall is that DMDD is characterized by *chronic* irritability without episodes. As indicated earlier, if irritability, increased goal-directed behavior/energy, or any of the symptoms included in the B criteria of mania are to be considered part of a manic or hypomanic episode, they must differ significantly from that child's baseline function. DMDD should be considered when these features are not different from that child's baseline behavior. DMDD is a much more likely diagnosis than bipolar disorder when irritability is consistently present most of the day, most days, for at least a year.

Clinicians should be mindful of several caveats in the diagnosis of DMDD. First, if there is any history of an episode of hypomania or mania, or if there is a clear episode of even 2 days' symptoms that would be sufficient for OSBP, then one should not diagnose DMDD. Thus, bipolar disorder or OSBP "trumps" DMDD. On the other hand, the diagnosis of DMDD "trumps" that of ODD. While most children with ODD do not have extreme irritability and hence do not meet criteria for DMDD, those with DMDD typically meet criteria for ODD. Thus, adding ODD to DMDD does not add meaningful information. Third, chronic irritability can be seen with other disorders, particularly major depression, autism spectrum, and posttraumatic stress disorders. When another diagnosis provides a better explanation for the irritability, DMDD is not given. For example, if severe irritability arose exclusively during a major depressive episode that lasted for a year, then DMDD would not be the appropriate diagnosis.

Whether DMDD will remain a valid construct remains to be seen. Only further study will determine whether DMDD is a distinct entity that warrants a separate diagnosis or is so closely related to ODD or other disruptive disorders that it would be more appropriately placed as a specifier with ODD or other disruptive disorders. This question can be answered only by additional neurobiological investigations and large prospective longitudinal studies comparing these conditions. The step taken by the *DSM-5* committee underscores that more research is needed in order to understand the course, treatment, and risks of this syndrome. Although DMDD has an estimated population prevalence of 3%,[7] clinicians have disappointingly meager data on psychological or pharmacological intervention to guide treatment of these people.

Psychosis in Bipolar Disorder Versus Schizophrenia

When a child's first presentation for psychiatric care includes psychosis, it may be difficult to differentiate between schizophrenia spectrum disorders (including schizophrenia, schizoaffective disorder, simple delusional disorders, and schizophreniform disorder) and mood disorders with psychotic features. Being mindful of several principles may assist the diagnostician.

One diagnostically crucial question is whether the psychotic symptoms are confined exclusively to a mood episode. When psychosis arises only during a major mood episode (depressive or manic), it establishes the diagnosis as major depression with psychotic features or a manic episode (and BP-1). However, when psychotic symptoms precede or extend beyond the mood episode, this temporal distinction suggests schizoaffective disorder or schizophrenia. In schizoaffective disorder, a major mood disorder coexists for a *majority* of the period of illness, but the psychotic symptoms extend for at least 2 weeks beyond the mood disorder. Admittedly, these distinctions can be difficult to make clinically, especially when they must be based on retrospective data.

For children and youth, the diagnostic implications of psychotic symptoms in the absence of a mood episode are less clear. Population studies suggest that psychotic symptoms are very common in children age 9–12 years (17%) and adolescents (7.5%).[55]

When children display psychotic symptoms that are subthreshold for schizophrenia (such as brief psychotic or schizophreniform disorders), the data are mixed on whether this increases the risk for ensuing bipolar disorder or schizophrenia.[56] Previous work led clinicians to consider such psychotic events as exclusively prodromal schizophrenia.[57] However, more recent longitudinal studies have suggested that psychotic symptoms without mood symptoms do not predict a specific outcome and may pose an equal risk for later depression, anxiety, or bipolar disorder.[56,58,59]

The clinical approach in deciding whether psychosis is part of a major mood disorder is to assess the entire array of mood symptoms in addition to the symptoms of psychosis. The most common way a psychotic mood disorder unfolds is with relatively mild mood symptoms that intensify before psychosis emerges. Generally, in psychotic depression or a manic episode, the mood symptoms are quite severe by the time that psychosis arises. It follows that generally, when a child has psychotic symptoms with equivocal or only mildly severe mood symptoms, it is less likely that he or she is experiencing a major depression with psychotic features or a manic episode.

Irritability as a Symptom

Irritability is a diagnostic criterion of at least 10 disorders, and a host of others are often accompanied by irritability even if it is not a diagnostic criterion. Thus, when a child presents with irritability, the diagnostician needs to consider a wide range of disorders that could account for it. One should not think of irritability as solely indicative of depressive or manic episodes, or of any condition, for that matter.

Perhaps the most frequent source of impairing irritability in children and youth is anxiety disorders. Among these, the criteria for generalized anxiety disorder include irritability associated with fears related to acceptance, performance, or competence.

Among the stress- and trauma-related disorders, reactive attachment disorder (RAD), PTSD, and acute stress disorder have an irritability criterion. Irritability usually is exhibited as a persistent negative affect that follows pathological care in the case of RAD, or exposure to actual or threatened death in PTSD. In addition, explosive angry outbursts can emerge as an alteration in arousal or hyperreactivity that are part of PTSD and acute stress disorder. In children and adolescents who have been exposed to stressful or life-threatening events, it can be difficult to confirm whether irritability or explosive outbursts emerged or only intensified following those experiences.

Among the disruptive and conduct disorders, ODD and intermittent explosive disorder specifically include irritability in their criteria. With conduct disorder, the criteria do not refer to irritability per se, but irritability is clearly described in the associated features. In addition, both reactive and instrumental aggression are usually part of the clinical picture in conduct disorder.[60]

Although irritability is not a diagnostic criterion for ADHD, it is clear that impulsive outbursts of frustration and anger are common among children with this disorder.[61,62]

Also, these impulsive angry reactions appear to be strongly associated with persistence of ADHD symptoms into adulthood.[61]

Other conditions that do not have irritability as a diagnostic criterion, but do describe irritability and extreme frustration as part of the clinical picture, are obsessive-compulsive disorder and autism spectrum disorders.[63,64] In both of these conditions, attempts to interrupt repetitive or ritualized acts or to interfere with patterned behaviors can arouse extreme irritability and outbursts. In children and adolescents this can reach levels of physical aggressive in reaction to limits or physical constraints on carrying out the activity.

Summary

The defining clinical feature of bipolar disorder is *episodes* of mania or hypomania. The diagnostic process centers on ascertaining a period when the child's mood and behavior was clearly different from his or her baseline and then determining whether B criteria appeared or intensified to a significant degree during this same time. Subjective and objective reports about the youth's behavior and functioning are needed to gain a reliable history.

Second, to identify an episode, the clinician must have a firm understanding of the person's baseline function. Only by having a good grasp of the child's baseline can the clinician begin to separate co-occurring symptoms that are part of other disorders from those that are part of bipolar disorder. This differentiation among conditions is particularly important when evaluating children who are young or immature, those with developmental disorders, and those with ODD or ADHD in order to best guide treatment.

The features of bipolar disorder may not be readily apparent in a single office visit or through observations over a few months. Often, taking time to follow a child and making systematic observations at regular intervals will reveal the clinical picture. This approach is essential when there is uncertainty about the diagnosis. Such longitudinal observation is of paramount importance for younger children with major depression, children and youth with major depression with psychotic features, and those with first-degree relatives who have bipolar disorder.

To reduce the morbidity and distress of bipolar disorder in children and youth, we must learn much more about treatments, course of illness, risk factors, epidemiology, and genetic contributions. All of these important endeavors rely on accurate diagnostic assessments and an appreciation of the phenomenology of this impairing disorder.

Author Disclosure

Drs. Towbin and Leibenluft have no conflicts to disclose. They are funded by the National Institute of Mental Health intramural program.

References

1. Mick E, Spencer T, Wozniak J, Biederman J. Heterogeneity of irritability in attention-deficit/hyperactivity disorder subjects with and without mood disorders. *Biol Psychiatry.* 2005;58(7):576–82.
2. Biederman J, Klein RG, Pine DS, Klein DF. Resolved: mania is mistaken for ADHD in prepubertal children. *J Am Acad Child Adolesc Psychiatry.* 1998;37:1091–9.
3. Geller B, Warner K, Williams M, Zimerman B. Prepubertal and young adolescent bipolarity versus ADHD: assessment and validity using the Wash-U-KSADS, CBCL, and TRF. *J Affect Disord* 1998;51:93–100.
4. Geller B, Tillman R, Bolhofner K. Proposed definitions of bipolar I disorder episodes and daily rapid cycling phenomena in preschoolers, school-aged children, adolescents, and adults. *J Child Adolesc Psychopharmacol.* 2007;17:217–22.
5. Moreno C, Laje G, Blanco C, Jiang H, Schmidt AB, Olfson M. National trends in the outpatient diagnosis and treatment of bipolar disorder in youth. *Arch Gen Psychiatry.* 2007;64(9):1032–9.
6. Blader JC, Carlson GA. Increased rates of bipolar disorder diagnoses among U.S. child, adolescent, and adult inpatients, 1996–2004. *Biol Psychiatry.* 2007;62(2):107–14.
7. Brotman MA, Schmajuk M, Rich BA, et al. Prevalence, clinical correlates, and longitudinal course of severe mood dys- regulation in children. *Biol Psychiatry.* 2006;60:991–7.
8. Costello EJ, Farmer EM, Angold A, Burns BJ, Erkanli A. Psychiatric disorders among American Indian and white youth in Appalachia: The Great Smoky Mountains Study. *Am J Pub Health.* 1997;87:827–32.
9. Leibenluft E. Severe mood dysregulation, irritability, and the diagnostic boundaries of bipolar disorder in youths. *Am J Psychiatry.* 2011;168(2):129–42.
10. American Psychiatric Association. *Diagnostic and Statistical Manual of Mental Disorders.* 5th ed. Arlington, VA: American Psychiatric Publishing; 2013.
11. American Psychiatric Association. *Diagnostic and Statistical Manual of Mental Disorders.* 4th ed. Text rev. Washington, DC: American Psychiatric Association; 2000.
12. Blakemore SJ, Robbins TW. Decision-making in the adolescent brain. *Nat Neurosci.* 2012;15(9):1184–91.
13. Spear LP. The adolescent brain and age-related behavioral manifestations. *Neurosci Biobehav Rev.* 2000;24(4):417–63.
14. Soto EC, Frederickson AM, Trivedi H, et al. Frequency and correlates of inappropriate pediatric psychiatric emergency room visits. *J Clin Psychiatry.* 2009;70(8):1164–77.
15. Tumuluru RV, Weller EB, Fristad MA, et al. Mania in six preschool children. *J Child Adolesc Psychopharmacol.* 2003;13(4):489–94.
16. Ferreira Maia AP, Boarati MA, Kleinman A, Fu-I L. Preschool bipolar disorder: Brazilian children case reports. *J Affect Disord.* 2007;104(1–3):237–43.
17. Luby J, Belden A. Defining and validating bipolar disorder in the preschool period. *Dev Psychopathol.* 2006;18(4):971–88.
18. Luby JL, Tandon M, Belden A. Preschool bipolar disorder. *Child Adolesc Psychiatr Clin N Am.* 2009;18(2):391–403.
19. McClellan J. Commentary: treatment guidelines for child and adolescent bipolar disorder. *J Am Acad Child Adolesc Psychiatry.* 2005;44(3):236–9.
20. Birmaher B, Axelson D, Strober M, et al. Clinical course of children and adolescents with bipolar spectrum disorders. *Arch Gen Psychiatry.* 2006;63:175–83.
21. Axelson DA, Birmaher B, Strober MA, et al. Course of subthreshold bipolar disorder in youth: diagnostic progression from bipolar disorder not otherwise specified. *J Am Acad Child Adolesc Psychiatry.* 2011;50(10):1001–16.
22. Towbin K, Axelson D, Leibenluft E, Birmaher B. Differentiating bipolar disorder-not otherwise specified and severe mood dysregulation. *J Am Acad Child Adolesc Psychiatry.* 2013;52(5):466–81.
23. Van Meter AR, Youngstrom EA, Findling RL. Cyclothymic disorder: a critical review. *Clin Psychol Rev.* 2012;32(4):229–43.
24. Cosgrove VE, Roybal D, Chang KD. Bipolar depression in pediatric populations: epidemiology and management. *Paediatr Drugs.* 2013;15(2):83–91.

25. Nandagopal JJ, DelBello MP, Kowatch R. Pharmacologic treatment of pediatric bipolar disorder. *Child Adolesc Psychiatr Clin N Am.* 2009;18(2):455–69.

26. Birmaher B, Axelson D, Goldstein B, et al. Four-year longitudinal course of children and adolescents with bipolar spectrum disorders: the Course and Outcome of Bipolar Youth (COBY) study. *Am J Psychiatry.* 2009;166(7):795–804.

27. DelBello MP, Hanseman D, Adler CM, Fleck DE, Strakowski SM. Twelve-month outcome of adolescents with bipolar disorder following first hospitalization for a manic or mixed episode. *Am J Psychiatry.* 2007;164:582–90.

28. Goldstein TR, Ha W, Axelson DA, et al. Predictors of prospectively examined suicide attempts among youth with bipolar disorder. *Arch Gen Psychiatry.* 2012;69(11):1113–22.

29. Copeland WE, Shanahan L, Costello EJ, Angold A. Childhood and adolescent psychiatric disorders as predictors of young adult disorders. *Arch Gen Psychiatry.* 2009;66:764–72.

30. Harrington R, Fudge H, Rutter M, Pickles A, Hill J. Adult outcomes of childhood and adolescent depression. I. Psychiatric status. *Arch Gen Psychiatry.* 1990;47(5):465–73.

31. Weissman MM, Wolk S, Goldstein RB, et al. Depressed adolescents grown up. *JAMA.* 1999;281(18):1707–13.

32. Beesdo K, Höfler M, Leibenluft E, Lieb R, Bauer M, Pfennig A. Mood episodes and mood disorders: patterns of incidence and conversion in the first three decades of life. *Bipolar Disord.* 2009;11(6):637–49.

33. Rao U, Ryan ND, Birmaher B, Dahl RE, Williamson DE, Kaufman J, et al. Unipolar depression in adolescents: clinical outcome in adulthood. *J Am Acad Child Adolesc Psychiatry.* 1995 May;34(5):566–78.

34. Perlis RH, Miyahara S, Marangell LB, et al.; STEP-BD Investigators. Long-term implications of early onset in bipolar disorder: data from the first 1000 participants in the systematic treatment enhancement program for bipolar disorder (STEP-BD). *Biol Psychiatry.* 2004;55(9):875–81.

35. Carlson GA, Bromet EJ, Sievers S. Phenomenology and outcome of subjects with early- and adult-onset psychotic mania. Am J Psychiatry. 2000;157(2):213–9.

36. Strober M, Lampert C, Schmidt S, Morrell W. The course of major depressive disorder in adolescents: I. Recovery and risk of manic switching in a follow-up of psychotic and non-psychotic subtypes. *J Am Acad Child Adolesc Psychiatry.* 1993;32:34–42.

37. DelBello MP, Carlson GA, Tohen M, Bromet EJ, Schwiers M, Strakowski SM. Rates and predictors of developing a manic or hypomanic episode 1 to 2 years following a first hospitalization for major depression with psychotic features. *J Child Adolesc Psychopharmacol.* 2003;13:173–85.

38. Strober M, Carlson G. Bipolar illness in adolescents with major depression: clinical, genetic, and psychopharmacologic predictors in a three- to four-year prospective follow-up investigation. *Arch Gen Psychiatry.* 1982;39(5):549–55.

39. Fiedorowicz JG, Endicott J, Leon AC, Solomon DA, Keller MB, Coryell WH. Subthreshold hypomanic symptoms in progression from unipolar major depression to bipolar disorder. *Am J Psychiatry.* 2011;168(1):40–8.

40. Zimmermann P, Brückl T, Nocon A, et al. Heterogeneity of DSM-IV major depressive disorder as a consequence of subthreshold bipolarity. *Arch Gen Psychiatry.* 2009;66(12):1341–52.

41. Axelson D, Birmaher B, Strober M, et al. Phenomenology of children and adolescents with bipolar spectrum disorders. *Arch Gen Psychiatry.* 2006;63(10):1139–48.

42. Hunt J, Birmaher B, Leonard H, et al. Irritability without elation in a large bipolar youth sample: frequency and clinical description. *J Am Acad Child Adolesc Psychiatry.* 2009;48(7):730–9.

43. Miklowitz DJ, Axelson DA, Birmaher B, George EL, Taylor DO, Schneck CD, Beresford CA, Dickinson LM, Craighead WE, Brent DA. Family-focused treatment for adolescents with bipolar disorder: results of a 2-year randomized trial. *Arch Gen Psychiatry.* 2008;65(9):1053–61.

44. Pavuluri MN, Graczyk PA, Henry DB, Carbray JA, Heidenreich J, Miklowitz DJ. Child- and family-focused cognitive-behavioral therapy for pediatric bipolar disorder: development and preliminary results. *J Am Acad Child Adolesc Psychiatry.* 2004;43(5):528–37.

45. Horwitz SM, Demeter CA, Pagano ME, et al. Longitudinal Assessment of Manic Symptoms (LAMS) study: background, design, and initial screening results. *J Clin Psychiatry.* 2010;71(11):1511–7.

46. Parens E, Johnston J, Carlson GA. Pediatric mental health care dysfunction disorder? *N Engl J Med.* 2010;362(20):1853–5.

47. Stringaris A, Cohen P, Pine DS, Leibenluft E. Adult outcomes of youth irritability: a 20-year prospective community-based study. *Am J Psychiatry.* 2009;166(9):1048–54.

48. Stringaris A, Zavos H, Leibenluft E, Maughan B, Eley TC. Adolescent irritability: phenotypic associations and genetic links with depressed mood. *Am J Psychiatry.* 2012;169(1):47–54.

49. Brotman MA, Kassem L, Reising MM, et al. Pa- rental diagnoses in youth with narrow phenotype bipolar disorder or severe mood dysregulation. *Am J Psychiatry.* 2007;164:1238–41.

50. Brotman MA, Rich BA, Guyer AE, et al. Amygdala activation during emotion processing of neutral faces in children with severe mood dysregulation versus ADHD or bipolar disorder. *Am J Psychiatry.* 2010;167:61–9.

51. Rich BA, Brotman MA, Dickstein DP, Mitchell DG, Blair RJ, Leibenluft E. Deficits in attention to emotional stimuli distin- guish youth with severe mood dysregulation from youth with bipolar disorder. *J Abnorm Child Psychol.* 2010;38:695–706.

52. Rich BA, Schmajuk M, Perez-Edgar KE, Fox NA, Pine DS, Leibenluft E. Different psychophysiological and behavioral responses elicited by frustration in pediatric bipolar disorder and severe mood dysregulation. *Am J Psychiatry.* 2007;164:309–17.

53. Guyer AE, McClure EB, Adler AD, et al. Specificity of facial expres- sion labeling deficits in childhood psychopathology. *J Child Psychol Psychiatry.* 2007;48:863–71.

54. Rich BA, Grimley ME, Schmajuk M, Blair KS, Blair RJR, Leibenluft E. Face emotion labeling deficits in children with bipolar disorder and severe mood dysregulation. *Dev Psychopathol.* 2008;20:529–46.

55. Kelleher I, Connor D, Clarke MC, Devlin N, Harley M, Cannon M. Prevalence of psychotic symptoms in childhood and adolescence: a systematic review and meta-analysis of population-based studies. *Psychol Med.* 2012;42(09):1857–63.

56. Kelleher I, Keeley H, Corcoran P, et al. Clinicopathological significance of psychotic experiences in non-psychotic young people: evidence from four population-based studies. *Br J Psychiatry.* 2012;201(1):26–32.

57. Volkmar FR. Childhood and adolescent psychosis: a review of the past 10 years. *J Am Acad Child Adolesc Psychiatry.* 1996;35(7):843–51.

58. Fisher HL, Caspi A, Poulton R, et al. Specificity of childhood psychotic symptoms for predicting schizophrenia by 38 years of age: a birth cohort study. *Psychol Med.* 2013;43(10):2077–86.

59. Murray GK, Jones PB. Psychotic symptoms in young people without psychotic illness: mechanisms and meaning. *Br J Psychiatry.* 2012;201:4–6.

60. Lahey BB, Waldman ID. Annual research review: phenotypic and causal structure of conduct disorder in the broader context of prevalent forms of psychopathology. *J Child Psychol Psychiatry.* 2012;53(5):536–57.

61. Barkley RA, Fischer M. The unique contribution of emotional impulsiveness to impairment in major life activities in hyperactive children as adults. *J Am Acad Child Adolesc Psychiatry.* 2010;49(5):503–13.

62. Martel MM. Research review: a new perspective on attentiondeficit/hyperactivity disorder: emotion dysregulation and trait models. *J Child Psychol Psychiatry.* 2009;50:1042–51.

63. Lecavalier L. Behavioral and emotional problems in young people with pervasive developmental disorders: relative prevalence, effects of subject characteristics, and empirical classification. *J Autism Dev Disord.* 2006;36(8):1101–14.

64. Storch EA, Jones AM, Lack CW, et al. Rage attacks in pediatric obsessive-compulsive disorder: phenomenology and clinical correlates. *J Am Acad Child Adolesc Psychiatry.* 2012;51(6):582–92.

Comorbid Conditions in Youth With and At Risk for Bipolar Disorder

Gagan Joshi and Timothy Wilens

Pediatric-Onset Bipolar Disorder

Pediatric-onset bipolar disorder seldom occurs in the absence of comorbid conditions. The co-occurrence of additional disorders complicates both the accurate diagnosis of bipolar disorder and its treatment. Bipolar disorder is one of the most debilitating psychiatric disorders, estimated to cost Americans $45 billion per year. It is not so infrequent as previously reported, with rates of bipolar spectrum disorder reaching an estimated 4%. Youth with bipolar disorder are among the most impaired populations, and the presence of comorbidity compounds disability, complicates treatment, and appears to worsen the prognosis in this population. Comorbid disorders may have a significant impact on various indices of bipolar disorder correlates. Knowledge of their comorbid presence with bipolar disorder could be informative in determining course, prognosis, and functional and therapeutic outcomes. Early identification and appropriate management may lead to improved functioning, prevention of impending emergence of comorbid disorders (e.g., oppositional defiant disorder, conduct disorder, substance use disorders), and attenuation of the untreated course of bipolar disorder.[1,2] On the other hand, if comorbidity is not appropriately acknowledged, then misattribution of impairing symptoms could lead to inappropriate therapeutic interventions such as unnecessary exposure to neuroleptics, worsening of symptoms, delayed diagnosis, and misuse of mental health resources.

Recognition of the co-occurrence of psychiatric and substance use disorders (referred to as comorbidity) is important as it has therapeutic implications such as (1) increased risk of mood destabilization that is inherent to the therapeutic options for the comorbidity, as is the case with antianxiety, antidepressant, or anti-attention-deficit/ hyperactivity disorder (ADHD) medications that may have the potential to induce mania; (2) atypical response (efficacy and tolerability) to psychotropics associated with certain disorders like autism spectrum disorder; or (3) less than expected antimanic response to thymoleptic agents in the presence of certain comorbid disorders (for instance, ADHD and obsessive-compulsive disorder).

Comorbid disorders may be challenging to diagnose due to overlapping symptoms and developmentally sensitive complicated patterns of symptom development. Several methods have been applied to understand comorbidity scientifically. Structured diagnostic interviews (for instance, Schedule for Affective Disorders and Schizophrenia-Epidemiological Fifth Version [K-SADS-E][3]) are helpful in parsing out clinically comorbid conditions as part of a comprehensive assessment of the spectrum of psychopathologies described in the *Diagnostic and Statistical Manual of Mental Disorders* (*DSM*), including past and present severity of symptoms. Diagnoses are considered positive only if the diagnostic criteria are met to a degree that would be considered clinically meaningful. "Clinically meaningful" means that the data collected from the structured interview indicated that the diagnosis should be a clinical concern due to the nature of the symptoms, the associated impairment, and the coherence of the clinical picture. For a given disorder the overlapping nonspecific symptoms are considered for the diagnosis if the respective cardinal symptoms are present and the disorder is cause for significant impairment. Furthermore, although *DSM* criteria do not permit comorbid presence of certain disorders and assign diagnoses based on hierarchy, in order to fully characterize the clinical picture a nonhierarchical diagnostic approach is taken to assess for comorbid disorders. Thus, the approach taken by structured interview objectively and comprehensively documents symptom presentation and minimizes diagnostic biases.

Perhaps the most compelling scientific method to examine comorbidity is familial risk analysis, which addresses uncertainties regarding complex phenotypes in probands by examining the transmission of comorbid disorders in families.[4,5] Therapeutic response has also provided evidence of the existence of separate conditions. For instance, in a review of clinical records in manic children, Biederman et al.[6] reported that whereas mood stabilizers significantly improved mania-like symptoms, antidepressants and stimulants did not; conversely, tricyclic antidepressants and not mood stabilizers were associated with improvement of ADHD symptoms. Finally, attributes of comorbidity can also be addressed by applying neurobiological probes to seek the existence of underlying changes commensurate with each comorbid disorder, either disorder, or neither disorder, indicating a unique subtype with distinct neurobiological attributes. The emerging proton magnetic resonance spectroscopic (HMRS)[7] imaging intervention research in youth with bipolar disorder is suggesting a profile of cerebral metabolites in a specific region of the brain that may facilitate understanding of neurochemical correlates of bipolar disorder in the context of comorbidity. For instance, the HMRS[7] profile of cerebral metabolites in the anterior cingulate cortex region of the brain in children with ADHD appears to have a significantly higher ratio of glutamate plus glutamine to myo-inositol-containing compounds than does the profile of children with comorbid bipolar disorder and ADHD.[8]

Present studies addressing comorbidity generally rely either on cross-sectional observations or on recall of disorders over the whole life course. Both of these approaches pose limitations. Longitudinal studies offer the best possibility for observing the developmental progression of the emergence of comorbid conditions.

Treatment guidelines for pediatric bipolar disorder indicate that the treatment plan must include treatment for each comorbid disorder, which may become a complex process of trial and error to find the most effective combination of medications.[9] These guidelines further recommend that in the absence of treatment trials specifically studying a population of children with bipolar disorder and specific comorbid disorders, clinicians should use psychopharmacological and psychosocial treatments that are generally recommended for each comorbid disorder when that disorder occurs as the primary problem. Although certain comorbid disorders associated with bipolar disorder respond to antimanic agents (e.g., disruptive behavior disorders, autism spectrum disorder), there are frequently co-occurring disorders (ADHD, anxiety disorders, depression) with typical onset prior to the emergence of mania that require treatment with agents that may have manicogenic potential. Available empirical evidence and clinical acumen dictate that treatment of comorbid conditions can be addressed only after the symptoms of bipolar disorder are stabilized.[10]

Comorbid conditions frequently associated with pediatric-onset bipolar disorder include ADHD, disruptive behavior disorders, substance use disorders, anxiety disorders (including panic disorder, posttraumatic stress disorder, and obsessive-compulsive disorder), and pervasive developmental disorders. A recent international World Health Organziation (WHO) survey of over 60,000 community adults from 11 countries demonstrated that despite varied rates of the prevalence of bipolar spectrum disorder, patterns of comorbidity were similar internationally.[11] In the following sections we will address the characteristics and management of frequently co-occurring disorders in children and adolescents with bipolar disorder.

Attention-Deficit/Hyperactivity Disorder

Systematic studies of pediatric populations with bipolar disorder show that the rates of comorbid ADHD range from 50% to 90% compared to nonbipolar samples in which the rates of ADHD are between 6% and 9% in children and 4% in adults.[12-17] While a high prevalence of ADHD is reported in youth with bipolar disorder, a lower risk for comorbid bipolar disorder (<22%) is reported in pediatric populations with ADHD.[18] Although the rates of ADHD in youth with bipolar disorder are universally high, the age at onset modifies the risk for comorbid ADHD. ADHD comorbidity is more often associated with early-onset bipolar disorder (<18 years).[17,19-21] Rates of ADHD are highest in those with onset of their bipolar disorder prepubertally and are relatively lower in those with adolescent-and adult-onset bipolar disorder.[17,22,23]

The National Comorbidity Survey Replication epidemiological study documented higher rates of bipolar disorder in adults with versus without ADHD (19.4% vs. 3.1%).[24] Consistent with the documented association of comorbid ADHD almost exclusively with early-onset bipolar disorder, a relatively lower lifetime prevalence (9.5% vs. 4.6% risk in general population)[24] of comorbid ADHD is reported in adults with bipolar disorder.[25] Winokur et al.[26] reported childhood hyperactivity in 21% of their 189 adults with bipolar disorder and in 19% of their first-degree adult relatives with bipolar disorder. Interestingly, when comorbid with ADHD, adults with bipolar disorder demonstrate the following features: the onset of their mood disorder approximately 5 years earlier, shorter periods of euthymia, more frequent depression, and a greater burden of additional comorbid psychiatric disorders—particularly anxiety disorders and substance use disorder.[25]

In a now-classic study, Wozniak et al.[27] demonstrated correlates of both ADHD and bipolar disorder in prepubertal children. Characteristic features of ADHD and associated neuropsychiatric correlates (e.g., additional help, learning disabilities) are identical to the presentation of ADHD without any major psychiatric or substance use comorbidities when ADHD is comorbid with bipolar disorder, suggesting that ADHD is an independent disorder when comorbid with bipolar disorder.[28,29] Given the concerns of symptomatic overlap, there is a risk of unintentional overdiagnosis of both disorders. Biederman et al.[30] have previously shown that even when eliminating overlapping symptoms, the majority of bipolar disorder plus ADHD children continued to meet criteria of both bipolar disorder and ADHD. Although limited information is available regarding the potential for different rates of comorbidity with bipolar disorder among the *DSM-IV/DSM-5* subtypes of ADHD, the rates of bipolar disorder are reported to be highest among youth with combined-type ADHD (26.5%) but also elevated among hyperactive-impulsive (14.3%) and inattentive (8.7%) youth.[31] In a group of adults with ADHD or ADHD plus bipolar disorder being treated pharmacologically,[32] ADHD adults with comorbid bipolar disorder shared the prototypic characteristics of both the disorders, but manifested higher rates of combined type ADHD, more ADHD symptoms, more anxiety, and poorer global functioning than ADHD alone.[32] While the mechanisms that mediate the association between bipolar disorder and ADHD remain unclear, it has been speculated that subforms of these disorders share common genes.[33] Relatives of ADHD children have an increased risk for bipolar disorder, and similarly, the children of bipolar disorder parents have an elevated risk for ADHD.[15]

In well-stabilized bipolar disorder youth with ADHD, ADHD symptoms often contribute dysfunction and become a target for treatment.[10] Inattentiveness, talkativeness, distractibility, hyperactivity, and impulsivity may not be identified as being connected with comorbid ADHD and may be targeted as being related to residual bipolar disorder. Conversely, the lack of acknowledgment of serious mood dysregulation and bipolar disorder in individuals with ADHD may result in ADHD treatments that further destabilize the mood.

The response to traditional mood stabilizers such as lithium has been reported to be less robust in the presence of ADHD comorbidity in youth with bipolar disorder,[34,35] suggesting that this subgroup of bipolar disorder may constitute a unique group with a differential treatment response. A systematic review of medical charts in children with bipolar disorder signaled that mood stabilizers improved bipolar disorder, whereas stimulants had no effect.[36] Furthermore, in children with bipolar disorder plus ADHD, the ADHD response only was manifested in the context of mood stabilization of the bipolar disorder.

The armementarium for ADHD appears useful in those with comorbid bipolar disorder, but only after stabilization of mania. Among first-line agents, stimulants have been reported to be efficacious in treating comorbid ADHD without precipitating (hypo)mania in mood-stabilized bipolar disorder youth in two controlled trials. In a placebo-controlled trial of stimulants as an adjunctive therapy for ADHD in bipolar disorder children stabilized on divalproex, low-dose mixed amphetamine salts improved ADHD without activating bipolar disorder.[37] Findling and colleagues[38] reported that in stabilized youth with bipolar disorder, concomitant methylphenidate improved ADHD in a dose-dependent manner without destabilization of mood. In contrast, Zeni et al.[39] found in stabilized children on aripiprazole no difference in efficacy or manic activation between methylphenidate and placebo. Furthermore, in an open trial of bupropion in adults with predominately stable bipolar II disorder and ADHD, we previously reported a significant improvement in ADHD without activation of mania.[40] Chang et al.[41] reported in children with well-stabilized bipolar disorder no increase in manic symptoms and improved ADHD when using atomoxetine administered in an open study. Of interest, in naturalistic evaluations of combined stimulants and antipsychotics, presumably for severe mood dysergulation and/or bipolar disorder in youth, improvements clinically have been reported with weight gain as the predominate adverse effect.[42,43]

Oppositional Defiant Disorder

High rates with bidirectional overlap of comorbid oppositional defiant disorder and bipolar disorder are reported by various studies. Rates of oppositional defiant disorder in the bipolar disorder population range from 47% to 88%[44-46] and conversely, 20% of children with oppositional defiant disorder are reported to have comorbid bipolar disorder.[47] A recent meta-analysis reported oppositional defiant disorder as the second most common comorbidity after ADHD, with a weighted rate of 53% among samples of children and adolescents with bipolar disorder.[9] Furthermore, Wozniak et al.[48] found that children with persistant bipolar I disorder had higher rates of comorbid oppositional defiant disorder compared to those children with nonpersistant bipolar disorder. Considering the high disability associated with oppositional defiant disorder, its association with persistant bipolar disorder adds to the severity of the clinical picture.

The diagnosis of oppositional defiant disorder in the context of bipolar disorder is challenging because nosologically oppositional defiant disorder shares overlapping symptoms with mania without any symptom specific to oppositional defiant disorder that could diagnostically differentiate it from mania. Because oppositional defiant disorder is so frequently comorbid with pediatric bipolar disorder, understanding of the relationship of oppositional defiant disorder with bipolar disorder ranges from oppositional defiant disorder being a secondary disorder as a consequence of bipolar illness or being a prodrome or early manifestation of bipolar disorder, to oppositional defiant disorder representing a "true independent" comorbid psychopathological phenomenon. However, many children with disruptive behavior disorders do not go on to develop bipolar disorder,[49] suggesting that different forms of disruptive behavior disorders may exist, one that could be prodromal to bipolar disorder and another form that is not. Additional work is needed in order to evaluate this issue further.

A clinical inquiry summarized eight reviews on treatments for children with oppositional defiant disorder and found improved behavior with a 20%–30% decrease in disruptive or aggressive behaviors with parenting interventions and behavioral therapy including cognitive-behavioral therapy, social problem-solving skills training, and parent management training involving the child and/or parent for 12–25 sessions.[50] Though treatment of oppositional defiant disorder is primarily behavioral in nature, when comorbid with other medication-responsive psychiatric conditions (bipolar disorder, ADHD), pharmacological treatment of the comorbid disorder often reduces overall symptoms of oppositional defiant disorder. While there are currently no data available on the treatment of oppositional defiant disorder in the context of bipolar disorder comorbidity, an emerging body of literature points to the role of thymoleptic agents in the treatment of disruptive behavior disorders (conduct disorder, oppositional defiant disorder, and disruptive behavior disorders-NOS), including oppositional defiant disorder in youth with significant aggression. Evidence suggests that pharmacotherapy may be effective in youth with disruptive behavior disorders, especially those experiencing problematic aggression, but response of the disruptive behavior disorders per se to these thymoleptics is understudied. Studies have examined the safety and efficacy of atypical antipsychotics (risperidone, olanzapine, quetiapine, and aripiprazole) in treating aggression in children with disruptive behavior disorders with results revealing atypical antipsychotics as being generally more efficacious than placebo.

To date, risperidone is the most extensively studied atypical antipsychotic for disruptive behavior disorders. Several trials indicate that risperidone can be useful for disruptive behavior disorders, especially for the aggressive features.[51–54] Short- and long-term efficacy and tolerability of risperidone as pharmacotherapy for disruptive behavior disorders in children with subaverage intelligence have been demonstrated in over 1,300 children and adolescents in the literature.[51–56] In two short-term (6-week) controlled trials

Aman and colleagues[57] studied the role of low dose risperidone (mean dose 1.16 and 0.98 mg/day) in borderline intellectual functioning (IQ of 36–84) disruptive behavior disorders youth ($n = 223$; ages 5–12 years) and reported an acceptable tolerability profile with significant improvement in aggression and behaviors associated with disruptive behavior disorders.[51,55] As the five long-term (1- to 3-year) follow-up trials suggest, a low dose of risperidone (mean dose ranged from 1.38 to 1.92 mg/day) was equally well tolerated and effective in controlling the disruptive behavior disorders and aggressive behaviors in this population.[52-54,56,58] Low-dose risperidone (0.02 mg/kg per day) is also reported to be well tolerated and efficacious in treating disruptive behavior disorders behaviors in youth with normal intelligence as suggested by short- and long-term trials.[58,59]

However, a post-hoc analysis of the data from the controlled trial of risperidone in disruptive behavior disorders conducted by Aman and colleagues[51] examined 24 candidate affective symptoms extracted from the 64-item Nisonger Child Behavior Rating Form.[60] These symptoms reflected the bipolar symptoms of explosive irritability, agitation, expansiveness, grandiosity, and depression. Risperidone was also effective in treating these putative symptoms of mania. This analysis raises the question of whether studies which examine the effects of antimanic agents on disruptive behavior disorders may include subjects with comorbid bipolar spectrum illness, and, further, whether the improvement in disruptive behavior disorders is a function in part of the improvement in bipolar disorder.

Quetiapine is the other most studied atypical antipsychotic for disruptive behavior disorders in youth. In youth with disruptive behavior disorders and ADHD who fail to respond to osmotic-release oral system methylphenidate monotherapy (at 54 mg/day dose), the addition of quetiapine (at a mean dose 329 mg/day) has been shown to be effective in controlling symptoms of oppositional defiant disorder and aggression.[61] Open-label and placebo-controlled studies suggest that divalproex is efficacious for the treatment of mood lability and explosive temper in children and adolescents with disruptive behavior disorders.[62,63] Further prospective studies addressing the course and treatment of oppositional defiant disorder when comorbid with bipolar disorder are warranted.

Conduct Disorder

In a comprehensive literature review, Geller[64] concluded that "Available data strongly suggest that prepubertal-onset bipolar disorder is a nonepisodic, chronic, rapid-cycling, mixed manic state that may be comorbid with attention-deficit hyperactivity disorder (ADHD) and conduct disorder or have features of ADHD and/or conduct disorder as initial manifestations." This observation is supported by a body of research documenting a bidirectional overlap between conduct disorder and bipolar disorder in children. As both conduct disorder and bipolar disorder are highly impairing conditions, their co-occurrence heralds a particularly severe clinical picture and raises important clinical questions. From a diagnostic standpoint, the question remains as to whether antisocial behaviors in a child with bipolar disorder, such as stealing, lying, or vandalizing, should be attributed to the disinhibition of mania with its attendant impulsivity, irritability and grandiosity or to comorbid conduct disorder. As for the treatment standpoint, the question further remains as to whether the symptoms of conduct disorder will diminish when the symptoms of bipolar disorder are adequately treated.

The association between conduct disorder and mania is consistent with the well-documented comorbidity between conduct disorder and major depression[65] and the frequently bipolar nature of juvenile depression.[66,67] Moreover, pediatric-onset bipolar disorder is frequently mixed (dysphoric) and commonly associated with "affective storms," with prolonged and aggressive temper outbursts.[68,69] These irritable outbursts often include threatening or attacking behaviors toward family members, children, adults, and teachers, behaviors that overlap with conduct disorder. For example, McGlashan et al.[70] reported that juvenile-onset bipolar disorder may be particularly explosive and disorganized and that children with mania tended to have more trouble with the law and more "psychotic assaultiveness" than adults with bipolar disorder. Kovacs[71] reported that some youngsters with mania showed serious acting-out behaviors, including burglary, stealing, vandalism, and a history of school suspensions. Although these aberrant behaviors are consistent with the diagnosis of conduct disorder, they may be due to the behavioral disinhibition that characterizes bipolar disorder. Thus, it is not surprising that youth with bipolar disorder frequently meet diagnostic criteria for conduct disorder. High rates of conduct disorder (55%–69%) are reported in youth with bipolar disorder,[17,71] and the comorbid presence of bipolar disorder and conduct disorder in youth heralds a more complicated course with high rates of hospitalization (42%).[72] Furthermore, conduct disorder is reported to be severe in the presence of comorbid bipolar disorder[73] with studies showing higher rates of global aggression and substance abuse.[17,74]

Epidemiologic studies report high rates of comorbidity between bipolar disorder and disruptive behavior disorders.[75,76] There seems to be an increase in the risk for bipolar disorder with a higher number of conduct disorder symptoms[76] and a nearly 7-fold increase in the risk for bipolar disorder in individuals with antisocial personality disorder.[77] The risk of conduct disorder is 3-fold higher in younger bipolar individuals (<30 years) with comorbid substance use disorder than those without substance use disorder (52% vs. 14.8%).[78]

Wilens et al.[17] reported in a case-controlled study of 105 adolescents with bipolar disorder and 98 adolescents without bipolar disorder the rate of comorbid conduct disorder was significantly higher for the cases compared to the non–mood disorder comparison subjects (55% vs. 8%). Furthermore, when they assessed substance use disorder in cases, they found a significant effect of bipolar disorder on risk for substance use disorder as well as a significant effect of conduct disorder.[17] However, they found that conduct disorder did not account for substance use disorder in the bipolar disorder sample, revealing that adolescents with bipolar disorder are at a heightened risk for the development of substance use disorder relative to non–mood disorder peers, independent of conduct disorder. Wilens et al.[79] previously found that the risk for substance use disorder associated with adolescent-onset bipolar disorder (9-fold) was reminiscent of the risk for substance use disorder associated with conduct disorder (6-fold), highlighting the importance of conduct disorder as a separate risk factor for substance use disorder. These findings support the notion that conduct disorder in conjunction with bipolar disorder only complicates and increases the severity of the clinical presentation.

Further evidence demonstrates the complicated relationship between conduct disorder and bipolar disorder. In a naturalistic study Masi et al.[74] assessed 307 adolescents (106 with conduct disorder without bipolar disorder, 108 with bipolar disorder without conduct disorder, and 92 with conduct disorder plus bipolar disorder) over a 6-month period. Findings revealed that the adolescents with conduct disorder plus bipolar disorder presented the highest rates of global aggression and substance use disorder. According to multiple scales, the adolescents with bipolar disorder without conduct disorder showed the best response to treatment, compared with conduct disorder youth.[74] The results of this study add to literature revealing the need for a deeper understanding of the implications of having comorbid conduct disorder and bipolar disorder.

Comorbid conduct disorder in bipolar disorder youth might confuse the clinical presentation of childhood bipolar disorder and possibly account for some of the documented failure to detect bipolar disorder in children. Isaac et al.[80] examined a group of adolescents found to be the most problematic, crisis prone, and treatment resistant in a special educational day school and treatment program. These authors found that two thirds of these youngsters satisfied *DSM-III-R* criteria for bipolar disorder, which had often been misdiagnosed as ADHD and conduct disorder. Most of the remaining youngsters showed significant bipolar features but did not fully satisfy *DSM-III-R* criteria for bipolar disorder. Considering the heterogeneity of bipolar disorder and that of conduct disorder, these findings may have important implications in helping to identify a subtype of bipolar disorder with early onset characterized by high levels of comorbid conduct disorder[71] and a subtype of conduct disorder with high levels of dysphoria and explosiveness.

In a large, well-characterized, prospective sample of children referred with ADHD,[81] ADHD children with comorbid bipolar disorder and conduct disorder reported higher familial and personal risk for mood disorders than youth with ADHD and conduct disorder alone, who were found to have higher personal risk for antisocial personality disorder. This observation suggests that the presence of bipolar disorder in some conduct disorder children could be clinically meaningful, at least in the context of ADHD. Further analysis of structured interview-derived data from a large sample of consecutive, clinic-referred children and adolescents showed again a large and symmetrical overlap between bipolar disorder and conduct disorder.[36] Examination of the clinical features, patterns of psychiatric comorbidity, and functioning in multiple domains showed that children with conduct disorder and bipolar disorder had similar features of each disorder irrespective of comorbidity with the other disorder. These findings further supported the hypothesis that children satisfying diagnostic criteria for bipolar disorder and conduct disorder suffer from both disorders, rather than one being misdiagnosed as the other, even outside the context of comorbid ADHD. These authors also documented that psychiatric hospitalizations among conduct disorder probands were almost entirely accounted for by those with comorbid bipolar disorder. This finding is consistent with the notion that conduct disorder plus bipolar disorder probands, along with other symptoms of conduct disorder, engage in a disorganized type of aggression associated with bipolar disorder. Since many children in psychiatric hospitals with the diagnosis of conduct disorder commonly have a profile of severe aggressiveness, it is likely that these children required psychiatric hospitalizations because of the manic picture and not necessarily due to the conduct disorder.

Further evidence that a subtype of conduct disorder linked to bipolar disorder could be identified derives from pilot familial risk analyses.[82,83] These results suggest that relatives of bipolar disorder probands were at an increased risk for bipolar disorder, but not conduct disorder. On the other hand, relatives of conduct disorder probands had an increased risk for conduct disorder, but not for bipolar disorder, while relatives of conduct disorder plus bipolar disorder probands had an elevated risk for both disorders.[83] Among relatives in this latter group, bipolar disorder and antisocial disorders showed significant cosegregation; that is, relatives with one disorder were highly likely to have the other. As a result of this cosegregation, conduct disorder plus bipolar disorder was significantly elevated among relatives of conduct disorder plus bipolar disorder probands, but it was rare among the relatives of the other proband groups. Probands with the combination of conduct disorder and bipolar disorder also had high rates of nonbipolar disorder conduct/antisocial disorders among the relatives, suggesting a genetic loading with two subtypes of conduct disorder: with and without bipolar disorder. These results provide compelling evidence that subtypes of conduct disorder and of bipolar disorder can be identified based on patterns of comorbidity with the other disorder, suggesting that their co-occurrence may correspond to a distinct familial syndrome.[15,31,82–84]

The delineation of a subgroup of manic conduct disorder children would have important clinical implications. It could lead to improvement in our efforts to ameliorate the guarded outcome of some conduct disorder youth. Since bipolar disorder may respond to specific pharmacological treatments, correctly identifying those conduct disorder children with bipolar disorder may afford the opportunity to introduce these medications in the treatment of antisocial and aggressive youth.

There is limited evidence from various trials of atypical antipsychotics in youth with bipolar disorder on the possible role of thymoleptics in managing conduct disorder when comorbid with bipolar disorder. In our open-label short-term (8-week) trials of risperidone ($n = 30$) and ziprasidone ($n = 21$) in children and adolescents aged 6–17 years with bipolar disorder, these atypical antipsychotics were associated not only with significant improvement in symptoms of pediatric bipolar disorder but also with improvement in the severity of comorbid conduct disorder (a CGI rating of much or very much improved) in the subset of bipolar disorder youth with comorbid conduct disorder.[85,86] Likewise, a similar response of comorbid conduct disorder to an open-label short-term trial (8-week) of risperidone (*n* = 16) and olanzapine (*n* = 15) is recorded in a younger population of preschool-age children (4–6 years) with bipolar disorder.[86] The promising role of atypical antipsychotics in treating comorbid conduct disorder in youth with bipolar disorder as suggested by these open trials requires further validation by conducting controlled studies that apply specific measures to assess the response of conduct disorder.

As discussed earlier under the role of thymoleptic agents in the disruptive behavior disorders population, potential pharmacotherapy for conduct disorder with marked aggression includes mood stabilizers, typical and atypical antipsychotics—the very medications most commonly recommended for the treatment of bipolar disorder. The antimanic agent lithium has been found to be an effective antiaggressive agent in youth with conduct disorder as reported by various studies conducted in ambulatory and hospitalized youth with conduct disorder.[1,87] A small literature suggests that typical antipsychotic medications such as haloperidol and molindone are helpful in decreasing aggression in youth with conduct disorder.[88-90] However, typical antipsychotic treatment was associated with a range of problematic adverse effects. This led to the use of the atypical antipsychotic agents in treating conduct disorder with aggressive features.

In an open-label short-term (8-week; N = 17) followed by long-term (18-week; N = 9) trial of quetiapine (at median dose 150 mg/day) in children aged 6–12 years with the primary diagnosis of conduct disorder, quetiapine was found to be effective in treating aggression and conduct problems by week 8; the benefit was sustained during long-term treatment with quetiapine in children who responded to an acute therapeutic trial of quetiapine.[38,91] In this trial, no subject developed extrapyramidal symptoms or discontinued the trial due to adverse events, suggesting that short- and long-term treatment with quetiapine was safe and well tolerated. More recently, in a controlled trial, quetiapine at 294 (±78) mg/day was reported to be superior to placebo in treating adolescents with conduct disorder (*n* = 9/10) on clinician-assessed measures of global severity but failed to separate from placebo on parent-assessed specific measures of aggression and conduct behaviors; this discrepancy could be attributed to small sample size, leading to diminished statistical power to detect differences.[92]

There is preliminary evidence on the role of olanzapine in treating aggression with conduct disorder from a retrospective chart review of adolescents with conduct disorder (*n* = 23) who were treated with olanzapine (mean dose of 8 ± 3.2 mg/day) for an extended period of time (6–12 months).[93] Treatment with olanzapine resulted in improvement of aggression but was also associated with a modest weight gain (4.6 ± 3 kg). The aforementioned empirical evidence from clinical trials exclusively conducted in conduct disorder populations in addition to the previous discussion of trials conducted in disruptive behavior disorders populations strongly suggest the role of atypical antipsychotics in managing behaviors related to conduct disorder and aggression. A preliminary open trial of child- and family-focused cognitive-behavioral therapy showed the possible benefits of psychotherapies for addressing bipolar disorder and conduct disorder in children and adolescents. Pavuluri et al.[94] studied 34 children and young adults and found that those who received child- and family-focused cognitive-behavioral therapy in conjunction with medication demonstrated reduced symptoms of aggression as well as higher global functioning scores.

Substance Use Disorders

In epidemiological and clinically based studies, substance use disorder is one of the most feared and unfortunately common comorbidities found in adolescents and young adults with bipolar disorder.[17,95–99] McElroy et al.[95] reported that drug and alcohol use disorders were found in 39% and 32% of bipolar disorder adults, respectively. Studies have shown that that bipolar disorder onset prior to adulthood was strongly and specifically related to substance use disorder development in young adults. Similarly, McElroy and colleagues[100] showed a retrospective association between early-onset bipolar disorder, mixed symptoms and comorbidity, and substance use disorder. Moreover, not surprisingly, substance use disorder exacerbates bipolar disorder course.[98,101]

Pediatric-onset bipolar disorder has been shown to be a major risk factor for substance use disorder.[17,97] The relationship appears to be bidirectional; bipolar disorder is overrepresented in adolescents with substance use disorder, and an excess of substance use disorder exists with bipolar disorder or prominent mood lability and dyscontrol.[17,102,103] Strober et al.[104] in a sample of inpatient adolescents reported an increase in the rates of substance use disorder from 10% at baseline (mean age 16 years) to 22% at 5-year follow-up and described a mixed presentation with highly relapsing course in the presence of comorbidity with substance use disorder.

Adolescents with substance use disorder referred to a child psychiatry outpatient clinic were more likely than those without substance use disorder to have comorbid bipolar disorder.[103] Prospective data from a sample of convenience (ADHD) signaled that adolescents with early-onset bipolar disorder were at the highest risk for substance use disorder[105] and were also found to be at higher risk for early initiation and higher rates of cigarette smoking.[106] Similarly, clinically referred adolescents with versus without bipolar disorder are at heightened risk for substance use disorder, independent of conduct disorder.[79]

Multiple prospective studies also show high rates of substance use disorder in adolescents with bipolar disorder. For instance, in a sample of 105 adolescents with bipolar disorder and 98 non-mood-disordered controls, we reported high rates of nicotine dependence (23% vs. 4%, respectively) and full substance use disorder (34% vs. 4%) that were independent of ADHD, conduct, or anxiety disorders.[17] We recently presented that at 5-year follow-up, over half of our now young adults with bipolar disorder manifested substance use disorder, which was significantly higher than the control group; and that substance use disorder was specifically associated with the persistence of the active bipolar disorder symptoms.[107] Geller et al.[108] in an 8-year follow-up of child-onset cases of bipolar disorder reported rates of substance use disorder of 34% at a mean age of 19 years with the majority meeting criteria for more severe dependence (30%). Similar, Goldstein et al.[97] reported from a large naturalistic study that 16% of adolescents with bipolar disorder had substance use disorder at a mean age of 15 years. In a 5-year follow-up of hospitalized adolescents with bipolar disorder, Strober et al.[104] reported that 9% of adolescents had substance use disorder at age 16 years. DelBello et al.[109] reported on a 12-month follow-up of previously hospitalized adolescents and found that 8% had a full alcohol use disorder. Wozniak et al.[48] found at 5-year follow-up that 30% of young adolescents with bipolar disorder manifested a substance use disorder. Kozloff et al.[99] in a community sample, showed that 42% of a young adult sample had substance use disorder, which was significantly greater than those without psychopathology.

Interestingly, similar to our findings, Goldstein and colleagues[97] found the high rates of substance use disorder in adolescents with bipolar spectrum disorders were linked to lack of treatment and bipolar disorder symptoms. Similarly, the 5-year follow-up of Wozniak et al.[48] using a similar definition of "persistence," reported an almost two-fold higher risk for substance use disorder and cigarette smoking in those with compared to without the persistence of the bipolar disorder into early adolescence. Along the same lines, Lewinsohn et al.[110] in a community sample showed a similar magnitude for a higher risk for alcohol and drug use in those with full bipolar disorder compared to subthreshold bipolar disorder.

Because conduct disorder is an important comorbidity of both bipolar disorder and a predictor of substance use disorder, we further examined the contribution of conduct disorder on later development of substance use disorder.[111] We found that while conduct disorder clearly increases the risk for substance use disorder in bipolar disorder, the risk of substance use disorder in bipolar disorder still remained significant with or without conduct disorder.

Mechanism of Risk for Substance Use Disorder in Bipolar Disorder

The reasons that juvenile bipolar disorder is a risk factor for substance use disorder in particular, and that adolescent- versus child-onset bipolar disorder confers a differential risk for substance use disorder remain unclear. Given the prominent genetic influences in both bipolar disorder and substance use disorder (as individual disorders and perhaps cosegregating[112]), it remains unclear whether substance use disorder in bipolar disorder youth represents a subtype of bipolar disorder and/or substance use disorder, or whether a vulnerability to substance use disorder development exists in these youth.

Among disturbances reported in bipolar disorder youth, severe affective and self-regulation problems appear to be an important mechanism for the development of substance use disorder.[93] By nature of their intrapsychic distress and behavioral disinhibition,

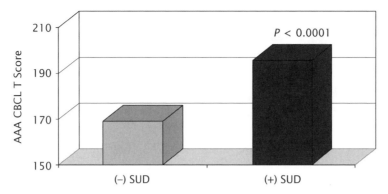

FIGURE 4.1 Using the aggregate AAA (Attention, Aggression, Anxiety) T-score from the Child Behavior Checklist (CBCL) as a proxy of emotional dysregulation, adolescents with substance use disorder (SUD) had higher rates of emotional dysregulation compared to those without a SUD. From Wilens et al. Difficulties in emotional regulation and substance use disorders: A controlled family study of bipolar adolescents. *Drug Alcohol Depend.* 2013;132(1–2):114–21.

these youth may try to modulate their irritable and labile mood with substances of abuse, as has been described in adults.[113,114] Moreover, deficits in emotional self-regulation have been posited to be critical in the development and maintenance of substance use disorder.[114] We examined this issue and found evidence that youth with bipolar disorder tended to initiate substances of abuse to attenuate mood relative to non-mood-disordered adolescents who reported using substance more often to get high.[115] Moreover, we recently reported a very strong association between deficits in emotional self-regulation and the risk for substance use disorder.[116] High rates of emotional dysregulation as measured by the Child Behavior Checklist were associated with both a higher risk and an earlier age of onset for substance use disorder.[116] In contrast, lower proxies of dysregulation were associated with lower risks for substance use disorder in our combined samples.[116] Conversely, individuals with substance use disorder, particularly with both drug and alcohol use disorder, had higher levels of dysregulation compared to those without substance use disorder[116] (see Fig. 4.1). Hence, these data highlight the importance of the mood symptoms within bipolar disorder that may be directly driving substance use disorder.

Genes and Adolescent Substance Use Disorder

Child- and adolescent-onset bipolar disorder may be etiologically distinct with a variable course and outcome, including the risk for substance use disorder. It may also be that adolescent-onset bipolar disorder and adolescent-onset substance use disorder may represent variable expressivity of a shared risk factor.[117,118] To better understand these competing influences, family studies are necessary. We reported that the parents of proband youth with bipolar disorder (without substance use disorder) and bipolar disorder with substance use disorder were more likely to develop bipolar disorder than the parents of controls.[112] Parents of adolescents with bipolar disorder and with bipolar disorder and substance use disorder were more likely than relatives of controls to develop substance use disorder; however, no differences emerged between the parents of the two bipolar groups. Within the parents of proband youth with bipolar disorder and substance use disorder, we found higher risk of substance use disorder in parents with bipolar disorder than in those without bipolar disorder, leading us to speculate that bipolar disorder and substance use disorder are prevalent in the first-degree relatives of adolescents with bipolar disorder, adults with bipolar disorder were more likely to manifest substance use disorder, and that bipolar disorder and substance use disorder cosegregated. Interestingly, work from our group identified a candidate gene for bipolar disorder—namely the dopamine transporter protein[119]—that has been linked with the development of early-onset substance use disorder. Of interest, we recently reported that having a parent with substance use disorder did not increase the risk for substance use disorder in our adolescents with bipolar disorder, in part because of the already very high risk bipolar disorder imparts on the development of substance use disorder in adolescents.[120]

Diagnostic and Treatment Considerations

Given the severity of comorbid bipolar disorder and substance use disorder in adolescents, clinicians need to consider initially the proper level of care. The simultaneous treatment of adolescents with bipolar disorder and substance use disorder appears necessary. Given limited, albeit important, data on the effects of medication treatment reducing substance use disorder in bipolar disorder, both psychosocial and medication strategies should be considered simultaneously in these comorbid adolescents.

There is evidence that pharmacological interventions are effective for youth with substance use disorder and bipolar disorder, and that these treatments should be utilized even in the context of an active addiction (e.g., help stabilize the bipolar disorder during substance use disorder). Three studies, including two randomized controlled studies, have reported that mood stabilizers and/or second-generation antipsychotics significantly reduced substance use in bipolar youth.[121] A controlled, 6-week study of treatment with lithium in youth with affective dysregulation and substance dependence by Geller et al.[121] reported a clinically significant decrease in the number of positive urines as well as a significant increase in overall global functioning. In a 5-week open trial of valproic acid in adolescent outpatients with marijuana abuse/dependence and "explosive mood disorder" (mood symptoms were not classified using the *DSM-IV*), Donovan et al.[62] reported significant improvement in their marijuana use and their affective symptoms. DelBello and colleagues[122] presented preliminary work indicating that the combination of quetiapine plus topiramate (an antiaddictive medication) was superior to quetiapine alone in reducing substance use disorder. Clearly, more work on the use of medications, structured therapies, and facilitated self-help groups alone and in combination are necessary in these difficult-to-treat youth.

Anxiety Disorders

The presence of anxiety disorders in individuals who suffer from bipolar disorder has been underrecognized and understudied. One reason for this lack of recognition could be the notion that it is counterintuitive to suggest that bipolar disorder, which is characterized by high levels of disinhibition, could coexist with anxiety, which is characterized by fear and inhibition. However, in the first paper to demonstrate the high frequency of bipolar disorder in an outpatient pediatric psychopharmacology clinic (16%), 56% of the children with bipolar disorder comorbidly suffered from two or more lifetime anxiety disorders (multiple anxiety disorders).[27] Furthermore, a recent detailed analysis of the comorbidity between pediatric bipolar disorder and anxiety disorders in a clinically referred population revealed that 76% of youth with bipolar disorder have one or more anxiety disorders comorbid with their bipolar disorder.[123] In a community sample, Lewinsohn et al.[75] reported that a third of nonreferred bipolar disorder adolescents had comorbid anxiety disorders, a significantly higher rate than that found in those without a history of bipolar disorder. Because anxiety disorders are heterogeneous (seven are included in the new *DSM-5*[124]) and often lumped together, uncertainties remain as to which specific anxiety disorders are associated with bipolar disorder. Various clinical and epidemiological studies in adult and pediatric populations have identified a wide range of anxiety disorders associated with bipolar disorder with rates ranging between 12.5% and 77.4%.[11,15,17,22,75,100,123,125–133]

Among anxiety disorders, certain phenotypes have been suggested to be specifically associated with youth.[127,134] A preponderance of investigators have suggested that a particular link exists between panic disorder and bipolar disorder in adults[11,135,136] and children.[134] Data from adult studies report a lifetime prevalence of panic disorder in 21%–33% of individuals with bipolar disorder[135–137] and, conversely, lifetime bipolar disorder in 6%–23% of individuals with panic disorder.[131,138] MacKinnon et al.[139,140] examined familial risk for panic disorder in 57 families with a high prevalence of bipolar disorder to argue that panic disorder with bipolar disorder is a genetic subtype of bipolar disorder. Savino et al.[141] systematically explored the intraepisodic and longitudinal comorbidity of 140 adults with panic disorder and reported comorbidity with bipolar disorder in 13.5% of the sample with panic disorder. They also note that an additional 34.3% met features of "hyperthymic temperament," a possible bipolar spectrum condition. Biederman et al. reported high rates of panic disorder (52%) among youth with bipolar disorder[129] consistent with the observation by Birmaher et al.[134] suggesting that the association between bipolar disorder and panic disorder in children and adolescents might be unique and specific. Recent emerging literature indicates a high prevalence of various anxiety disorders—including but not limited to panic disorder—in pediatric[123,125,126,142,143] and adult[100,144,145] populations with bipolar disorder, challenging the notion of a sole specific link between bipolar disorder and panic disorder. More information is needed to elucidate the etiologic basis of the association between bipolar disorder and anxiety disorders in youth and investigate whether the connection is differentially dependent on specific anxiety disorder diagnoses or is more trait-based.

In the presence of high levels of anxiety, adults with bipolar disorder experience greater symptom severity, increased risk for suicide and alcohol abuse, higher frequency of polypharmacy, more severe adverse effects, poor treatment response, and higher rates of nonremission with poor course and functioning.[130,146–148] Olvera et al.[149] found that children with bipolar disorder and multiple anxiety disorders displayed manic symptoms at an earlier age and were more likely to have been hospitalized for their illness. Anxiety disorders in adolescents with bipolar disorder have been associated with a poorer course of bipolar disorder and lower global functioning.[150]

Improving understanding of the relationships between anxiety disorders and bipolar disorder in youth has important treatment implications. Masi et al.[126] reported high rates of pharmacologically induced hypo/mania in bipolar disorder youth with anxiety disorders, with the mean age of onset for anxiety disorders preceding that for bipolar disorder. Other studies have also demonstrated that anxiety disorders tend to predate bipolar disorder onset.[142,150,151] These findings suggest caution when considering antidepressant pharmacotherapy in a pediatric population with multiple anxiety disorders, given that antidepressants can have manicogenic effects.[152,153]

Considering that typical bipolar disorder treatment options such as traditional mood stabilizers do not generally treat anxiety disorders and that treatment of anxiety disorders with selective serotonin reuptake inhibitors (SSRIs) can aggravate bipolar disorder, the pharmacological approach to treating bipolar children with comorbid anxiety disorders needs to be defined. As bipolar disorder and anxiety disorders respond to different treatments, identification of the comorbid state is essential for proper treatment and for achieving optimal functioning.

The treatment of anxiety disorders in the context of bipolar comorbidity is understudied.[154] Treatment trials for pediatric anxiety disorders typically exclude children with bipolar disorder by protocol design, and similarly, children with a bipolar disorder diagnosis are typically excluded from trials of treatment for both depression and anxiety.

One open-label trial has assessed response of co-occurring panic attacks and generalized anxiety disorder in adults with bipolar disorder, reporting a significant decrease in or remission of anxiety symptoms with divalproex therapy.[155] The majority of treatment studies for comorbid anxiety disorders and bipolar disorder, however, are case studies.[154] Corroborative evidence for the anxiolytic effect of mood stabilizers comes from various open-label and controlled trials in adult populations with anxiety disorders that suggest valproate to be effective in treating panic disorder and posttraumatic stress disorder.[156–162] An antianxiety response of certain mood stabilizers could be specific to certain anxiety disorder(s). For instance, although carbamazepine is effective in treating certain symptoms of posttraumatic stress disorder, it is found to be ineffective in treating other anxiety disorders in adults—namely panic disorder and obsessive-compulsive disorder.[163–167] Preliminary results of nonpharmacological treatment research suggest that cognitive-behavioral therapy can effectively treat anxiety disorders in populations with comorbid bipolar disorder.[168]

Obsessive-Compulsive Disorder

Clinical descriptions of obsessive-compulsive disorder symptoms in bipolar patients date back to the 19th century.[169] Most data on comorbid obsessive-compulsive disorder and bipolar disorder are not based on systematic studies[170,171] but result from naturalistic studies. In adults, evidence of a significant overlap between obsessive-compulsive disorder and bipolar disorder first came from the landmark Epidemiological Catchment Area (ECA) study, in which 23% of those with bipolar disorder also met criteria for obsessive-compulsive disorder.[76] Subsequent studies have consistently found an overlap between obsessive-compulsive disorder and bipolar disorder at rates as high as 15%–35%.[17,135,172] When comorbid with bipolar disorder, obsessive-compulsive disorder in adults has a more episodic course, often featuring higher rates of sexual and religious obsessions, lower rates of checking rituals, and greater frequency of concurrent major depressive episodes and panic disorder. Adults with comorbid obsessive-compulsive disorder and bipolar disorder also exhibit increased rates of suicidality and more frequent hospitalizations, requiring more complex pharmacological interventions than those without bipolar disorder.[135,172–174] A recent survey conducted among the French Association of individuals with obsessive-compulsive disorder provides corroborating evidence for this comorbidity in subjects giving retrospective childhood reports. Reporting a high prevalence of comorbid lifetime bipolarity, Hantouche and colleagues also noted that many of these subjects had a juvenile onset of their obsessive-compulsive disorder.[175,176]

While the available literature suggests the co-occurrence of bipolar disorder and obsessive-compulsive disorder in youth substantially impacts clinical presentation, global functioning, and treatment decisions,[132,177] the nature of this relationship is not clearly delineated. For example, the agitation, racing thoughts, and feelings of distress that can be associated with severe obsessive-compulsive disorder could mimic a bipolar presentation; conversely, the manic symptom of increased goal-directed activity ("mission mode" behavior) or repetitive, unwanted hypersexual thoughts in a child or adolescent with bipolar disorder could mimic an obsessive-compulsive disorder presentation. In one of few studies that addresses this question of comorbid presentation, Masi et al.[132] reported that in comparison to obsessive-compulsive disorder, comorbid obsessive-compulsive disorder and bipolar disorder youth were significantly more impaired, had an earlier age of onset of obsessive-compulsive disorder, and had more frequent existential, philosophical, odd, and/or superstitious obsessions, indicating that comorbidity with bipolar disorder may have a clinically relevant influence on the symptom expression of obsessive-compulsive disorder. Half of the comorbid population in this study had type II bipolar disorder and one third experienced pharmacologically induced hypomania. The high risk of (hypo) manic switches reported with antidepressant treatment in pediatric obsessive-compulsive disorder is suggestive of a bipolar diathesis.[178,179] A later naturalistic retrospective study of obsessive-compulsive disorder children and adolescents by Masi et al. confirmed earlier outcomes and found those with comorbid obsessive-compulsive disorder and bipolar disorder to have more frequent hoarding obsessions and compulsions, providing further evidence for the specific impact of bipolar disorder on the clinical presentation of obsessive-compulsive disorder.[177]

In another study of youth ascertained for a family genetic study of bipolar disorder and obsessive-compulsive disorder, we previously documented a significant and symmetrical bidirectional overlap between bipolar disorder and obsessive-compulsive disorder (21% of the bipolar disorder cohort and 15% of the obsessive-compulsive disorder cohort satisfied criteria for both bipolar disorder and obsessive-compulsive disorder).[180] In the presence of comorbid bipolar disorder, youth with obsessive-compulsive disorder more often presented with the symptom of hoarding/saving, experienced a higher prevalence of other comorbid disorders (especially oppositional defiant disorder, major depressive disorder, and psychosis), suffered from poorer psychosocial functioning, and required hospitalization at a greater frequency. Higher prevalence of comorbidity with multiple anxiety disorders, especially generalized anxiety disorder and social phobia, was observed in youth with comorbid obsessive-compulsive disorder and bipolar disorder than when either disorder occurred alone in youth. Limited family genetic data suggest a genetic linkage between obsessive-compulsive disorder and bipolar disorder. Coryell[181] reported an equal incidence (2.3%) of bipolar disorder in families of probands with obsessive-compulsive disorder and in families with bipolar disorder. Similarly, an increased incidence of obsessional traits has been reported in the offspring of bipolar probands.[182]

Although, to date, no systematic data are available that address the therapeutic response of bipolar disorder in the presence of comorbid anxiety disorders, Joshi et al.[183] conducted a secondary data analysis to examine the antimanic effect of olanzapine in bipolar disorder youth with comorbid obsessive-compulsive disorder and generalized

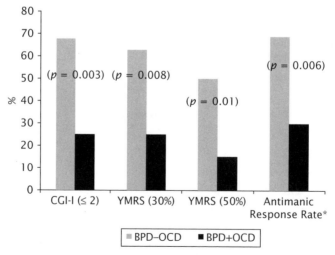

FIGURE 4.2 Comparison of improvement associated with olanzapine monotherapy in bipolar disorder (BPD) youth with and without comorbid obsessive-compulsive disorder (OCD). From Joshi G et al., Impact of obsessive-compulsive disorder on the antimanic response to olanzapine therapy in youth with bipolar disorder. *Bipolar Disord.* 2010;12(2):196-204. doi: 10.1111/j.1399-5618.2010.00789.x.

anxiety disorder and concluded that in children and adolescents with bipolar disorder the comorbid presence of lifetime obsessive-compulsive disorder, but not generalized anxiety disorder, is associated with poor antimanic response (see Fig. 4.2). This finding suggests that when comorbid with bipolar disorder, certain anxiety disorders may have a larger mediating effect on bipolar disorder treatment outcome than others.

Similarly, the presence of bipolar disorder with anxiety disorders may have a negative effect on the treatment outcome of the anxiety disorder treatment. For instance, compared to obsessive-compulsive disorder youth without comorbid bipolar disorder, children and adolescents with comorbid obsessive-compulsive disorder and bipolar disorder have been reported to show poor response to psychotropic medications and are more frequently on a combined pharmacy regimen.[184] Nonpharmacological treatments such as cognitive-behavioral therapy have been found to be useful and should be instituted when possible, along with any of the pharmacological alternatives to selective serotonin reuptake inhibitors (SSRIs).

Posttraumatic Stress Disorder

Individuals who work with trauma victims make the clinical observation that mood swings are common in such populations. Although considerable literature implicates psychosocial stresses in the onset and recurrence of bipolar disorder,[185-187] there is a paucity of research on the association of posttraumatic stress disorder and bipolar disorder. While Breslau et al.[188] reported that 40%–76% of children had been exposed to a traumatic event by age 17,[189] the estimated lifetime prevalence of the full syndromatic posttraumatic stress disorder in the general population is between 1% and 14%, and its prevalence in children is around 6%.[189] By contrast, reported rates of posttraumatic stress disorder comorbidity in adults with bipolar disorder have varied widely from 7% to 50%. Overlap between bipolar disorder and posttraumatic stress disorder has also been demonstrated in community samples; the National Comorbidity Survey identified posttraumatic stress disorder in 39% of bipolar disorder individuals surveyed.[190]

Rates of substance use disorder are substantially higher in youth who had a lifetime diagnosis of posttraumatic stress disorder before age 18 compared to youth who had never experienced a trauma.[72] Given the increasing recognition of substance use disorder in bipolar disorder and posttraumatic stress disorder, we further examined the relationship of bipolar disorder, substance use disorder, and posttraumatic stress disorder in an older group of adolescents with bipolar disorder. We found significantly more posttraumatic stress disorder in adolescents with bipolar disorder compared to non-mood-disordered controls. Sixteen percent of youth with bipolar disorder had broad posttraumatic stress disorder compared to 4% of comparison subjects. Moreover, a higher risk of substance use disorder was found in bipolar disorder adolescents with posttraumatic stress disorder. While exploratory in nature, interesting temporal patterns emerged, suggesting an initial onset of bipolar disorder followed by substance use, trauma, posttraumatic stress disorder, and then finally full substance use disorder. These data highlight the high risk of posttraumatic stress disorder in bipolar disorder adolescents that appears to be related to substance use disorder in these youth.

Although many studies have looked at possible links between early traumatic events and development of psychopathology over the life span,[191–194] few studies have examined the potential role of early traumatic life stresses on the development of bipolar disorder and posttraumatic stress disorder. Emerging evidence suggests that trauma significantly compromises the course of bipolar disorder. Leverich et al.[195] evaluated 631 outpatients with bipolar disorder and reported that nearly half of the females (49%) and one third of the males (36%) reported early sexual and physical abuse. Those who endorsed a history of child or adolescent physical or sexual abuse, compared with those who did not, had significantly higher rates of comorbid posttraumatic stress disorder, a history of an earlier onset of bipolar illness, and a higher rate of suicide attempts. Garno et al.[196] studied 100 adults with bipolar disorder, and half (51%) reported a history of abuse while a quarter suffered from comorbid posttraumatic stress disorder (24%). Similarly, 32% of bipolar disorder youth treated in a community clinic experienced three or more adverse life events such as neglect, abuse, and foster care placement, and adverse event exposure was associated with poorer bipolar disorder prognosis.[197] In a sample of adolescent inpatients, Havens et al.[198] reported that those with probable posttraumatic stress disorder were three times as likely to have a bipolar disorder diagnosis.

Despite concerns that pediatric bipolar disorder may be inappropriately diagnosed in youth with high rates of trauma and emotional dysregulation,[199] evidence suggests that bipolar disorder and posttraumatic stress disorder are etiologically distinct and can truly co-occur. Geller et al.[45] reported high rates (43%) of the symptom of hypersexuality (higher in pubertal versus prepubertal bipolar disorder population) and low rates (<1%) of history of sexual abuse in their prepubertal and early adolescent bipolar disorder cohort, suggesting that the symptom of hypersexuality in pediatric bipolar disorder is etiologically unrelated to sexual abuse and more reflective of mania and puberty. Our group recently compared patterns of familial aggregation of bipolar disorder in bipolar disorder children with and without posttraumatic stress disorder and found that irrespective of posttraumatic stress disorder comorbidity, the clinical features of bipolar disorder did not significantly differ between groups.[200] Children with bipolar disorder and posttraumatic stress disorder matched bipolar disorder children without posttraumatic stress disorder when comparing mean age of onset, mean number of episodes, and profiles of individual mania symptoms, in addition to patterns of psychiatric comorbidity and cognitive and psychosocial functioning. Familial risk analysis found that relatives of bipolar disorder probands had a similarly increased risk for bipolar disorder compared to controls, regardless of proband posttraumatic stress disorder comorbidity (see Fig. 4.3). These findings suggest that the clinical expression of bipolar disorder comorbid with posttraumatic stress disorder does not reflect a traumatically derived phenotype, but rather, represents the true co-occurrence of bipolar disorder and posttraumatic stress disorder.

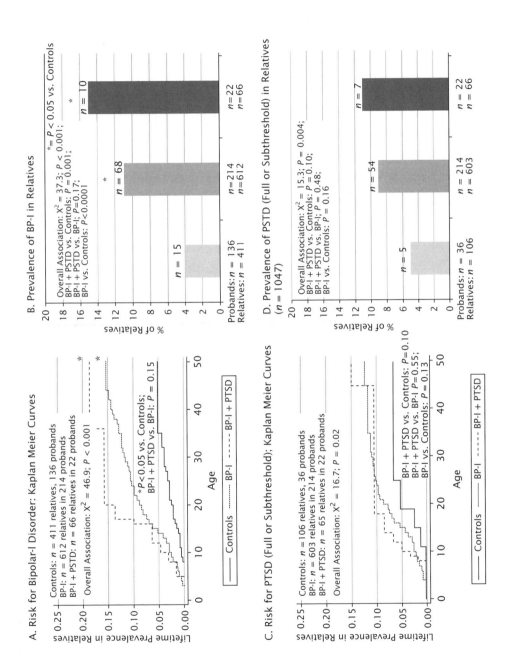

FIGURE 4.3 Risk for disorders in first-degree relatives. From Biederman J et al., Can pediatric bipolar-I disorder be diagnosed in the context of posttraumatic stress disorder? A familial risk analysis. *Psychiatry Res.* 2013. http://dx.doi.org/10.1016/j.psychres.2013.05.011.

A report by Wozniak et al. raises the question as to whether a diagnosis of bipolar disorder may pose a risk factor for trauma. Using data from a large longitudinal sample of well-characterized boys with and without ADHD, these authors failed to find meaningful associations between ADHD, trauma, and posttraumatic stress disorder. Instead, they identified early bipolar disorder as an important antecedent for later trauma. When traumatized children present with severe irritability and mood lability, there may be a tendency to associate these symptoms with the trauma. On the contrary, these longitudinal results suggest that, rather than a consequence, bipolar disorder may be an antecedent risk factor for later trauma (possibly because of the attendant reckless, disinhibited state). If confirmed, these results could help dispel the commonly held notion that mania-like symptoms in youths represent a reaction to trauma and would further suggest that children with bipolar disorder should be adequately treated and monitored closely to avoid trauma.

Although no empirical evidence is available for the treatment of comorbid bipolar disorder and posttraumatic stress disorder, corroborative evidence comes from trials of mood stabilizers in adult populations suggesting valproate to be effective in treating certain combat-related (but not non-combat-related) posttraumatic stress disorder symptoms.[156,159–162] Certain mood stabilizers have shown promise in treating specific symptoms of posttraumatic stress disorder. Several open trials report that carbamazepine may be useful for treating posttraumatic stress disorder symptoms of flashbacks, nightmares, and intrusive thoughts.[164–166] In a preliminary controlled trial, lamotrigine exhibited potential efficacy in the treatment of posttraumatic stress disorder symptoms of re-experiencing, avoidance, and numbing in adults.[201] There is a dearth of literature addressing the beneficial role of psychotherapies as treatment for comorbid bipolar disorder and posttraumatic stress disorder. To date, there has been a handful of studies that have assessed the role of psychotherapy to address those with posttraumatic stress disorder and severe mental illness (not specifically bipolar disorder).[202–204] These studies did find that therapy reduced symptoms of posttraumatic stress disorder; however, they did not specially study those with comorbid bipolar disorder.

Autism Spectrum Disorder

Recently, there has been immense interest in the overlap of bipolar disorder and autism spectrum disorder. A limited literature exists on the diagnosis and treatment of comorbid bipolar disorder and autism spectrum disorder in children and adolescents. In the absence of systematic research on comorbid bipolar disorder and autism spectrum disorder, indirect evidence suggestive of comorbid bipolar disorder in pediatric populations with autism spectrum disorder comes from high rates of aggressive behaviors documented in children with autism spectrum disorder, a high incidence of bipolar disorder in family members of children with autism spectrum disorder, and from a small literature documenting the presence of bipolar disorder comorbidity in autism spectrum disorder populations.

High rates of aggressive behaviors and severe mood disturbances are documented in children with autism spectrum disorder.[205–208] There is considerable evidence suggesting that a subset of autism spectrum disorder youth with extreme disturbance of mood suffer from a symptom cluster that is phenomenologically consistent with bipolar disorder. In a study of a group of children with Asperger's disorder who were followed into adolescence, Wing et al.[209] found that nearly one half of the children developed affective disorders. Conversely, high rates of autism spectrum disorder or autism spectrum disorder traits are reported in children and adolescents with bipolar disorder. Presence of significant autism spectrum disorder traits are reported to be as high as 62% in pediatric mood and anxiety disorder research populations.[210]

In the first study to use accepted operationalized criteria, our group assessed clinically referred children and adolescents ($n = 727$) using a comprehensive diagnostic battery including structured diagnostic interview. We reported a bidirectional overlap; bipolar disorder occurred in 21% of autism spectrum disorder youth, and autism spectrum disorder occurred in 11% of bipolar disorder youth.[211] There was striking homology in the clinical characteristics of autism spectrum disorder and bipolar disorder when clinical features were compared based on the presence or absence of reciprocal comorbidity. Bipolar disorder and autism spectrum disorder, irrespective of reciprocal comorbidity, were similar in phenotypic features, including symptom profile, pattern of comorbidity, and measures of functioning. This work suggests that bipolar disorder and autism spectrum disorder are bona fide independent disorders when they co-occur in youth.

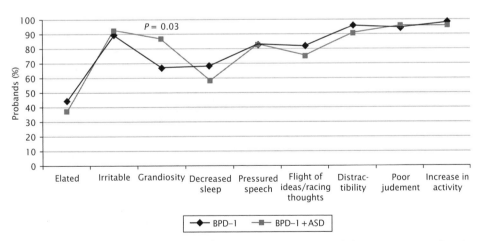

FIGURE 4.4 Presentation of mania symptomatology in youth with comorbid autism spectrum disorder (ASD) and bipolar disorder (BPD). Adapted from Joshi G et al., Examining the comorbidity of bipolar disorder and autism spectrum disorders: a large controlled analysis of phenotypic and familial correlates in a referred population of youth with bipolar I disorder with and without autism spectrum disorders. *J Clin Psychiatry.* 2013;74(6):578–86. doi: 10.4088/JCP.12m07392.

Recently we replicated our earlier findings and reported that one third of our clinically referred population of children and adolescents with autism spectrum disorder also received the diagnosis of bipolar disorder via structured diagnostic interviews.[212] Similarly, we found consistently high rates of comorbid autism spectrum disorder (15%) in our research populations of children and adolescents with bipolar disorder, irrespective of the aims for ascertainment—family genetic study or treatment trials of bipolar disorder.[213,214] In a secondary analysis of data from a family study of bipolar I disorder youth, comorbid autism spectrum disorder was present in 30.3% of bipolar I disorder probands.[215] Supporting our previous findings of similar clinical presentations irrespective of comorbidity, bipolar disorder youth with and without autism spectrum disorder demonstrated analogous profiles of mania symptomatology (see Fig. 4.4). In the presence of comorbid autism spectrum disorder, youth with bipolar disorder experience an earlier age of onset and increased severity of bipolar disorder with a poorer level of functioning.[212-215] Furthermore, autism spectrum disorder youth with a family history of bipolar disorder are more often high functioning, and their mood disturbance is characterized by a severe cycling pattern, agitation, and aggression along with neurovegetative disturbances.[216] There is an accumulating body of literature from family genetic studies suggesting a higher-than-expected incidence of bipolar disorder in first-degree relatives of about one third of the population with autism spectrum disorder.[216-218]

Treatment response to psychotropics in youth with autism spectrum disorder is noted to be less robust with higher rates of adverse effects to both medication and placebo.[57,219,220] Thus, due to an atypical response and higher susceptibility to adverse effects, it is advisable to initiate and titrate psychotropics at a lower dose and titrate upward in smaller increments in this population. Although there is substantial evidence documenting the role of pharmacotherapy for the management of extreme mood difficulties, there is minimal published literature and no systematic data on the treatment of comorbid bipolar disorder in pediatric autism spectrum disorder populations. Limited literature on the treatment of comorbid bipolar disorder in children with autism spectrum disorder suggests that first-generation antipsychotics (haloperidol, chlorpromazine, thioridazine) and traditional mood stabilizers (lithium, carbamazepine) are minimally effective for the treatment of mania.[221] On the contrary, in a recent secondary analysis of acute atypical antipsychotic monotherapy trials in bipolar disorder youth, we reported acceptable tolerability and robust antimanic response to atypical antipsychotics (risperidone, olanzapine, quetiapine, ziprasidone, or aripiprazole) in the presence of autism spectrum disorder comorbidity.[213] No difference was observed in the rate of antimanic response and tolerability with the exception that autism spectrum disorder youth were more susceptible to the adverse effect of slurred speech and teary eyes. Furthermore, compared to other atypical antipsychotics, risperidone had a superior antimanic response in bipolar disorder youth with comorbid autism spectrum disorder. However, this study is limited by the retrospective nature of post-hoc analysis and lack of direct measures of autism spectrum disorder symptomatology.

There is evidence from treatment trials of risperidone, aripiprazole, and ziprasidone that second-generation neuroleptics are well tolerated and efficacious in treating symptoms of irritability and aggression in youth with autism spectrum disorder, a spectrum of symptoms suggestive of bipolar disorder. Controlled trials of risperidone consistently report a favorable safety, tolerability, and efficacy profile for treating symptoms of irritability and aggression in youth with autism spectrum disorder.[222,223] Although risperidone is the only atypical antipsychotic that is FDA-approved for the treatment of irritability and aggression in autistic children, weight gain associated with risperidone is a significant adverse effect that often limits continuation of treatment in this population. In contrast, results from recent short-term open-label trials with newer atypical antipsychotics—aripiprazole and ziprasidone—show promise as treatment for irritability in children with autism spectrum disorder and are associated with negligible weight gain.[224,225] Contrary to the encouraging response observed with the aforementioned atypical antipsychotics, quetiapine and olanzapine—also atypical antipsychotics—are noted to be ineffective in treating symptoms of irritability and aggression in this population.[226–228]

Thus, in choosing a thymoleptic agent for the treatment of bipolar disorder in youth with comorbid autism spectrum disorder, consideration should be given to those antimanic agents that are also shown to be efficacious in treating associated and core features of autism spectrum disorder. Furthermore, due to higher susceptibility to adverse effects, it is advisable to initiate and titrate psychotropics at a lower dose in this population. As the aforementioned empirical evidence suggests, risperidone appears to be efficacious in treating both core and associated features of autism spectrum disorder and may be superior to other atypical antipsychotics as an antimanic agent in youth with autism spectrum disorder. Youth should be closely monitored for adverse effects, especially weight gain, as it remains a concern in short- and long-term therapy with risperidone. Recent research has examined the use of metformin to mitigate weight gain and abnormal glucose metabolism following treatment with second-generation antipsychotics.[229] A review of these studies found metformin treatment to significantly reduce body weight in both adults and children treated with atypical antipsychotics.[230] Only case reports have documented the use of metformin's mitigation effectiveness with weight gain secondary to antipsychotic use in the autism spectrum disorder population.[231]

Summary

The diagnosis and treatment of bipolar disorder needs to address psychiatric comorbidity given its ubiquitous nature. ADHD comorbidity is particularly associated with very early-onset bipolar disorder, whereas the risk of substance use disorder comorbidity is much higher for adolescent-onset versus child-onset bipolar disorder. Onset of pediatric bipolar disorder is generally either prior or simultaneous to the onset of substance use disorder, and severity of both disorders is worse in the comorbid state. A higher than expected prevalence of anxiety disorders is documented in individuals with bipolar disorder. In the presence of an anxiety disorder, individuals with bipolar disorder experience greater symptom severity, poorer treatment response, and poorer course and functioning. Hypersexuality in pediatric bipolar disorder is etiologically unrelated to sexual abuse and more reflective of dysregulation related to mania and puberty. Bipolar disorder may be an antecedent risk factor for later trauma and subsequent posttraumatic stress disorder and not merely represent a reaction to any trauma experienced. There is an accumulating body of literature that suggests that a subset of autism spectrum disorder youth with extreme disturbance of mood suffer from a symptom cluster that is phenomenologically consistent with the syndrome of bipolar disorder, and this is equally substantiated by family genetic studies that document a higher than expected incidence of bipolar disorder in first-degree relatives of youth with autism spectrum disorder.

In general, the presence of comorbid disorders with bipolar disorder results in a more severe clinical condition. Earlier onset bipolar disorder seems to be related to additional comorbidity and more severe episodes and cycle acceleration. Identifying and treating these co-occurring psychiatric conditions may help alleviate the severity of impairment and duration of mood episodes in bipolar disorder.

Knowledge of the impact of comorbid disorders on the therapeutic response in youth with bipolar disorder is growing rapidly. Bipolar disorder response to lithium is less robust in the presence of ADHD comorbidity. Stimulants are safe and efficacious for the treatment of comorbid ADHD once mania is stabilized in youth with bipolar disorder. Treatment of bipolar disorder with lithium or valproic acid results in attenuation of active substance use disorder. In youth with bipolar disorder, the comorbid presence of lifetime obsessive-compulsive disorder, but not generalized anxiety disorder, is associated with poor antimanic response. Response to psychotropics in autism spectrum disorder youth with mood dysregulation is noted to be less robust with higher susceptibility to adverse effects.

The scientific interface between bipolar disorder and comorbidities remains unclear. Comorbidity may represent an important genetic and clinical subtype with distinct psychopathology, familiality, and cognitive, neural, and genetic underpinnings. Future longitudinal studies addressing the impact of comorbidity on the clinical presentation, course, and response to treatment along with studies examining the cognitive correlates, genetic-candidate genes, and neurobiological overlap would assist in further clarifying the relationship of bipolar disorder with its comorbidities.

Author Disclosures

Dr. Wilens receives or has received grant support from the following sources: National Institutes of Health (National Institute on Drug Abuse) and Shire. He is or has been a consultant for Euthymics/Neurovance, and Shire. He has published *Straight Talk*

About Psychiatric Medications for Kids and coedited *ADHD in Children and Adults* and *Comprehensive Clinical Psychiatry*.

Dr. Wilens is director of the Center for Addiction Medicine at Massachusetts General Hospital. He serves as a consultant to the US National Football League (ERM Associates), US Minor/Major League Baseball, and Bay Cove Human Services (Clinical Services).

Dr. Joshi has received research support from Forest Research Laboratories, Duke University, Bristol Myers Squibb, and Glaxo Smith Kline as a principal investigator on multisite clinical trials.

Acknowledgments

This work was supported by the K24 DA016264[2] and the Pediatric Psychopharmacology Council Fund.[1] The authors thank Courtney Zulauf, BA, and Stephannie Furtak, BA, for their help with the chapter.

References

1. Campbell M, Cueva JE. Psychopharmacology in child and adolescent psychiatry: a review of the past seven years. part II. *J Am Acad Child Adolesc Psychiatry*. 1995;34(10):1262–72.
2. Tarter R. Evaluation and treatment of adolescent substance abuse: a decision tree method. *J Am Acad Child Adolesc Psychiatry*. 1990;42:1486.
3. Ambrosini PJ. Historical development and present status of the schedule for affective disorders and schizophrenia for school-age children (K-SADS). *J Am Acad Child Adolesc Psychiatry*. 2000;39(1):49–58.
4. Faraone SV, Tsuang MT. Methods in psychiatric genetics. In: Tohen M, Tsuang MT, Zahner GEP, eds. *Textbook in Psychiatric Epidemiology*. New York, NY: Wiley; 1995:81–134.
5. Faraone SV, Tsuang MT, Tsuang D. *Genetics and Mental Disorders: A Guide for Students, Clinicians, and Researchers*. New York, NY: Guilford Press; 1999.
6. Biederman J, Klein RG, Pine DS, Klein DF. Resolved: mania is mistaken for ADHD in prepubertal children. *J Am Acad Child Adolesc Psychiatry*. 1998;37(10):1091–6; discussion 1096–9.
7. American Psychiatric Association. *Diagnostic and Statistical Manual of Mental Disorders* 4th ed. Washington, DC: American Psychiatric Association; 1994.
8. Moore CM, Biederman J, Wozniak J, et al. Differences in brain chemistry in children and adolescents with attention deficit hyperactivity disorder with and without comorbid bipolar disorder: a proton magnetic resonance spectroscopy study. *Am J Psychiatry*. 2006;163(2):316–8.
9. Kowatch RA, Fristad M, Birmaher B, Wagner KD, Findling RL, Hellander M. Treatment guidelines for children and adolescents with bipolar disorder. *J Am Acad Child Adolesc Psychiatry*. 2005;44(3):213–35.
10. Wozniak J, Biederman J. A pharmacological approach to the quagmire of comorbidity in juvenile mania. *J Am Acad Child Adolesc Psychiatry*. 1996;35(6):826–28.
11. Merikangas KR, Jin R, He JP, et al. Prevalence and correlates of bipolar spectrum disorder in the world mental health survey initiative. *Arch Gen Psychiatry*. 2011;68(3):241–51.
12. Geller B, Sun K, Zimmerman B, Luby J, Frazier J, Williams M. Complex and rapid-cycling in bipolar children and adolescents: a preliminary study. *J Affect Disord*. 1995;34:259–68.
13. West S, McElroy S, Strakowski S, Keck P, McConville B. Attention deficit hyperactivity disorder in adolescent mania. *Am J Psychiatry*. 1995;152(2):271–73.
14. Geller D, Biederman J, Jones J, et al. Is juvenile obsessive-compulsive disorder a developmental subtype of the disorder? A review of the pediatric literature. *J Am Acad Child Adolesc Psychiatry*. 1998;37(4):420–7.

15. Faraone SV, Biederman J, Mennin D, Wozniak J, Spencer T. Attention-deficit hyperactivity disorder with bipolar disorder: a familial subtype? *J Am Acad Child Adolesc Psychiatry.* 1997;36(10):1378–7; discussion 1387–90.

16. Axelson D, Birmaher B, Strober M, et al. Phenomenology of children and adolescents with bipolar spectrum disorders. *Arch Gen Psychiatry.* 2006;63(10):1139–48.

17. Wilens TE, Biederman J, Adamson JJ, et al. Further evidence of an association between adolescent bipolar disorder with smoking and substance use disorders: a controlled study. *Drug Alcohol Depend.* 2008;95(3):188–98.

18. Biederman J, Faraone S, Kiely K. Comorbidity in outcome of attention-deficit hyperactivity disorder. In: Hechtman L, ed. *Do They Grow Out of It? Long Term Outcome of Childhood Disorders.* Washington, DC: American Psychiatric Press; 1996:39–76.

19. Sachs GS, Baldassano CF, Truman CJ, Guille C. Comorbidity of attention deficit hyperactivity disorder with early- and late-onset bipolar disorder. *Am J Psychiatry.* 2000;157(3):466–68.

20. Chang KD, Steiner H, Ketter TA. Psychiatric phenomenology of child and adolescent bipolar offspring. *J Am Acad Child Adolesc Psychiatry.* 2000;39(4):453–60.

21. Perlis RH, Miyahara S, Marangell LB, et al. Long-term implications of early onset in bipolar disorder: data from the first 1000 participants in the systematic treatment enhancement program for bipolar disorder (STEP-BD). *Biol Psychiatry.* 2004;55(9):875–881.

22. Faraone SV, Biederman J, Wozniak J, Mundy E, Mennin D, O'Donnell D. Is comorbidity with ADHD a marker for juvenile onset mania? *J Am Acad Child Adolesc Psychiatry.* 1997;36(8):1046–55.

23. Biederman J, Petty C, Faraone SV, et al. Moderating effects of major depression on patterns of comorbidity in referred adults with panic disorder: a controlled study. *Psychiatry Res.* 2004;126(2):143–9.

24. Kessler RC, Adler L, Barkley R, et al. The prevalence and correlates of adult ADHD in the United States: results from the National Comorbidity Survey Replication. *Am J Psychiatry.* 2006;163(4):716–23.

25. Nierenberg AA, Miyahara S, Spencer T, et al. Clinical and diagnostic implications of lifetime attention-deficit/hyperactivity disorder comorbidity in adults with bipolar disorder: data from the first 1000 STEP-BD participants. *Biol Psychiatry.* 2005;57(11):1467–73.

26. Winokur G, Coryell W, Keller M, Endicott J, Akiskal H. A prospective follow-up of patients with bipolar and primary unipolar affective disorder. *Arch Gen Psychiatry.* 1993;50(6):457–66.

27. Wozniak J, Biederman J, Kiely K, et al. Mania-like symptoms suggestive of childhood onset bipolar disorder in clinically referred children. *J Am Acad Child Adolesc Psychiatry.* 1995;34(7):867–6.

28. Biederman J, Mick E, Bostic J, et al. The naturalistic course of pharmacologic treatment of children with manic-like symptoms: a systematic chart review. *J Clin Psychiatry.* 1998;59(11):628–37; quiz 638.

29. Geller B, Williams M, Zimerman B, Frazier J, Beringer L, Warner K. Prepubertal and early adolescent bipolarity differentiate from ADHD by manic symptoms, grandiose delusions, ultra-rapid or ultradian cycling. *J Affect Disord.* 1998;51:81–91.

30. Biederman J, Faraone S, Mick E, et al. Attention-deficit hyperactivity disorder and juvenile mania: an overlooked comorbidity? *J Am Acad Child Adolesc Psychiatry.* 1996;35(8):997–1008.

31. Faraone SV, Biederman J, Mennin D, Russell RL. Bipolar and antisocial disorders among relatives of ADHD children: parsing familial subtypes of illness. *Am J Med Genet.* 1998;81(1):108–116.

32. Wilens T, Biederman J, Forkner P, et al. Patterns of comorbidity and dysfunction in clinically referred preschoolers with bipolar disorder. *J Child Adolesc Psychopharmacol.* 2003;13(4):495–505.

33. Faraone S, Glatt S, Tsuang M. The genetics of pediatric onset bipolar disorder. *Biol Psychiatry.* 2003;53(11):970–77.

34. Strober M, DeAntonio M, Schmidt-Lackner S, Freeman R, Lampert C, Diamond J. Early childhood attention deficit hyperactivity disorder predicts poorer response to acute lithium therapy in adolescent mania. *J Affect Disord.* 1998;51:145–51.

35. State RC, Frye MA, Altshuler LL, et al. Chart review of the impact of attention-deficit/hyperactivity disorder comorbidity on response to lithium or divalproex sodium in adolescent mania. *J Clin Psychiatry.* 2004;65(8):1057–63.

36. Biederman J, Faraone SV, Chu MP, Wozniak J. Further evidence of a bidirectional overlap between juvenile mania and conduct disorder in children. *J Am Acad Child Adolesc Psychiatry.* 1999;38(4):468–76.

37. Scheffer RE, Kowatch RA, Carmody T, Rush AJ. Randomized, placebo-controlled trial of mixed amphetamine salts for symptoms of comorbid ADHD in pediatric bipolar disorder after mood stabilization with divalproex sodium. *Am J Psychiatry*. 2005;162(1):58–64.

38. Findling RL, Short EJ, McNamara NK, et al. Methylphenidate in the treatment of children and adolescents with bipolar disorder and attention-deficit/hyperactivity disorder. *J Am Acad Child Adoles Psychiatry*. 2007;46(11):1445–53.

39. Zeni CP, Tramontina S, Ketzer CR, Pheula GF, Rohde LA. Methylphenidate combined with aripiprazole in children and adolescents with bipolar disorder and attention-deficit/hyperactivity disorder: a randomized crossover trial. *J Child Adolesc Psychopharmacol*. 2009;19(5):553–61.

40. Wilens T, Prince J, Spencer T, et al. An open trial of bupropion for the treatment of adults with attention deficit hyperactivity disorder and bipolar disorder. *Biol Psychiatry*. 2003;54(1):9–16.

41. Chang K, Nayar D, Howe M, Rana M. Atomoxetine as an adjunt therapy in the treatment of co-morbid attention-deficit/hyperactivity disorder in children and adolescents with bipolar I or II disorder. *J Child Adolesc Psychopharacol*. 2009;19(5):547–51.

42. Weiss M, Panagiotopoulos C, Giles L, et al. A naturalistic study of predictors and risks of atypical antipsychotic use in an attention-deficit/hyperactivity disorder clinic. *J Child Adolesc Psychopharmacol*. 2009;19(5):575–82.

43. Penzner JB, Dudas M, Saito E, et al. Lack of effect of stimulant combination with second-generation antipsychotics on weight gain, metabolic changes, prolactin levels, and sedation in youth with clinically relevant aggression or oppositionality. *J Child Adolesc Psychopharmacol*. 2009;19(5):563–73.

44. Findling RL, Gracious BL, McNamara NK, et al. Rapid, continuous cycling and psychiatric co-morbidity in pediatric bipolar I disorder. *Bipolar Disord*. 2001;3(4):202–10.

45. Geller B, Zimerman B, Williams M, et al. Diagnostic characteristics of 93 cases of a prepubertal and early adolescent bipolar disorder phenotype by gender, puberty and comorbid attention deficit hyperactivity disorder. *J Child Adolesc Psychopharmacol*. 2000;10(3):157–64.

46. Birmaher B, Axelson D, Strober M, et al. Comparison of manic and depressive symptoms between children and adolescents with bipolar spectrum disorders. *Bipolar Disord*. 2009;11(1):52–62.

47. Greene RW, Doyle AE. Toward a transactional conceptualization of oppositional defiand disorder: implications for assessment and treatment. *Clin Child Fam Psychol Rev*. 1999;2(3):129–48.

48. Wozniak J, Petty CR, Schreck M, Moses A, Faraone SV, Biederman J. High level of persistence of pediatric bipolar-I disorder from childhood onto adolescent years: a four year prospective longitudinal follow-up study. *J Psychiatr Res*. 2011;45(10):1273–82.

49. Biederman J, Faraone SV, Milberger S, et al. Is childhood oppositional defiant disorder a precursor to adolescent conduct disorder? Findings from a four-year follow-up study of children with ADHD. *J Am Acad Child Adolesc Psychiatry*. 1996;35(9):1193–204.

50. Farley SE, Adams JS, Lutton ME, Scoville C, Fulkerson RC, Webb AR. Clinical inquiries. What are effective treatments for oppositional and defiant behaviors in preadolescents? *J Fam Pract*. 2005;54(2):162, 164–5.

51. Aman MG, De Smedt G, Derivan A, Lyons B, Findling RL. Double-blind, placebo-controlled study of risperidone for the treatment of disruptive behaviors in children with subaverage intelligence. *Am J Psychiatry*. 2002;159(8):1337–46.

52. Findling RL, Aman MG, Eerdekens M, Derivan A, Lyons B. Long-term, open-label study of risperidone in children with severe disruptive behaviors and below-average IQ. *Am J Psychiatry*. 2004;161(4):677–84.

53. Croonenberghs J, Fegert JM, Findling RL, De Smedt G, Van Dongen S. Risperidone in children with disruptive behavior disorders and subaverage intelligence: a 1-year, open-label study of 504 patients. *J Am Acad Child Adolesc Psychiatry*. 2005;44(1):64–72.

54. Turgay A, Binder C, Snyder R, Fisman S. Long-term safety and efficacy of risperidone for the treatment of disruptive behavior disorders in children with subaverage IQs. *Pediatrics*. 2002;110(3):e34.

55. Snyder SH. Forty years of neurotransmitters: a personal account. *Arch Gen Psychiatry*. 2002;59(11):983–94.

56. Reyes M, Olah R, Csaba K, Augustyns I, Eerdekens M. Long-term safety and efficacy of risperidone in children with disruptive behaviour disorders. Results of a 2-year extension study. *Eur Child Adolesc Psychiatry*. 2006;15(2):97–104.

57. Aman MG, Arnold MDL, McDougle CJ, et al. Acute and long-term safety and tolerability of risperidone in children with autism. *J Child Adolesc Psychopharmacol*. 2005;15(6):869–84.

58. Reyes M, Buitelaar J, Toren P, Augustyns I, Eerdekens M. A randomized, double-blind, placebo-controlled study of risperidone maintenance treatment in children and adolescents with disruptive behavior disorders. *Am J Psychiatry*. 2006;163(3):402–10.

59. Haas M, Karcher K, Pandina GJ. Treating disruptive behavior disorders with risperidone: a 1-year, open-label safety study in children and adolescents. *J Child Adolesc Psychopharmacol*. 2008;18(4):337–45.

60. Biederman J, Mick E, Faraone SV, Wozniak J, Spencer T, Pandina G. Risperidone in the treatment of affective symptoms: a secondary analysis of a randomized clinical trial in children with disruptive behavior disorder. *Clinical therapeutics*. 2006;28(5):794–800.

61. Kronenberger WG, Giauque AL, Lafata DE, Bohnstedt BN, Maxey LE, Dunn DW. Quetiapine addition in methylphenidate treatment-resistant adolescents with comorbid ADHD, conduct/oppositional-defiant disorder, and aggression: a prospective, open-label study. *J Child Adolesc Psychopharmacol*. 2007;17(3):334–47.

62. Donovan S, Susser E, Nunes E, Stewart J, Quitkin F, Klein D. Divalproex treatment of disruptive adolescents: a report of 1 cases. *J Clin Psychiatry*. 1997;58(1):12–5.

63. Donovan SJ, Stewart JW, Nunes EV, et al. Divalproex treatment for youth with explosive temper and mood lability: a double-blind, placebo-controlled crossover design. *Am J Psychiatry*. 2000;157(5):818–20.

64. Geller B, Luby J. Child and adolescent bipolar disorder: a review of the past 10 years. *J Am Acad Child Adolesc Psychiatry*. 1997;36(Sept.):1168–76.

65. Angold A, Costello EJ. Depressive comorbidity in children and adolescents: empirical, theoretical and methodological issues. *Am J Psychiatry*. 1993;150(12):1779–91.

66. Geller B, Fox L, Clark K. Rate and predictors of prepubertal bipolarity during follow-up of 6-to 12-year-old depressed children. *J Am Acad Child Adolesc Psychiatry*. 1994;33(4):461–468.

67. Strober M, Carlson G. Bipolar illness in adolescents with major depression: clinical, genetic, and psychopharmacologic predictors in a three- to four-year prospective follow-up investigation. *Arch Gen Psychiatry*. 1982;39:549–5.

68. Davis RE. Manic-depressive variant syndrome of childhood: a preliminary report. *Am J Psychiatry*. 1979;136(5):702–6.

69. Carlson GA. Classification issues of bipolar disorders in childhood. *Psychiatric Developments*. 1984;2(4):273–85.

70. McGlashan T. Adolescent versus adult onset of mania. *Am J Psychiatry*. 1988;145(2):221–3.

71. Kovacs M, Pollock M. Bipolar disorder and comorbid conduct disorder in childhood and adolescence. *J Am Acad Child Adolesc Psychiatry*. 1995;34(6):715–23.

72. Kutcher SP, Marton P, Korenblum M. Relationship between psychiatric illness and conduct disorder in adolescents. *Can J Psychiatry*. 1989;34(6):526–29.

73. Moore JM Jr., Thompson-Pope SK, Whited RM. MMPI-A profiles of adolescent boys with a history of firesetting. *J Pers Assess*. 1996;67(1):116–26.

74. Masi G, Milone A, Manfredi A, Pari C, Paziente A, Millepiedi S. Comorbidity of conduct disorder and bipolar disorder in clinically referred children and adolescents. *J Child Adolesc Psychopharmacol*. 2008;18(3):271–9.

75. Lewinsohn P, Klein D, Seeley J. Bipolar disorders in a community sample of older adolescents: prevalence, phenomenology, comorbidity, and course. *J Am Acad Child Adolesc Psychiatry*. 1995;34(4):454–63.

76. Robins L, Price R. Adult disorders predicted by childhood conduct problems: results from the NIMH epidemiologic catchment area project. *Psychiatry*. 1991;54(2):116–32.

77. Boyd JH, Burke JD, Gruenberg E, et al. Exclusion criteria of DSM-III: a study of co-occurrence of hierarchy-free syndromes. *Arch Gen Psychiatry*. 1984;41:983–989.

78. Carlson GA, Kelly KL. Manic symptoms in psychiatrically hospitalized children—what do they mean? *J Affect Disord*. 1998;51(2):123–35.

79. Wilens T, Biederman J, Millstein R, Wozniak J, Hahsey A, Spencer T. Risk for substance use disorders in youths with child- and adolescent-onset bipolar disorder. *J Am Acad Child Adolesc Psychiatry*. 1999;38(6):680–85.

80. Isaac G. Misdiagnosed bipolar disorder in adolescents in a special educational school and treatment program. *J Clin Psychiatry*. 1992;53(4):133–6.

81. Biederman J, Faraone S, Hatch M, Mennin D, Taylor A, George P. Conduct disorder with and without mania in a referred sample of ADHD children. *J Affect Disord*. 1997;44(2–3):177–88.

82. Biederman J, Faraone SV, Wozniak J, Monuteaux MC. Parsing the association between bipolar, conduct, and substance use disorders: a familial risk analysis. *Biol Psychiatry*. 2000;48(11):1037–44.

83. Wozniak J, Biederman J, Faraone SV, Blier H, Monuteaux MC. Heterogeneity of childhood conduct disorder: further evidence of a subtype of conduct disorder linked to bipolar disorder. *J Affect Disord*. 2001;64(2–3):121–31.

84. Faraone SV, Biederman J, Monuteaux MC. Attention deficit hyperactivity disorder with bipolar disorder in girls: further evidence for a familial subtype? *J Affect Disord*. 2001;64(1):19–26.

85. Joshi G, Biederman J, Wozniak J, et al. Response to second generation antipsychotics in youth with comorbid bipolar disorder and autism spectrum disorder. *CNS Neurosci Ther*. 2012;18(1):28–33.

86. Biederman J, Mick E, Hammerness P, et al. Open-label, 8-week trial of olanzapine and risperidone for the treatment of bipolar disorder in preschool-aged children. *Biol Psychiatry*. 2005;58(7):589–94.

87. Sheard MH. Lithium in the treatment of aggression. *J Nerv Mental Dis*. 1975;160(2–1):108–18.

88. Campbell M, Anderson LT, Green WH. Behavior-disordered and aggressive children: new advances in pharmacotherapy. *J Dev Behav Pediatrics*. 1983;4(4):265–71.

89. Greenhill LL, Solomon M, Pleak R, Ambrosini P. Molindone hydrochloride treatment of hospitalized children with conduct disorder. *J Clin Psychiatry*. 1985;46(8):20–25.

90. Campbell M, Small AM, Green WH, et al. Behavioral efficacy of haloperidol and lithium carbonate: a comparison in hospitalized aggressive children with conduct disorder. *Arch Gen Psychiatry*. 1984;41(7):650–56.

91. Findling RL, Reed MD, O'Riordan MA, Demeter CA, Stansbrey RJ, McNamara NK. Effectiveness, safety, and pharmacokinetics of quetiapine in aggressive children with conduct disorder. *J Am Acad Child Adolesc Psychiatry*. 2006;45(7):792–800.

92. Connor DF, McLaughlin TJ, Jeffers-Terry M. Randomized controlled pilot study of quetiapine in the treatment of adolescent conduct disorder. *J Child Adolesc Psychopharmacol*. 2008;18(2):140–56.

93. Masi G, Milone A, Canepa G, Millepiedi S, Mucci M, Muratori F. Olanzapine treatment in adolescents with severe conduct disorder. *Eur Psychiatry*. 2006;21(1):51–7.

94. Pavuluri MN, Graczyk PA, Henry DB, Carbray JA, Heidenreich J, Miklowitz DJ. Child- and family-focused cognitive-behavioral therapy for pediatric bipolar disorder: development and preliminary results. *J Am Acad Child Adolesc Psychiatry*. 2004;43(5):528–37.

95. McElroy SL, Strakowski SM, Keck PE, Tugrul KL, West SA, Lonczak HS. Differences and similarities in mixed and pure mania. *Compr Psychiatry*. 1995;36(3):187–94.

96. Winokur G, Coryell W, Akiskal HS, et al. Alcoholism in manic-depressive (bipolar) illness: familial ilness, course of illness, and the primary-secondary distinction. *Am J Psychiatry*. 1995;152:365–72.

97. Goldstein BI, Strober MA, Birmaher B, et al. Substance use disorders among adolescents with bipolar spectrum disorders. *Bipolar Disord*. 2008;10(4):469–78.

98. Strakowski SM, DelBello MP, Fleck DE, et al. Effects of co-occurring cannabis use disorders on the course of bipolar disorder after a first hospitalization for mania. *Arch Gen Psychiatry*. 2007;64(1):57–64.

99. Kozloff N, Cheung AH, Schaffer A, et al. Bipolar disorder among adolescents and young adults: results from an epidemiological sample. *J Affect Disord*. 2010;125(1–3):350–4.

100. McElroy SL, Altshuler LL, Suppes T, et al. Axis I psychiatric comorbidity and Its relationship to historical illness variables in 288 patients with bipolar disorder. *Am J Psychiatry*. 2001;158(3):420–6.

101. Strakowski SM, DelBello MP, Fleck DE, et al. Effects of co-occurring alcohol abuse on the course of bipolar disorder following a first hospitalization for mania. *Arch Gen Psychiatry*. 2005;62(8):851–8.

102. West SA, Strakowski SM, Sax KW, McElroy SL, Keck PE, McConville BJ. Phenomenology and comorbidity of adolescents hospitalized for the treatment of acute mania. *Biol Psychiatry*. 1996;39:458–60.

103. Wilens T, Biederman J, Abrantes AM, Spencer TJ. Clinical characteristics of psychiatrically referred adolescent outpatients with substance use disorder. *J Am Acad Child Adolesc Psychiatry*. 1997;36(7):941–7.

104. Strober M, Schmidt-Lackner S, Freeman R, Bower S, Lampert C, DeAntonio M. Recovery and relapse in adolescents with bipolar affective illness: a five-year naturalistic, prospective follow-up. *J Am Acad Child Adolesc Psychiatry*. 1995;34(6):724–31.

105. Biederman J, Wilens T, Mick E, et al. Is ADHD a risk factor for psychoactive substance use disorders? Findings from a four-year prospective follow-up study. *J Am Acad Child Adolesc Psychiatry*. 1997;36(1):21–9.

106. Wilens TE, Biederman J, Milberger S, et al. Is bipolar disorder a risk for cigarette smoking in ADHD youth? *Am J Addict*. 2000;9(3):187–95.

107. Wilens T. Development of substance use disorders in adolescents with bipolar disorder: a 5 year follow-up study. Paper presented at: American Academy of Child and Adolescent Psychiatry; October 23–28, 2012; San Francisco, CA.

108. Geller B, Tillman R, Bolhofner K, Zimerman B. Child bipolar I disorder: prospective continuity with adult bipolar I disorder; characteristics of second and third episodes; predictors of 8-year outcome. *Arch Gen Psychiatry*. 2008;65(10):1125–33.

109. Delbello MP, Hanseman D, Adler CM, Fleck DE, Strakowski SM. Twelve-month outcome of adolescents with bipolar disorder following first hospitalization for a manic or mixed episode. *Am J Psychiatry*. 2007;164(4):582–90.

110. Lewinsohn PM, Klein DN, Seeley JR. Bipolar disorder during adolescence and young adulthood in a community sample. *Bipolar Disorders*. 2000;2:281–93.

111. Wilens TE, Martelon M, Kruesi MJ, et al. Does conduct disorder mediate the development of substance use disorders in adolescents with bipolar disorder? A case-control family study. *J Clin Psychiatry*. 2009;70(2):259–65.

112. Wilens T, Biederman J, Adamson JJ, et al. Association of bipolar and substance use disorders in parents of adolescents with bipolar disorder. *Biol Psychiatry*. 2007;62(2):129–34.

113. Khantzian EJ. Reflections on treating addictive disorders: a psychodynamic perspective. *Am J Addict*. 2012;21(3):274–9; discussion 279.

114. Cheetham A, Allen NB, Yucel M, Lubman DI. The role of affective dysregulation in drug addiction. *Clin Psychol Rev*. 2010;30(6):621–34.

115. Lorberg B, Martelon M, Parcell T, Wilens T. Self medication in BPD adolescents. Paper presented at: American Academy of Child and Adolescent Psychiatry; October 28–November 3, 2008; Chicago, IL.

116. Wilens TE, Martelon M, Anderson JP, Shelley-Abrahamson R, Biederman J. Difficulties in emotional regulation and substance use disorders: A controlled family study of bipolar adolescents. *Drug Alcohol Depend*. 2013;132(1–2):114–21.

117. Comings DE, Comings BG, Muhleman D, et al. The dopamine D2 receptor locus as a modifying gene in neuropsychiatric disorders. *JAMA*. 1991;266(13):1793–800.

118. Ebstein RP, Novick O, Umansky R, et al. Dopamine D4 receptor (D4DR) exon III polymorphism associated with the human personality trait of novelty seeking. *Nat Genet*. 1996;12:78–80.

119. Mick E, Kim JW, Biederman J, et al. Family based association study of pediatric bipolar disorder and the dopamine transporter gene (SLC6A3). *Am J Med Genet B Neuropsychiatr Genet*. 2008;147B(7):1182–5.

120. Wilens T, Yule A, Martelon M, Zulauf C, Faraone SV. Parental history of substance use disorders (SUD) and SUD in offspring: a controlled family study of bipolar disorder. *Am J Addict*. 2014. doi: 10.1111/j.1521-0391.2014.12125.x.

121. Geller B, Cooper T, Sun K, et al. Double-blind and placebo-controlled study of lithium for adolescent bipolar disorders with secondary substance dependency. *J Am Acad Child Adolesc Psychiatry*. 1998;37(2):171–8.

122. DelBello MP, Kowatch RA, Warner J, et al. Adjunctive topiramate treatment for pediatric bipolar disorder: a retrospective chart review. *J Child Adolesc Psychopharmacol*. 2002;12(4):323–30.

123. Harpold T, Biederman J, Kwon A, Gilbert J, Wood J, Smith L. Examining the association between pediatric bipolar disorder and anxiety disorders in psychiatrically-referred children and adolescents.

Paper presented at: 158th Annual Meeting of the American Psyciatric Association; May 21–26, 2005; Atlanta, GA.

124. American Psychiatric Association. *Diagnostic and Statistical Manual of Mental Disorders*. 5th ed. Washington, DC: American Psychiatric Publishing; 2013.

125. Johnson JG, Cohen P, Brook JS. Associations between bipolar disorder and other psychiatric disorders during adolescence and early adulthood: a community-based longitudinal investigation. *Am J Psychiatry*. 2000;157(10):1679–81.

126. Masi G, Toni C, Perugi G, Mucci M, Millepiedi S, Akiskal HS. Anxiety disorders in children and adolescents with bipolar disorder: a neglected comorbidity. *Can J Psychiatry*. 2001;46(9):797–802.

127. Tillman R, Geller B, Bolhofner K, Craney JL, Williams M, Zimerman B. Ages of onset and rates of syndromal and subsyndromal comorbid DSM-IV diagnoses in a prepubertal and early adolescent bipolar disorder phenotype. *J Am Acad Child Adolesc Psychiatry*. 2003;42(12):1486–93.

128. Wozniak J, Biederman J, Monuteaux MC, Richards J, Faraone SV. Parsing the comorbidity between bipolar disorder and anxiety disorders: a familial risk analysis. *J Child Adolesc Psychopharmacol*. 2002;12(2):101–11.

129. Biederman J, Faraone SV, Marrs A, et al. Panic disorder and agoraphobia in consecutively referred children and adolescents. *J Am Acad Child Adolesc Psychiatry*. 1997;36(2):214–23.

130. Feske U, Frank E, Mallinger AG, et al. Anxiety as a correlate of response to the acute treatment of bipolar I disorder. *Am J Psychiatry*. 2000;157(6):956–62.

131. Perugi G. Depressive comorbidity of panic, social phobic, and obsessive compulsive disorders re-examined: is there a bipolarII connection? *J Psychiatric Res*. 1999;33:53–61.

132. Masi G, Perugi G, Toni C, et al. Obsessive-compulsive bipolar comorbidity: focus on children and adolescents. *J Affect Disord*. 2004;78:175–83.

133. Dickstein DP, Rich BA, Binstock AB, et al. Comorbid anxiety in phenotypes of pediatric bipolar disorder. *J Child Adolesc Psychopharmacol*. 2005;15(4):534–48.

134. Birmaher B, Kennah A, Brent D, Ehmann M, Bridge J, Axelson D. Is bipolar disorder specifically associated with panic disorder in youths? *J Clin Psychiatry*. 2002;63(5):414–9.

135. Chen Y, Dilsaver S. Comorbidity of panic disorder in bipolar illness: evidence from the epidemiologic catchment area survey. *Am J Psychiatry*. 1995;152(2):280–3.

136. Goodwin RD, Hoven CW. Bipolar-panic comorbidity in the general population: prevalence and associated morbidity. *J Affect Disord*. 2002;70(1):27–33.

137. Kessler RC, Stang PE, Wittchen HV, Ustun TB, Roy-Burne PP, Walters EE. Lifetime panic-depression comorbidity in the National Comorbidity Survey. *Arch Gen Psychiatry*. 1998;55:801–8.

138. Bowen R, South M, Hawkes J. Mood swings in patients with panic disorder. *Can J Psychiatry*. 1994; 39(2):91–4.

139. MacKinnon D, Xu J, McMahon F, et al. Bipolar disorder and panic disorder in families: an analysis of chromosome 18 data. *Am J Psychiatry*. 1998;155(6):829–31.

140. MacKinnon DF, Zandi PP, Cooper J, et al. Comorbid bipolar disorder and panic disorder in families with a high prevalence of bipolar disorder. *Am J Psychiatry*. 2002;159(1):30–5.

141. Savino M, Perugi G, Simonini E, Soriani A, Cassano G, Akiskal H. Affective comorbidity in panic disorder: is there a bipolar connection? *J Affect Disord*. 1993;28(3):155–63.

142. Sala R, Axelson DA, Castro-Fornieles J, et al. Comorbid anxiety in children and adolescents with bipolar spectrum disorders: prevalence and clinical correlates. *J Clin Psychiatry*. 2010;71(10):1344–50.

143. Simon NM, Smoller JW, Fava M, et al. Comparing anxiety disorders and anxiety-related traits in bipolar disorder and unipolar depression. *J Psychiatr Res*. 2003;37(3):187–92.

144. Freeman MP. The comorbidity of bipolar and anxiety disorders: prevalence, psychobiology, and treatment issues. *J Affect Disord*. 2002;68:1–23.

145. Cassano GB, Pini S, Saettoni M, Dell'Osso L. Multiple anxiety disorder comorbidity in patients with mood spectrum disorders with psychotic features. *Am J Psychiatry*. 1999;156(3):474–6.

146. Young L, Cooke R, Robb J, Levitt A, Joffe R. Anxious and non-anxious bipolar disorder. *J Affect Disord*. 1993;29(1):49–52.

147. Gaudiano BA, Miller IW. Anxiety disorder comobidity in bipolar I disorder: relationship to depression severity and treatment outcome. *Depress Anxiety*. 2005;21(2):71–7.

148. Otto MW, Simon NM, Wisniewski SR, et al. Prospective 12-month course of bipolar disorder in out-patients with and without comorbid anxiety disorders. *Br J Psychiatry.* 2006;189:20–5.

149. Olvera RL, Hunter K, Fonseca M, et al. Juvenile onset bipolar disorder and comorbid anxiety. Paper presented at: The 52nd Annual Meeting of American Academy of Child and Adolescent Psychiatry; October 18–23, 2005; Toronto, Ontario, Canada.

150. Ratheesh A, Srinath S, Reddy YC, et al. Are anxiety disorders associated with a more severe form of bipolar disorder in adolescents? *Ind J Psychiatry.* 2011;53(4):312–8.

151. Dineen Wagner K. Bipolar disorder and comorbid anxiety disorders in children and adolescents. *J Clin Psychiatry.* 2006;67(Suppl.)1:16–20.

152. Sasson Y, Chopra M, Harrari E, Amitai K, Zohar J. Bipolar comorbidity: from diagnostic dilemmas to therapeutic challenge. *Int J Neuropsychopharmacol.* 2003;6(2):139–44.

153. Ghaemi SN, Hsu DJ, Soldani F, Goodwin FK. Antidepressants in bipolar disorder: the case for caution. *Bipolar Disord.* 2003;5(6):421–33.

154. Provencher MD, Guimond AJ, Hawke LD. Comorbid anxiety in bipolar spectrum disorders: a neglected research and treatment issue? *J Affect Disord.* 2012;137(1–3):161–4.

155. Calabrese J, Delucchi G. Spectrum of efficacy of valproate in 55 patients with rapid-cycling bipolar disorder. *Am J Psychiatry.* 1990;147(4):431–4.

156. Baetz M, Bowen RC. Efficacy of divalproex sodium in patients with panic disorder and mood instability who have not responded to conventional therapy. *Can J Psychiatry.* 1998;43(1):73–7.

157. McElroy SL, Keck PE, Jr., Lawrence JM. Treatment of panic disorder and benzodiazepine withdrawal with valproate. *J Neuropsychiatry Clin Neurosci.* 1991;3(2):232–3.

158. Lum M, Fontaine R, Elie R, Ontiveros A. Divalproex sodium's anti-panic effect in panic disorder: a placebo-controlled study. *Biol Psychiatry.* 1990;27:164A–5A.

159. Fesler FA. Valproate in combat-related posttraumatic stress disorder. *J Clin Psychiatry.* 1991;52(9):361–4.

160. Clark RD, Canive JM, Calais LA, Qualls CR, Tuason VB. Divalproex in posttraumatic stress disorder: an open-label clinical trial. *J Traumatic Stress.* 1999;12(2):395–401.

161. Petty F, Davis LL, Nugent AL, et al. Valproate therapy for chronic, combat-induced posttraumatic stress disorder. *J Clin Psychopharmacol.* 2002;22(1):100–1.

162. Otte C, Wiedemann K, Yassouridis A, Kellner M. Valproate monotherapy in the treatment of civilian patients with non-combat-related posttraumatic stress disorder: an open-label study. *J Clin Psychopharmacol.* 2004;24(1):106–8.

163. Tondo L, Burrai C, Scamonatti L, et al. Carbamazepine in panic disorder. *Am J Psychiatry.* 1989;146(4):558–9.

164. Wolf ME, Alavi A, Mosnaim AD. Posttraumatic stress disorder in Vietnam veterans clinical and EEG findings; possible therapeutic effects of carbamazepine. *Biol Psychiatry.* 1988;23(6):642–4.

165. Looff D, Grimley P, Kuller F, Martin A, Shonfield L. Carbamazepine for PTSD. *J Am Acad Child Adolesc Psychiatry.* 1995;34(6):703–4.

166. Stewart JT, Bartucci RJ. Posttraumatic stress disorder and partial complex seizures. *Am J Psychiatry.* 1986;143(1):113–4.

167. Joffe RT, Swinson RP. Carbamazepine in obsessive-compulsive disorder. *Biol Psychiatry.* 1987;22(9):1169–71.

168. Provencher MD, Hawke LD, Thienot E. Psychotherapies for comorbid anxiety in bipolar spectrum disorders. *J Affect Disord.* 2011;133(3):371–80.

169. Morel BA. *Traite de Maladies Metales.* Paris, France: Libairie Victor Masson; 1860.

170. Goodwin F, Jamison K. *Manic-Depressive Illness.* New York, NY: Oxford University Press; 1990.

171. Rasmussen S, Eisen J. The epidemiology and differential diagnosis of obsessive compulsive disorder. *J Clin Psychiatry.* 1992;53(April Suppl.):4–10.

172. Perugi G, Akiskal HS, Pfanner C, et al. The clinical impact of bipolar and unipolar affective comorbidity on obsessive-compulsive disorder. *J Affect Disord.* 1997;46(1):15–23.

173. Perugi G, Toni C, Frare F, Travierso MC, Hantouche E, Akiskal HS. Obsessive-compulsive-bipolar comorbidity: a systematic exploration of clinical features and treatment outcome. *J Clin Psychiatry.* 2002;63(12):1129–34.

174. Centorrino F, Hennen J, Mallya G, Egli S, Clark T, Baldessarini RJ. Clinical outcome in patients with bipolar I disorder, obsessive compulsive disorder or both. *Hum Psychopharmacol.* 2006;21(3):189–93.

175. Hantouche EG, Demonfaucon C, Angst J, Perugi G, Allilaire JF, Akiskal HS. [Cyclothymic obsessive-compulsive disorder. Clinical characteristics of a neglected and under-recognized entity]. *Presse Med.* 2002;31(14):644–8.

176. Kochman FJ, Hantouche EG, Millet B, et al. Trouble obsessionnel compulsif et bipolarite attenuee chez l'enfant et l'adolescent: re sultants de l'enquete "ABC-TOC." *Neuropsychiatr Enface Adolesc.* 2002;50:1–7.

177. Masi G, Perugi G, Millepiedi S, et al. Bipolar co-morbidity in pediatric obsessive-compulsive disorder: clinical and treatment implications. *J Child Adolesc Psychopharmacol.* 2007;17(4):475–86.

178. Diler RS, Avci A. SSRI-induced mania in obsessive-compulsive disorder. *J Am Acad Child Adolesc Psychiatry.* 1999;38(1):6–7.

179. King RA, Riddle MA, Chappel PB, et al. Case study: emergence of self-destructive phenomena in children and adolescents during fluoxetine treatment. *J Am Acad Child Adolesc Psychiatry.* 1991;30(2):179–86.

180. Joshi G, Wozniak J, Geller D, Petty C, Vivas F, Biederman J. Clinical characteristics of comorbid obsessive-compulsive disorder and bipolar disorder in children and adolescents. Paper presented at: The 52nd Annual Meeting of American Academy of Child and Adolescent Psychiatry; October 18–23, 2005; Toronto, Ontario, Canada.

181. Coryell W. Obsessive-compulsive disorder and primary unipolar depression. Comparisons of background, family history, course, and mortality. *J Nervous Mental Dis.* 1981;169(4):220–4.

182. Klein D, Depue R, Slater J. Cyclothymia in the adolescent offspring of parents with bipolar affective disorder. *J Abnorm Psychol.* 1985;94(2):115–27.

183. Joshi G, Mick E, Wozniak J, et al. Impact of obsessive-compulsive disorder on the antimanic response to olanzapine therapy in youth with bipolar disorder. *Bipolar Disord.* Mar 2010;12(2):196–204.

184. Masi G, Millepiedi S, Mucci M, Bertini N, Milantoni L, Arcangeli F. A naturalistic study of referred children and adolescents with obsessive-compulsive disorder. *J Am Acad Child Adolesc Psychiatry.* 2005;44(7):673–81.

185. Kraepelin E. *Manic-Depressive Insanity and Paranoia.* Edinburgh, UK: E. and S. Livingstone; 1921.

186. Brown GW, Harris T. Disease, distress and depression. A comment. *J Affect Disord.* 1982;4(1):1–8.

187. Hlastala SA, Frank E, Kowalski J, et al. Stressful life events, bipolar disorder, and the "kindling model." *J Abnorm Psychol.* 2000;109(4):777–86.

188. Breslau N, Lucia VC, Alvarado GF. Intelligence and other predisposing factors in exposure to trauma and posttraumatic stress disorder: a follow-up study at age 17 years. *Arch Gen Psychiatry.* 2006;63(11):1238–45.

189. Giaconia RM, Reinherz HZ, Silverman AB, Pakiz B, Frost AK, Cohen E. Traumas and posttraumatic stress disorder in a community population of older adolescents. *J Am Acad Child Adolesc Psychiatry.* 1995;34(10):1369–80.

190. Kessler RC, Rubinow DR, Holmes C, Abelson JM, Zhao S. The epidemiology of DSM-III-R bipolar I disorder in a general population survey. *Psychol Med.* 1997;27(5):1079–89.

191. Grilo CM, Sanislow C, Fehon DC, Martino S, McGlashan TH. Psychological and behavioral functioning in adolescent psychiatric inpatients who report histories of childhood abuse. *Am J Psychiatry.* 1999;156(4):538–43.

192. Kaplan SJ, Pelcovitz D, Salzinger S, et al. Adolescent physical abuse: risk for adolescent psychiatric disorders. *Am J Psychiatry.* 1998;155(7):954–9.

193. Kessler RC, Davis CG, Kendler KS. Childhood adversity and adult psychiatric disorder in the US National Comorbidity Survey. *Psychol Med.* 1997;27(5):1101–19.

194. Read J, Perry BD, Moskowitz A, Connolly J. The contribution of early traumatic events to schizophrenia in some patients: a traumagenic neurodevelopmental model. *Psychiatry.* 2001;64(4):319–45.

195. Leverich GS, Altshuler LL, Frye MA, et al. Risk of switch in mood polarity to hypomania or mania in patients with bipolar depression during acute and continuation trials of venlafaxine, sertraline, and bupropion as adjuncts to mood stabilizers. *Am J Psychiatry.* 2006;163(2):232–9.

196. Garno JL, Goldberg JF, Ramirez PM, Ritzler BA. Impact of childhood abuse on the clinical course of bipolar disorder. *Br J Psychiatry.* 2005;186:121–5.

197. Marchand WR, Wirth L, Simon C. Adverse life events and pediatric bipolar disorder in a community mental health setting. *Comm Mental Health J.* 2005;41(1):67–75.

198. Havens JF, Gudino OG, Biggs EA, Diamond UN, Weis JR, Cloitre M. Identification of trauma exposure and PTSD in adolescent psychiatric inpatients: an exploratory study. *J Traumatic Stress.* 2012;25(2):171–8.

199. Parens E, Johnston J, Carlson GA. Pediatric mental health care dysfunction disorder? *N Engl J Med.* 2010;362(20):1853–5.

200. Biederman J, Wozniak J, Martel MM, et al. Can pediatric bipolar-I disorder be diagnosed in the context of posttraumatic stress disorder? A familial risk analysis. Paper presented at: Psychiatry Research May 11, 2013; Boston, MA.

201. Hertzberg MA, Butterfield MI, Feldman ME, et al. A preliminary study of lamotrigine for the treatment of posttraumatic stress disorder. *Biol Psychiatry.* 1999;45(9):1226–9.

202. Rosenberg SD, Mueser KT, Jankowski MK, Salyers MP, Acker K. Cognitive-behavioral treatmenzt of PTSD in severe mental illness: results of a pilot study. *Am J Psychiatric Rehabilitation.* 2004;7(2):171–86.

203. Mueser KT, Bolton E, Carty PC, et al. The trauma recovery group: a cognitive-behavioral program for post-traumatic stress disorder in persons with severe mental illness. *Comm Mental Health J.* 2007;43(3):281–304.

204. Mueser KT, Rosenberg SD, Xie H, et al. A randomized controlled trial of cognitive-behavioral treatment for posttraumatic stress disorder in severe mental illness. *J Consult Clin Psychol.* 2008;76(2):259.

205. Kerbeshian J, Burd L. Case study: comorbidity among Tourette's syndrome, autistic disorder, and bipolar disorder. *J Am Acad Child Adolesc Psychiatry.* 1996;35(5):681–5.

206. Komoto J, Seigo U, Hirata J. Infantile autism and affective disorder. *J Autism Dev Disord.* 1984;14(1):81–4.

207. Sovner R, Hurley AD. Do the mentally retarded suffer from affective illness? *Arch Gen Psychiatry.* 1983;40(1):61–7.

208. Steingard R, Biederman J. Lithium responsive manic-like symptoms in two individuals with autism and mental retardation. *J Am Acad Child Adolesc Psychiatry.* 1987;26(6):932–5.

209. Wing L. Asperger's syndrome: a clinical account. *Psychol Med.* 1981;11(1):115–29.

210. Towbin KE, Pradella A, Gorrindo T, Pine DS, Leibenluft E. Autism spectrum traits in children with mood and anxiety disorders. *J Child Adolesc Psychopharmacol.* 2005;15(3):452–64.

211. Wozniak J, Biederman J, Faraone SV, et al. Mania in children with pervasive developmental disorder revisited. *J Am Acad Child Adolesc Psychiatry.* 1997;36(11):1552–9; discussion 1559–1560.

212. Joshi G, Morrow EM, Wozniak J, et al. Prevalence amd clinical correlates of pervasive developmental disorders in clinically referred population of children and adolescents. Paper presented at: 6th International Meeting for Autism Research; May 3–5, 2007; Seattle, WA.

213. Joshi G, Biederman J, Wozniak J, et al. Response to second generation neuroleptics in youth with comorbid bipolar disorder and pervasive developmental disorders. Paper presented at: 161st American Psychiatric Association Annual Meeting; May 3–8, 2008; Washington, DC.

214. Joshi G, Wozniak J, Wilens T, Petty C, MacPherson H, Biederman J. Clinical characteristics of youth with comorbid bipolar disorder and autism spectrum disorders. Paper presented at: NIMH-MGH-The Ryan Licht Sang Bipolar Foundation Annual Pediatric Bipolar Conference; March 28–29, 2008; Cambridge, MA.

215. Joshi G, Biederman J, Petty C, Goldin RL, Furtak SL, Wozniak J. Examining the comorbidity of bipolar disorder and autism spectrum disorders: a large controlled analysis of phenotypic and familial correlates in a referred population of youth with bipolar I disorder with and without autism spectrum disorders. *J Clin Psychiatry.* 2013;74(6):578–86.

216. DeLong GR, Nohria C. Psychiatric family history and neurological disease in autistic spectrum disorders. *Dev Med Child Neurol.* 1994;36:441–8.

217. Herzberg B. The families of autistic children. In: Coleman M, ed. *The Autistic Syndromes.* Amsterdam, The Netherlands: North Holland; 1976:151–72.

218. DeLong GR, Dwyer JT. Correlation of family history with specific autistic subgroups: Asperger's syndrome and bipolar affective disease. *J Autism Dev Disord.* 1988;18(4):593–600.

219. Posey DJ, Wiegand RE, Wilkerson J, Maynard M, Stigler KA, McDougle CJ. Open-label atomoxetine for attention-deficit/ hyperactivity disorder symptoms associated with high-functioning pervasive developmental disorders. *J Child Adolesc Psychopharmacol.* 2006;16(5):599–610.

220. Research Units on Pediatric Psychopharmacology Autism Network. Randomized, controlled, cross-over trial of methylphenidate in pervasive developmental disorders with hyperactivity. *Arch Gen Psychiatry.* 2005;62(11):1266–74.

221. Lainhart JE, Folstein SE. Affective disorders in people with autism: a review of published cases. *J Autism Dev Disord.* 1994;24(5):587–601.

222. Nagaraj R, Singhi P, Malhi P. Risperidone in children with autism: randomized, placebo controlled, double-blind study. *J Child Neurol.* 2006;21:450–5.

223. Shea S, Turgay A, Carroll A, et al. Risperidone in the treatment of disruptive behavioral symptoms in children with autistic and other pervasive developmental disorders. *Pediatrics.* 2004;114(5):e634–641.

224. Malone RP, Delaney MA, Hyman SB, Cater JR. Ziprasidone in adolescents with autism: an open-label pilot study. *J Child Adolesc Psychopharmacol.* 2007;17(6):779–90.

225. Stigler KA, Diener JT, Kohn AE, Erickson CA, Posey DJ, McDougle CJ. A prospective, open-label study of aripiprazole in youth with Asperger's disorder and pervasive development disorder not otherwise specified. *Neuropscyhopharmacology.* 2006;31:S194.

226. Hollander E, Wasserman S, Swanson EN, et al. A double-blind placebo-controlled pilot study of olanzapine in childhood/adolescent pervasive developmental disorder. *J Child Adolesc Psychopharmacol.* 2006;16(5):541–8.

227. Findling RL, McNamara NK, Gracious BL, et al. Quetiapine in nine youths with autistic disorder. *J Child Adolesc Psychopharmacol.* 2004;14(2):287–94.

228. Martin A, Koenig K, Scahill L, Bregman J. Open-label quetiapine in the treatment of children and adolescents with autistic disorder. *J Child Adolesc Psychopharmacol.* 1999;9(2):99–107.

229. Klein DJ, Cottingham EM, Sorter M, Barton BA, Morrison JA. A randomized, double-blind, placebo-controlled trial of metformin treatment of weight gain associated with initiation of atypical antipsychotic therapy in children and adolescents. *Am J Psychiatry.* 2006;163(12):2072–9.

230. Bjorkhem-Bergman L, Asplund AB, Lindh JD. Metformin for weight reduction in non-diabetic patients on antipsychotic drugs: a systematic review and meta-analysis. *J Psychopharmacol.* 2011;25(3):299–305.

231. Gutkovich ZA, Carlson GA, Carlson HE, Coffey B, Wieland N. Asperger's disorder and co-morbid bipolar disorder: diagnostic and treatment challenges. *J Child Adolesc Psychopharmacol.* 2007;17(2):247–55.

Heritability of Bipolar Disorder

Katie Mahon, Katherine E. Burdick,
and Anil K. Malhotra

Bipolar disorder, like all neuropsychiatric diseases, is a complex disorder with many interacting genetic and environmental factors contributing to the development and expression of the full clinical phenotype. Early expectations that a small number of genetic variants would be identified that would explain much of the variance in liability to developing the disorder have been abandoned; nevertheless, a large body of evidence demonstrates that bipolar disorder is highly heritable and the expression of the illness is under strong genetic control.

One of the biggest challenges in seeking to understand the genetics of bipolar disorder is the phenotypic heterogeneity that exists among individuals. Individuals with bipolar disorder vary in terms of the age at onset of the disorder, the predominant mood episode (i.e., depressed, manic, or mixed), the degree of altered circadian functioning, the frequency of mood episodes, the level of neurocognitive impairment, and the extent of interepisode recovery, among other variables. Large-scale molecular genetic studies, which have been focused on gene discovery, have not typically collected detailed phenotypic data; this omission generally limits the utility of the results. The interpretation of data from different studies seeking to understand the genetic mechanisms underlying bipolar disorder are complicated by the inclusion of what may be genetically distinct subtypes of the disorder. However, despite these complications, robust and replicable evidence has begun to elucidate the genetic underpinnings of bipolar disorder.

Family Studies

Family studies seek to understand whether relatives of individuals with bipolar disorder have an increased risk for developing the disorder themselves compared to individuals who are not closely related to someone with bipolar disorder. Many family studies have been conducted to date and demonstrate conclusively that relatives of probands with bipolar disorder have a greater chance of developing the disorder than members of the general population.[1-3] In the largest population-based family study, Lichtenstein and colleagues (2009) found that children of a parent with bipolar disorder have a more than 6-fold increased risk (relative risk = 6.4) for developing the disorder; the risk for the sibling of a proband was nearly 8-fold (relative risk = 7.9). Previous studies found that the relative risk for first-degree relatives is approximately 9.0 when using a population risk of 1%–2%.[4]

Given the wealth of evidence demonstrating that bipolar disorder runs in families, twin studies have provided the next step in determining the heritability of the disorder. By examining the concordance rate for bipolar disorder in monozygotic and dizygotic twin pairs, the influence of genetics and environment can begin to be examined. Twin studies have consistently found that monozygotic twins, who are approximately genetically identical, have a significantly higher concordance rate for bipolar disorder (38.5%–43%) than do dizygotic twins (4.5%–5.6%), who share approximately half of their genes.[4-7] The higher concordance rate in monozygotic versus dizygotic twins demonstrates that the development of bipolar disorder is under strong genetic control. Heritability estimates (the proportion of risk for the disorder that is explained by genetic factors as opposed to other factors) derived from these studies range from 79% to 93%. As noted by Barnett and Smoller (2009), these heritability estimates are higher than those for many medical disorders for which specific susceptibility genes have already been identified. Importantly, twin studies generally do not find a substantial role for shared familial environment in contributing to risk for bipolar disorder,[2,4] suggesting that factors such as parenting style, if applied consistently to each child within a family, do not appear to affect the liability to develop bipolar disorder. Several studies have found significant, albeit small, estimates of effect for nonshared environmental factors, as addressed extensively in Chapter 6. Although limited in number, several adoption studies, in which the risk of developing bipolar disorder is examined among the biological and adoptive relatives of patients, have also demonstrated that genetic factors rather than shared environmental factors contribute most strongly to the development of the disorder.[2] Most recently, Lichtenstein and colleagues (2009) found that adopted children with a biological parent with bipolar disorder had a relative risk of 4.3 for developing the disorder, whereas adopted children whose biological parents were free from bipolar disorder had a relative risk of 1.3 for developing the disorder.

An earlier age at illness onset has long been recognized as a potential marker of a more severe disease course, as well as an indication of a stronger genetic component as compared with later (adult)-onset forms of the disorder.[4,8] Many studies have demonstrated an increased familial risk for developing an affective illness (either bipolar or unipolar disorder) for early-onset forms of the disorder compared to later onset subtypes.[9-16] Such findings led to the hypothesis that early-onset forms of bipolar disorder, and in particular prepubertal onset of the disorder, may be a distinct genetic subtype. Unfortunately, few genetic studies have distinguished between early- and late-onset forms of the disorder.

Family studies provide strong evidence that bipolar disorder is highly heritable and that certain phenotypic aspects of the disorder tend to run in families. The next step in investigating the genetic underpinnings of the disorder is to try to identify regions within the genome that may confer risk for developing the clinical phenotype.

Linkage Analysis

In a linkage analysis study, genetic information is typically collected from pedigrees (multiple family members with and without the disorder) to try to identify the chromosomal region wherein susceptibility genes may be located. To do this, hundreds to thousands of markers spread across the genome are examined, with the goal of identifying genomic areas that appear to be inherited along with the disorder within each family. This methodology is particularly well suited to identifying the genetic causes of disorders in which a small number of genes contribute to a large degree of risk for developing the disorder across families. Bipolar disorder, like other complex neuropsychiatric disorders, does not appear to be inherited in this fashion in most families and, thus, evidence from the many linkage analysis studies that have been performed to date in bipolar disorder has been largely inconclusive.[4,17,18]

Recently, the largest linkage analysis ever conducted in bipolar disorder was performed; no strong positive findings resulted from an analysis of 972 pedigrees, including 2,782 individuals with bipolar disorder.[19] The lack of compelling findings from decades of linkage analysis studies suggests that, for most cases of bipolar disorder, the genetic architecture is likely to involve many different genes in which each contributes a small effect toward risk for developing the disorder. However, the lack of findings from linkage analysis to date does not preclude the possibility that for some families, bipolar disorder is the result of a small number of genes contributing a large effect. It may be that such genes are specific to certain families or small populations, which would not allow for these genes to be identified through linkage analysis.

Association Studies
Candidate Gene Association Studies

In candidate gene association studies, a single or small number of genes that have been selected a priori based on biological hypotheses of the disorder are examined in cases and controls. Evidence from candidate gene association studies has been inconsistent and there is little persuasive support for any one candidate gene.[20] A recent meta-analysis of 487 candidate gene studies in bipolar disorder failed to find any genes that were significantly associated with bipolar disorder after correction for multiple comparisons, most likely a result of methodological limitations, such as small sample sizes, the lack of a strong pathophysiological understanding of the disorder upon which to select candidate genes, and the improbability that single genes of large effect account for much of the variance in risk for bipolar disorder.[20] Nevertheless, it may be useful to examine candidate genes and their association with discrete phenotypic aspects of bipolar disorder, as will be discussed later in this chapter.

Genome-Wide Association Studies

Technological advancements have resulted in the ability to perform genome-wide association studies (GWAS) in bipolar disorder, in which hundreds of thousands of single-nucleotide polymorphisms (SNPs) are simultaneously genotyped in tens of thousands of people.[21,22] In contrast to candidate gene studies, GWAS is unbiased in that it identifies potentially relevant sequence variation based on its position within the genome rather than on any *a priori* biological theory. GWAS approaches are well suited to the notion that bipolar disorder may be the result of many different common SNPs, each with a very small effect on risk for developing the disorder. This methodology is limited, however, in that it is not likely to detect rare genetic variations (found in less than 1% of the population), which may play a critical role in many cases of bipolar disorder. Sequencing studies are likely to be necessary to gain a further understanding of the contribution of rare SNPs in susceptibility to bipolar disorder.

To date, approximately 12 GWAS have been conducted in bipolar disorder, of which half have identified SNPs that have reached genome-wide significance (see Table 5.1). Many of these studies have included individuals with both bipolar I and bipolar II

TABLE 5.1 Genome-Wide Significant Findings in Bipolar Disorder

Study	Cases	Controls	Top SNP(s)	Nearest Gene	p-Value
Baum et al., 2008	1233	1429	rs1012053	*DGKH*	1.5×10^{-8}
Ferreira et al., 2008	4387	6209	rs10994336	*ANK3*	9.1×10^{-9}
Cichon et al., 2011	8441	35362	rs1064395	*NCAN*	2.14×10^{-9}
PGC-BD, 2011	11974	51792	rs4765913	*CACNA1C*	1.52×10^{-8}
			rs12576775	*ODZ4*	4.40×10^{-8}
Green et al., 2012	1218	2913	rs7296288	*RHEBL1; DHH*	8.97×10^{-9}
			rs3818253	*TRPC4AP*	3.88×10^{-8}
Chen et al., 2013[a]	7773	9883	rs9834970	*TRANK1*	1.48×10^{-12}
			rs2271893	*LMAN2L*	2.2×10^{-10}
			rs4650608	*PTGFR*	$<5 \times 10^{-8}$
			rs4948418	*ANK3*	$<5 \times 10^{-8}$
			rs7618915	—	$<5 \times 10^{-8}$

[a]Sample included Asian cases and controls.
ANK3, ankyrin3; CACNA1C, calcium channel, voltage-dependent, L type, alpha 1C subunit; DGKH, diacylglycerol kinase, eta; DHH, desert hedgehog; LMAN2L, lectin, mannose-binding 2-like; NCAN, neurocan; ODZ4, odz; PGC-BD, Psychiatric Genome-Wide Association Study (GWAS) Consortium Bipolar Disorder Working Group; PTGFR, prostaglandin F receptor; RHEBL1, ras homolog enriched in brain like-1; TRPC4AP, transient receptor potential cation channel, subfamily C, member 4; TRANK1, tetratricopeptide repeat and ankyrin repeat containing 1.

disorders, as well as people with schizoaffective disorder, bipolar type. The majority of subjects included in these studies have been of European ancestry, limiting the ability to generalize these results to non-European samples (although studies including samples of African American and Asian participants have recently been conducted).[23–25] As has been the case for GWAS in other neuropsychiatric disorders, results from several initial GWAS in bipolar disorder were negative[25–27]; however, with larger samples, more robust positive findings have emerged.[28–31] Given the many SNPs that are tested in GWAS (up to about a million in most studies), a conservative and generally accepted statistical criterion for genome-wide significance is a p-value $< 5 \times 10^{-8}$. This stringent threshold, in combination with the fact that most common SNPs have small to modest effect sizes,[18,21] suggests that in order to have enough power to detect a significant association, a very large sample size (>10,000 cases and controls) must be studied. As sample sizes have increased and researchers have either replicated their most promising results in independent samples or have conducted meta-analyses, several SNPs have been found to be significantly associated with bipolar disorder at this conservative threshold.

One of the earliest genome-wide significant findings was an association between bipolar disorder and the gene DGKH, encoding diacylglycerol kinase eta[32]; this finding, however, has not been replicated in subsequent studies. CACNA1C, which encodes for the alpha subunit of the L-type calcium channel, has now been identified in two large bipolar GWAS,[31,33] providing compelling support that this region is associated with bipolar disorder. Ferreira and colleagues (2008) identified the region of ANK3 (encoding ankyrin 3), and this finding was subsequently independently replicated in the stage 1 findings of another large GWAS.[31] However, in the replication portion of that study, ANK3 did not survive statistical correction; this failure may mean that the effect size for ANK3 is smaller than originally estimated and will require even larger sample sizes to consistently reach genome-wide significance. In another GWAS, NCAN (encoding neurocan) attained genome-wide significance,[28] although this finding has not been replicated. The largest GWAS ever conducted in bipolar disorder identified two genome-wide significant loci: CACNA1C as well as ODZ4, which is likely involved with neuronal path finding and cell surface signaling.[31] A subsequent GWAS provided support for findings near these two loci and identified a significant and novel locus between DHH and RHEBL1 as well as an additional significant locus on the gene TRPC4AP.[29] More recently, another large GWAS provided support for previous findings near ANK3 as well as three novel loci near TRANK3, LMAN2L, and PTGFR.[23] Interestingly, mRNA expression of TRANK3 was found to be markedly increased upon administration of valproic acid,[23] providing further support that this gene may be involved in the pathogenesis of bipolar disorder.

As GWAS sample sizes increase, more SNPs will undoubtedly be identified. Just how many common SNPs can we expect to find that are associated with bipolar disorder? Chen and colleagues (2013) employed a discovery trajectory model to understand how many more common SNPs are currently undiscovered and what sample size would be required in order to identify them. Their results suggest that there are likely to be at least ~150 common SNPs that confer significant risk for bipolar disorder, but that in order to identify these loci, samples sizes would need to reach at least ~63,000.[23] Their model further estimated that common SNPs account for approximately 5.5% of the variance in genetic risk for developing bipolar disorder.[23] These results should be considered with some caution, as there are currently only a handful of SNPs that have been found to be associated with bipolar disorder; the discovery trajectory model will improve and become more reliable as more SNPs are identified. Nevertheless, these results suggest that complementary molecular genetic approaches, such as deep sequencing to identify rare and structural variation, will be required to elucidate more fully the genetic basis of bipolar disorder.

In addition to examining each SNP individually, the PGC-BD study also performed an analysis in which all potential risk variants were aggregated and compared between cases and controls. This type of analysis allows for signals arising from individual SNPs of very small effect to combine such that a significant effect may be detected. As had previously been demonstrated in a sample comprised of patients with schizophrenia and patients with bipolar disorder, the PGC-BD group demonstrated a significant "polygenic" signal ($p < 10^{-8}$) arising from many risk variants of small effect, providing direct evidence for a polygenic component in bipolar disorder.[31] In other words, this significant effect demonstrates that at least some of the genetic risk for bipolar disorder arises from small effects from many different genes. As these genes are likely to interact with one another and with other genes within molecular networks, it is also important to consider approaches that take these biological pathways into account.

Pathway Analysis

Pathway analysis is another method of analyzing data arising from GWASs and allows for the investigation of biologically related genes, such as those that are involved in specific biochemical functions. In bipolar disorder, pathway analysis has revealed significant enrichment in three calcium channel subunits (CACNA1C, CACNA1D, and CACNB3) within the gene ontology (GO) category of voltage-gated calcium channel activity.[31] This finding is intriguing, as two of these (CACNA1C and CACNA1D) encode for the major L-type alpha subunits in the brain, and there is some evidence that L-type calcium channel blockers are effective in the treatment of bipolar disorder.[34]

Structural Variation

An alternative (or complementary) approach to investigating the genetics of bipolar disorder is to examine structural alterations in the genome. These alterations are expected to be rare but also to contribute a greater effect on risk for the disorder than common SNPs. In disorders such as schizophrenia and autism spectrum disorders (ASDs), structural variation in the form of copy number variations (CNVs) has been found to play a role in the pathogenesis of each illness.[35] To date, few studies have examined structural variation in bipolar disorder, but the evidence that has emerged suggests that although CNVs do play a role in the development of bipolar disorder, that role may be more limited than it is in other neuropsychiatric disorders.[36]

There appears to be an enrichment of rare CNVs among patients with bipolar disorder compared to controls,[37–39] although the effects reported are small (odds ratios are approximately 1.5) compared to results for schizophrenia and ASDs and several studies have reported negative findings.[40,41] Family-based studies are able to investigate the rate of de novo CNVs (present in an individual but not present in either parent). To date, one study has measured the rate of de novo CNVs in bipolar disorder, and the results indicate that individuals with bipolar disorder do indeed show an increase (4.3%) compared to unaffected individuals (0.9%).[37] Across studies, bipolar subjects with an early-onset form of the disorder appear to have a greater burden of both inherited and de novo CNVs.[37–39] In fact, the rate of de novo CNVs in people with an early-onset form of the disorder was comparable to that found for individuals with schizophrenia.[36] This evidence adds to the wealth of data suggesting that early-onset forms of the disorder may be genetically distinct from later onset forms and that early-onset forms have a stronger genetic basis.

Phenotypic Considerations

As technological advances have made it possible to perform more expansive and complicated molecular genetics studies, the heterogeneity of the bipolar phenotype remains problematic in seeking to understand the genetic causes of what are likely multiple, distinct disorders. Given that the clinical definition of bipolar disorder has evolved over time and remains relatively unstable at present, individuals diagnosed with the disorder represent an exceedingly heterogeneous group. To date, large-scale molecular genetics studies have not been able to incorporate detailed phenotypic information due to the sheer number of subjects recruited. As noted previously, evidence from candidate gene studies has been inconsistent and no single gene has emerged as being definitively associated with the disorder based on these studies. Nevertheless, linking genetic variation with specific phenotypic aspects of the disorder may be useful in seeking to narrow the genetic complexity of the disorder and to begin to understand how certain genes may affect specific features of the disorder, rather than risk for the disorder itself. As such, two main strategies to try to address this variation are to search for intermediate phenotypes and to study people at high risk for developing the disorder.

Intermediate phenotypes, or endophenotypes, are discrete traits or characteristics that are believed to index biological function more closely than the complex diagnostic syndrome. Several endophenotypes have been proposed for bipolar disorder, including circadian rhythm disruption, neurocognitive impairment, and temperament.

Unaffected offspring of parents with bipolar disorder demonstrate disrupted sleep/activity levels versus healthy subjects without a family history of the disorder,[42] suggesting that circadian abnormalities may be a genetically mediated, central feature of the disorder. Supporting this hypothesis, there is some evidence that several genes that are known to regulate circadian functions (e.g., CLOCK, PERIOD, VIP) may be risk loci for bipolar disorder.[43–45] A CLOCK gene polymorphism may moderate features of the illness such as diurnal preference,[46] levels of evening activity, and delayed sleep onset in bipolar disorder.[47] These data suggest that genes involved in circadian functioning are relevant to the pathophysiology of bipolar disorder, although further work in larger samples is required.

Neurocognitive impairment is another potential endophenotype in bipolar disorder, as both individuals with bipolar disorder and their first-degree relatives demonstrate impairment in multiple domains.[48] A recent cognitive genomics study by Glahn et al.[49] included 660 members of extended multiplex bipolar disorder pedigrees, of which 230 individuals had the disorder. Heritability estimates and genetic correlations were calculated, indicating strong evidence for a genetic influence on tasks of processing speed, working memory, and declarative memory within bipolar disorder families. Genetic correlations between neurocognition and risk for illness were high (up to 0.80), indicative of a partially shared underlying genetic etiology. Thus, there is evidence that genetic factors influence cognitive functioning in people with bipolar disorder; however, very few studies to date have attempted to identify specific molecular genetic markers associated with these features of the disorder. One such study demonstrated an association between variation in the COMT gene and risk for developing bipolar disorder as well as neurocognitive impairment.[50] Further studies linking genetic variation and specific aspects of neurocognition in bipolar disorder are required.

Several studies have demonstrated the heritability of affective temperaments,[51,52] pervasive personality styles that feature affective traits common to bipolar disorder (e.g., cyclothymia, depression, irritability).[53–58] More recently, heritability estimates for the various identified affective temperaments were estimated to range from ~20% (for hyperthymic temperament) to ~50% (for irritable temperament) and suggestive linkage to specific SNPs was demonstrated.[59] In particular, hyperthymic temperament was associated with SNPs located on chromosomes 1q44, 2p16, 6q16, and 14q23; dysthymic temperament was linked with findings on chromosomes 3p21 and 13q34, and irritable temperament was associated with chromosome 6q24.

Another recent study examined mood-incongruent psychotic symptoms and found suggestive evidence for an association between this aspect of the disorder and three loci (6q14.2, 3p22.2, and 14q24.2).[60] Negative mood delusions are another phenotypic aspect recently investigated through GWAS. Results indicated that rs9875793, a SNP located in an intergenic region on 3q26.1, was significantly associated with a delusional dimension identified through factor analysis.[61] Perlis and colleagues (2010) recently completed a GWAS of suicidality in patients with either bipolar disorder or major depression; no single locus met criteria for genome-wide significance in bipolar disorder, although several loci provided suggestive evidence of association (SNPs within TBL1XR1, CAPN13, and IRX2).[62] These preliminary studies using GWAS to investigate symptom dimensions within bipolar samples must be interpreted with caution, as sample sizes were small and few SNPs attained genome-wide significance. However, it is intriguing that molecular genetics methods, such as GWAS, can be applied to further understand dimensional aspects of bipolar disorder. Although replication with larger samples is required, these data suggest that further delineating the phenotype will help to elucidate the genetic mechanisms underlying the disorder.

In addition to the molecular genetic evidence for psychosis and suicidality previously described, family studies also suggest that these symptoms tend to aggregate in families.[63–65] Other phenotypic aspects of the disorder that have been found to cluster in families include the frequency of mood episodes,[66,67] response to lithium,[68,69] polarity of mood episode at illness onset,[70] and comorbid panic disorder.[68,71–73] Such familial clustering suggests that these aspects of the disorder have a strong genetic basis.

Distinction Between Bipolar Subtypes

There is some evidence that bipolar I and bipolar II disorders represent at least partially distinct genetic subtypes of the disorder, as several family studies have demonstrated that relatives of probands with bipolar II disorder have a higher risk of developing this subtype of the disorder than do relatives of probands with bipolar I disorder.[74,75] There is also evidence, however, that the risk of developing bipolar I disorder is increased in relatives of patients with bipolar II disorder.[2] Complicating this picture is the consistent finding that relatives of people with bipolar I or bipolar II disorder have higher rates of unipolar depression than is found in the general population. It must also be kept in mind that, given the higher base rate of unipolar depression in the general population relative to that of bipolar disorder, relatives of individuals with bipolar disorder are more likely to develop unipolar depression than bipolar disorder.[4] Taken together, the evidence suggests that perhaps some cases of bipolar II disorder are more genetically related to bipolar I disorder, some are more genetically related to unipolar depression, and that there also may exist a distinct genetic entity of bipolar II disorder that aggregates within families.[2] Finally, the possibility that developmental aspects of these disorders play a role in their heritability must be considered, and age at onset and other factors may mediate these relationships.

Overlap With Other Neuropsychiatric Disorders

Bipolar disorder appears to share some genetic overlap with other neuropsychiatric diseases such as schizophrenia, attention-deficit/hyperactivity disorder, unipolar depression, and autism.[76] Early studies suggested that bipolar disorder and schizophrenia "breed true" within families such that although both are substantially heritable, the enhanced risk within families is specific to the disorder present within the family (Kendler et al.,

1993). More recent data from very large samples argue strongly against this notion. Lichtenstein et al.[1] identified more than 9 million individuals from more than 2 million nuclear families and assessed recurrence risks (RR) within families both within and across diagnoses (SZ and BD). Heritability estimates were high for both schizophrenia (64%) and bipolar disorder (59%) and *within*-disorder RR were consistent with prior reports (schizophrenia sibling RR = 9.0; bipolar disorder sibling RR = 7.9). Importantly, this study provided compelling evidence of overlapping genetic risk, as a sibling of a proband with schizophrenia was shown to have a 4-fold increased risk for developing bipolar disorder, and likewise, a sibling of a proband with bipolar disorder was at 4-fold increased risk for developing schizophrenia. The comorbidity between disorders within families was largely explained (64% variance) by additive genetic effects common to both disorders.

More recently, the largest GWAS ever conducted on psychiatric disorders identified four SNPs that attained genome-wide significance in a sample comprised of patients with ADHD, ASD, bipolar disorder, major depressive disorder, and schizophrenia.[76] Three of these four SNPs were found to have shared effects on each of the

TABLE 5.2 Genome-Wide Significant Findings Across Disorders

Nearest Gene/Region	SNP	Associated Phenotype	Study
ZNF804A	rs1344706	BPD and SCZ combined	O'Donovan et al., 2008; Williams et al., 2011
	rs1344706	SCZ alone	Williams et al., 2011
ANK3	rs10994359	BPD and SCZ combined	SCZ-PGC, 2011
	rs10994359	BPD alone	Ferreira et al., 2008
CACNA1C	rs4765905	BPD and SCZ combined	SCZ-PGC, 2011
	rs4765905	BPD alone	PGC-BD, 2011
	rs4765905	SCZ alone	Hamshere et al., 2013
	rs1024582	BPD, SCZ, MDD, ASD, and ADHD combined	CDG-PGC, 2013
3p21.1	rs2251219	BPD and MDD combined	Akula et al., 2010
	rs2535629	BPD, SCZ, MDD, ASD, and ADHD combined	CDG-PGC, 2013
		BPD and SCZ combined	SCZ-PGC, 2011
	rs2239547	SCZ alone	Hamshere et al., 2013
AS3MT (plus others)	rs11191454	BPD, SCZ, MDD, ASD, and ADHD combined	CDG-PGC, 2013
CACNB2	rs2799573	BPD, SCZ, MDD, ASD, and ADHD combined	CDG-PGC, 2013

ADHD, attention-deficit/hyperactivity disorder; ANK3, ankyrin3; ASD, autism spectrum disorder; AS3MT, arsenic methyltransferase; BPD, bipolar disorder; CACNA1C, calcium channel, voltage-dependent, L type, alpha 1C subunit; CACNB2, calcium channel, voltage-dependent, beta 2 subunit; CDG-PGC, Cross-Disorder Group of the Psychiatric Genetics Consortium; MDD, major depressive disorder; PGC-BD, Psychiatric Genome-Wide Association Study Consortium Bipolar Disorder Working Group; SCZ, schizophrenia; SCZ-PGC, Schizophrenia Psychiatric Genome-Wide Association Study Consortium; ZNF804A, zinc finger protein 804A.

five disorders, whereas one SNP (rs1024582) was found to be associated mainly with bipolar disorder and schizophrenia. Two of the SNPs (CACNA1C and CACNB2) were located within genes that encode L-type voltage-gated calcium-channel subunits, suggesting that genes involved in brain-expressed ion channels are relevant not only to bipolar disorder but also to other psychiatric illnesses. Several other studies combining samples of people with bipolar disorder and with schizophrenia have been conducted and have identified SNPs that are associated with both disorders[77–80] (see Table 5.2). In addition, studies that have combined samples of patients with bipolar disorder and unipolar depression have identified SNPs that confer risk for both disorders.[81–83] Such cross-disorder effects challenge current diagnostic classifications and suggest that bipolar disorder and other major psychiatric illnesses may be less genetically distinct than previously thought.

Summary

The genetic architecture of bipolar disorder is complex; several approaches focusing on common genomic variation have highlighted its polygenic nature. Recent large-scale GWASs have contributed important initial evidence of replicable, common, single-locus risk alleles for bipolar disorder.[31] Consistent with the family-based evidence of considerable genetic overlap, many of the variants identified as predisposing to bipolar disorder have also been associated with risk for other neuropsychiatric phenotypes,[76] suggesting that many genetic risk loci will have broad effects on brain functioning that ultimately place an individual at risk for a number of psychiatric disorders. Beyond those variants that rise to the level of statistical significance, a substantial polygenic component has been shown to underlie risk for bipolar disorder, involving thousands of common alleles, in aggregate, each with very small effect but together accounting for up to 30% of the genetic variance for the illness.[84] The importance of these variants is likely to be amplified when more complex analyses incorporate multiple common loci within sets of relevant molecular pathways. Of particular importance for future work, many if not most of the identified risk variants are currently of unknown function. Future studies focusing on the functional relevance of these variants and their associated pathways with regard to brain function will be critical to gaining a complete understanding of the genetic architecture of bipolar disorder.

Author Disclosures

Dr. Mahon has no conflicts to disclose.

Dr. Burdick has no conflicts to disclose. She is funded by the National Institute of Mental Health and the U.S. Department of Veterans Affairs only.

Dr. Malhotra is a paid consultant for Genomind, Inc.

References

1. Lichtenstein P, Yip BH, Björk C, et al. Common genetic determinants of schizophrenia and bipolar disorder in Swedish families: a population-based study. *Lancet*. 2009;373(9659):234–9.
2. Smoller JW, Finn CT. Family, twin, and adoption studies of bipolar disorder. *Am J Med Genet C Semin Med Genet*. 2003;123C(1):48–58.
3. Wozniak J, Biederman J, Martelon MK, Hernandez M, Yvonne Woodworth K, Faraone SV. Does sex moderate the clinical correlates of pediatric bipolar-I disorder? Results from a large controlled family-genetic study. *J Affect Disord*. 2013;149(1–3):269–76.
4. Barnett JH, Smoller JW. The genetics of bipolar disorder. *Neuroscience*. 2009;164(1):331–43.
5. Kendler KS, Pedersen NL, Neale MC, Mathé AA. A pilot Swedish twin study of affective illness including hospital- and population-ascertained subsamples: results of model fitting. *Behav Genet*. 1995;25(3):217–32.
6. Kieseppä T, Partonen T, Haukka J, Kaprio J, Lönnqvist J. High concordance of bipolar I disorder in a nationwide sample of twins. *Am J Psychiatry*. 2004;161(10):1814–21.
7. McGuffin P, Rijsdijk F, Andrew M, Sham P, Katz R, Cardno A. The heritability of bipolar affective disorder and the genetic relationship to unipolar depression. *Arch Gen Psychiatry*. 2003;60(5):497–502.
8. Faraone SV, Glatt SJ, Tsuang MT. The genetics of pediatric-onset bipolar disorder. *Biol Psychiatry*. 2003;53(11):970–7.
9. Geller B, Tillman R, Bolhofner K, Zimerman B, Strauss NA, Kaufmann P. Controlled, blindly rated, direct-interview family study of a prepubertal and early-adolescent bipolar I disorder phenotype: morbid risk, age at onset, and comorbidity. *Arch Gen Psychiatry*. 2006;63(10):1130–8.
10. Grigoroiu-Serbanescu M, Martinez M, Nöthen MM, Grinberg M, Sima D, Propping P, et al. Different familial transmission patterns in bipolar I disorder with onset before and after age 25. *Am J Med Genet*. 2001;105(8):765–73.
11. James NM. Early- and late-onset bipolar affective disorder. A genetic study. *Arch Gen Psychiatry*. 1977;34(6):715–7.
12. Neuman RJ, Geller B, Rice JP, Todd RD. Increased prevalence and earlier onset of mood disorders among relatives of prepubertal versus adult probands. *J Am Acad Child Adolesc Psychiatry*. 1997 Apr;36(4):466–73.
13. Pauls DL, Morton LA, Egeland JA. Risks of affective illness among first-degree relatives of bipolar I old-order Amish probands. *Arch Gen Psychiatry*. 1992;49(9):703–8.
14. Rice J, Reich T, Andreasen NC, et al. The familial transmission of bipolar illness. *Arch Gen Psychiatry*. 1987;44(5):441–7.
15. Somanath CP, Jain S, Reddy YCJ. A family study of early-onset bipolar I disorder. *J Affect Disord*. 2002;70(1):91–4.
16. Strober M, Morrell W, Burroughs J, Lampert C, Danforth H, Freeman R. A family study of bipolar I disorder in adolescence. Early onset of symptoms linked to increased familial loading and lithium resistance. *J Affect Disord*. 1988;15(3):255–68.
17. Craddock N, Sklar P. Genetics of bipolar disorder: successful start to a long journey. *Trends Genet*. 2009;25(2):99–105.
18. Craddock N, Sklar P. Genetics of bipolar disorder. *Lancet*. 201311;381(9878):1654–62.
19. Badner JA, Koller D, Foroud T, et al. Genome-wide linkage analysis of 972 bipolar pedigrees using single-nucleotide polymorphisms. *Mol Psychiatry*. 2012;17(8):818–26.
20. Seifuddin F, Mahon PB, Judy J, et al. Meta-analysis of genetic association studies on bipolar disorder. *Am J Med Genet B Neuropsychiatr Genet*. 2012;159B(5):508–18.
21. Psychiatric GWAS Consortium Coordinating Committee, Cichon S, Craddock N, et al. Genomewide association studies: history, rationale, and prospects for psychiatric disorders. *Am J Psychiatry*. 2009;166(5):540–56.
22. Sullivan PF, Daly MJ, O'Donovan M. Genetic architectures of psychiatric disorders: the emerging picture and its implications. *Nat Rev Genet*. 2012;13(8):537–51.
23. Chen DT, Jiang X, Akula N, et al. Genome-wide association study meta-analysis of European and Asian-ancestry samples identifies three novel loci associated with bipolar disorder. *Mol Psychiatry*. 2013;18(2):195–205.

24. Lee MTM, Chen CH, Lee CS, et al. Genome-wide association study of bipolar I disorder in the Han Chinese population. *Mol Psychiatry*. 2011;16(5):548–56.
25. Smith EN, Bloss CS, Badner JA, et al. Genome-wide association study of bipolar disorder in European American and African American individuals. *Mol Psychiatry*. 2009;14(8):755–63.
26. Scott LJ, Muglia P, Kong XQ, et al. Genome-wide association and meta-analysis of bipolar disorder in individuals of European ancestry. *Proc Natl Acad Sci USA*. 2009;106(18):7501–6.
27. Sklar P, Smoller JW, Fan J, et al. Whole-genome association study of bipolar disorder. *Mol Psychiatry*. 2008;13(6):558–69.
28. Cichon S, Mühleisen TW, Degenhardt FA, et al. Genome-wide association study identifies genetic variation in neurocan as a susceptibility factor for bipolar disorder. *Am J Hum Genet*. 2011;88(3):372–81.
29. Green EK, Hamshere M, Forty L, et al. Replication of bipolar disorder susceptibility alleles and identification of two novel genome-wide significant associations in a new bipolar disorder case-control sample. *Mol Psychiatry*. 2012;18(12):1302–7.
30. Hamshere ML, Walters JTR, Smith R, et al. Genome-wide significant associations in schizophrenia to ITIH3/4, CACNA1C and SDCCAG8, and extensive replication of associations reported by the Schizophrenia PGC. *Mol Psychiatry*. 2013;18(6):708–12.
31. Psychiatric GWAS Consortium Bipolar Disorder Working Group. Large-scale genome-wide association analysis of bipolar disorder identifies a new susceptibility locus near ODZ4. *Nat Genet*. 2011;43(10):977–83.
32. Baum AE, Akula N, Cabanero M, et al. A genome-wide association study implicates diacylglycerol kinase eta (DGKH) and several other genes in the etiology of bipolar disorder. *Mol Psychiatry*. 2008;13(2):197–207.
33. Ferreira MAR, O'Donovan MC, Meng YA, et al. Collaborative genome-wide association analysis supports a role for ANK3 and CACNA1C in bipolar disorder. *Nat Genet*. 2008;40(9):1056–8.
34. Casamassima F, Hay AC, Benedetti A, Lattanzi L, Cassano GB, Perlis RH. L-type calcium channels and psychiatric disorders: a brief review. *Am J Med Genet B Neuropsychiatr Genet*. 2010;153B(8):1373–90.
35. Merikangas AK, Corvin AP, Gallagher L. Copy-number variants in neurodevelopmental disorders: promises and challenges. *Trends Genet*. 2009;25(12):536–44.
36. Malhotra D, Sebat J. CNVs: harbingers of a rare variant revolution in psychiatric genetics. *Cell*. 2012;148(6):1223–41.
37. Malhotra D, McCarthy S, Michaelson JJ, et al. High frequencies of de novo CNVs in bipolar disorder and schizophrenia. *Neuron*. 2011;72(6):951–63.
38. Priebe L, Degenhardt FA, Herms S, et al. Genome-wide survey implicates the influence of copy number variants (CNVs) in the development of early-onset bipolar disorder. *Mol Psychiatry*. 2012;17(4):421–32.
39. Zhang D, Cheng L, Qian Y, et al. Singleton deletions throughout the genome increase risk of bipolar disorder. *Mol Psychiatry*. 2009;14(4):376–80.
40. Grozeva D, Kirov G, Ivanov D, et al. Rare copy number variants: a point of rarity in genetic risk for bipolar disorder and schizophrenia. *Arch Gen Psychiatry*. 2010;67(4):318–27.
41. McQuillin A, Bass N, Anjorin A, et al. Analysis of genetic deletions and duplications in the University College London bipolar disorder case control sample. *Eur J Hum Genet*. 2011;19(5):588–92.
42. Ankers D, Jones SH. Objective assessment of circadian activity and sleep patterns in individuals at behavioural risk of hypomania. *J Clin Psychol*. 2009;65(10):1071–86.
43. Dallaspezia S, Benedetti F. Melatonin, circadian rhythms, and the clock genes in bipolar disorder. *Curr Psychiatry Rep*. 2009;11(6):488–93.
44. Shi J, Wittke-Thompson JK, Badner JA, et al. Clock genes may influence bipolar disorder susceptibility and dysfunctional circadian rhythm. *Am J Med Genet B Neuropsychiatr Genet*. 2008;147B(7):1047–55.
45. Soria V, Martínez-Amorós E, Escaramís G, et al. Differential association of circadian genes with mood disorders: CRY1 and NPAS2 are associated with unipolar major depression and CLOCK and VIP with bipolar disorder. *Neuropsychopharmacology*. 2010;35(6):1279–89.
46. Katzenberg D, Young T, Finn L, et al. A CLOCK polymorphism associated with human diurnal preference. *Sleep*. 1998;21(6):569–76.

47. Benedetti F, Dallaspezia S, Fulgosi MC, et al. Actimetric evidence that CLOCK 3111 T/C SNP influences sleep and activity patterns in patients affected by bipolar depression. *Am J Med Genet B Neuropsychiatr Genet*. 2007;144B(5):631–5.

48. Bora E, Yucel M, Pantelis C. Cognitive endophenotypes of bipolar disorder: a meta-analysis of neuropsychological deficits in euthymic patients and their first-degree relatives. *J Affect Disord*. 2009;113(1–2):1–20.

49. Glahn DC, Almasy L, Barguil M, et al. Neurocognitive endophenotypes for bipolar disorder identified in multiplex multigenerational families. *Arch Gen Psychiatry*. 2010; 67(2):168–77.

50. Burdick KE, Funke B, Goldberg JF, et al. COMT genotype increases risk for bipolar I disorder and influences neurocognitive performance. *Bipolar Disord*. 2007;9(4):370–6.

51. Akiskal HS, Mallya G. Criteria for the "soft" bipolar spectrum: treatment implications. *Psychopharmacol Bull*. 1987;23(1):68–73.

52. Cassano GB, Akiskal HS, Perugi G, Musetti L, Savino M. The importance of measures of affective temperaments in genetic studies of mood disorders. *J Psychiatr Res*. 1992;26(4):257–68.

53. Evans L, Akiskal HS, Keck PE Jr, et al. Familiality of temperament in bipolar disorder: support for a genetic spectrum. *J Affect Disord*. 2005;85(1–2):153–68.

54. Gandotra S, Ram D, Kour J, Praharaj SK. Association between affective temperaments and bipolar spectrum disorders: preliminary perspectives from a controlled family study. *Psychopathology*. 2011;44(4):216–24.

55. Kesebir S, Vahip S, Akdeniz F, Yüncü Z, Alkan M, Akiskal H. Affective temperaments as measured by TEMPS-A in patients with bipolar I disorder and their first-degree relatives: a controlled study. *J Affect Disord*. 2005;85(1–2):127–33.

56. Mendlowicz MV, Jean-Louis G, Kelsoe JR, Akiskal HS. A comparison of recovered bipolar patients, healthy relatives of bipolar probands, and normal controls using the short TEMPS-A. *J Affect Disord*. 2005;85(1–2):147–51.

57. Savitz J, van der Merwe L, Ramesar R. Hypomanic, cyclothymic and hostile personality traits in bipolar spectrum illness: a family-based study. *J Psychiatr Res*. 2008;42(11):920–9.

58. Vázquez GH, Kahn C, Schiavo CE, et al. Bipolar disorders and affective temperaments: a national family study testing the "endophenotype" and "subaffective" theses using the TEMPS-A Buenos Aires. *J Affect Disord*. 2008;108(1–2):25–32.

59. Greenwood TA, Akiskal HS, Akiskal KK, Kelsoe JR. Genome-wide association study of temperament in bipolar disorder reveals significant associations with three novel loci. *Biol Psychiatry*. 2012;72(4):303–10.

60. Goes FS, Hamshere ML, Seifuddin F, et al. Genome-wide association of mood-incongruent psychotic bipolar disorder. *Transl Psychiatry*. 2012;2:e180.

61. Meier S, Mattheisen M, Vassos E, et al. Genome-wide significant association between a "negative mood delusions" dimension in bipolar disorder and genetic variation on chromosome 3q26.1. *Transl Psychiatry*. 2012;2:e165.

62. Perlis RH, Huang J, Purcell S, et al. Genome-wide association study of suicide attempts in mood disorder patients. *Am J Psychiatry*. 2010;167(12):1499–507.

63. O'Mahony E, Corvin A, O'Connell R, et al. Sibling pairs with affective disorders: resemblance of demographic and clinical features. *Psychol Med*. 2002;32(1):55–61.

64. Potash JB, Willour VL, Chiu YF, et al. The familial aggregation of psychotic symptoms in bipolar disorder pedigrees. *Am J Psychiatry*. 2001;158(8):1258–64.

65. Potash JB, Chiu Y-F, MacKinnon DF, et al. Familial aggregation of psychotic symptoms in a replication set of 69 bipolar disorder pedigrees. *Am J Med Genet B Neuropsychiatr Genet*. 2003;116B(1):90–7.

66. Fisfalen ME, Schulze TG, DePaulo JR Jr, DeGroot LJ, Badner JA, McMahon FJ. Familial variation in episode frequency in bipolar affective disorder. *Am J Psychiatry*. 2005;162(7):1266–72.

67. Saunders EH, Scott LJ, McInnis MG, Burmeister M. Familiality and diagnostic patterns of subphenotypes in the National Institutes of Mental Health bipolar sample. *Am J Med Genet B Neuropsychiatr Genet*. 2008;147B(1):18–26.

68. Duffy A, Alda M, Kutcher S, et al. A prospective study of the offspring of bipolar parents responsive and nonresponsive to lithium treatment. *J Clin Psychiatry*. 2002;63(12):1171–8.

69. Grof P, Duffy A, Cavazzoni P, et al. Is response to prophylactic lithium a familial trait? *J Clin Psychiatry*. 2002;63(10):942–7.

70. Kassem L, Lopez V, Hedeker D, et al. Familiality of polarity at illness onset in bipolar affective disorder. *Am J Psychiatry*. 2006;163(10):1754–9.

71. Goes FS, McCusker MG, Bienvenu OJ, et al. Co-morbid anxiety disorders in bipolar disorder and major depression: familial aggregation and clinical characteristics of co-morbid panic disorder, social phobia, specific phobia and obsessive-compulsive disorder. *Psychol Med*. 2012;42(7):1449–59.

72. MacKinnon DF, McMahon FJ, Simpson SG, McInnis MG, DePaulo JR. Panic disorder with familial bipolar disorder. *Biol Psychiatry*. 1997;42(2):90–5.

73. MacKinnon DF, Zandi PP, Cooper J, et al. Comorbid bipolar disorder and panic disorder in families with a high prevalence of bipolar disorder. *Am J Psychiatry*. 2002;159(1):30–5.

74. Andreasen NC, Rice J, Endicott J, Coryell W, Grove WM, Reich T. Familial rates of affective disorder. A report from the National Institute of Mental Health Collaborative Study. *Arch Gen Psychiatry*. 1987;44(5):461–9.

75. Heun R, Maier W. The distinction of bipolar II disorder from bipolar I and recurrent unipolar depression: results of a controlled family study. *Acta Psychiatr Scand*. 1993;87(4):279–84.

76. Cross-Disorder Group of the Psychiatric Genomics Consortium, Smoller JW, Craddock N, et al. Identification of risk loci with shared effects on five major psychiatric disorders: a genome-wide analysis. *Lancet*. 2013;381(9875):1371–9.

77. O'Donovan MC, Craddock N, Norton N, et al. Identification of loci associated with schizophrenia by genome-wide association and follow-up. *Nat Genet*. 2008;40(9):1053–5.

78. Schizophrenia Psychiatric Genome-Wide Association Study (GWAS) Consortium. Genome-wide association study identifies five new schizophrenia loci. *Nat Genet*. 2011;43(10):969–76.

79. Steinberg S, de Jong S, Mattheisen M, et al. Common variant at 16p11.2 conferring risk of psychosis. *Mol Psychiatry*. 2014;19(1):108–14.

80. Williams HJ, Norton N, Dwyer S, et al. Fine mapping of ZNF804A and genome-wide significant evidence for its involvement in schizophrenia and bipolar disorder. *Mol Psychiatry*. 2011;16(4):429–41.

81. Green EK, Grozeva D, Jones I, et al. The bipolar disorder risk allele at CACNA1C also confers risk of recurrent major depression and of schizophrenia. *Mol Psychiatry*. 2010;15(10):1016–22.

82. Green EK, Grozeva D, Forty L, et al. Association at SYNE1 in both bipolar disorder and recurrent major depression. *Mol Psychiatry*. 2013;18(5):614–7.

83. McMahon FJ, Akula N, Schulze TG, et al. Meta-analysis of genome-wide association data identifies a risk locus for major mood disorders on 3p21.1. *Nat Genet*. 2010;42(2):128–31.

84. The International Schizophrenia Consortium. Common polygenic variation contributes to risk of schizophrenia and bipolar disorder. *Nature*. 2009;460:748–752.

Nonheritable Risk Factors for Bipolar Disorder

Robert K. McNamara and Jeffrey R. Strawn

Overview

Bipolar disorder is a chronic psychiatric disorder typically characterized by recurrent episodes of mania and depression, as well as interepisode periods of euthymia.[1] Untreated patients with bipolar disorder typically exhibit progressive increases in the frequency and severity of manic and depressive episodes over time, particularly early in the course of illness. The initial onset of mania, and by definition bipolar I disorder, most frequently occurs during childhood and adolescence.[2] Retrospective and prospective longitudinal studies suggest that mood symptoms, including subsyndromal depression and major depressive disorder (MDD),[3,4] as well as deficits in attention,[5] frequently precede the first episode of mania. Outcome data further indicate that bipolar disorder is associated with significant psychosocial morbidity and excess premature mortality primarily attributable to suicide and cardiovascular-related diseases.[6,7] Bipolar disorder has a significant economic impact, estimated at $25–45 billion per year due in part to excess health care utilization.[8,9] Therefore, there is an urgent need to elucidate risk and resilience mechanisms associated with the pathoetiology of bipolar disorder to inform early intervention and prevention strategies.

Heritability estimates for bipolar disorder range from 60% to 87%[10] and there have been extensive efforts devoted to identify susceptibility genes for bipolar disorder using linkage and genome-wide association approaches. However, a robust and consistent pattern has yet to emerge, suggesting that the etiology of bipolar disorder is polygenic and multifactorial.[11] Although heritability for bipolar disorder is high, it is not 100% indicating that nongenetic environmental risk factors must contribute to illness onset and progression.[10] Moreover, while there is strong evidence for familial transmission of bipolar disorder,[10,12] shared environmental influences including myriad sociocultural factors may moderate risk[13] and have not been considered in previous linkage analyses. Therefore, identifying environmental risk factors for bipolar disorder may provide new insights into pathogenic mechanisms and inform novel strategies to increase resilience.

Because environmental risk factors are amenable to modification, there is an increasing appreciation for developing a clearer understanding of their role in the etiology of bipolar disorder and how they interact with genotype either directly[14] or through epigenetic effects (i.e., DNA methylation)[15,16] to increase risk. The objective of this chapter is to provide an overview of candidate environmental factors that have been investigated as potential risk factors for bipolar disorder. These candidate risk factors are critically evaluated within the framework of established epidemiological risk factor criteria, including consistency, response to treatment, prediction, specificity, and biological plausibility.[17] We also rank environmental risk factors according to their amenability to modification, and discuss the potential contribution of gene–environmental interactions to endophenotypes.

Perinatal and Childhood Developmental Factors

Maternal Infection or Stress During Pregnancy

There is abundant evidence from rodent studies indicating that prenatal maternal infection or stress has an enduring negative impact on brain development and behaviors relevant to bipolar disorder.[18,19] Although one study found a significant association between bipolar disorder and exposure to influenza epidemic during the second trimester,[20] other studies have not replicated this association.[12,21,22] For example, in a population-based cohort of 2.1 million individuals in the Danish Civil Registration System linked with the Danish Psychiatric Central Register, rates of influenza during the in utero period were not associated with increased risk of developing bipolar affective disorder after adjusting for a family history of mental illness.[12] Although additional research is needed, these data suggest that infection during pregnancy is not a significant risk factor for bipolar disorder.

Regarding maternal stress during pregnancy, a large population study found that bereavement stress prior to conception or postnatally was not associated with increased risk of developing bipolar disorder before and after adjusting for familial history of psychopathology.[23] A retrospective study found that offspring in their first trimester, and most robustly during the third month in utero, during the Arab-Israeli war of June 1967, were more likely to subsequently be admitted to hospitals for bipolar disorder (OR: 2.4).[24] However, a second retrospective study found that the incidence of bipolar disorder in children who were in the second (OR: 1.4) and third (OR: 1.3) trimesters during the winter famine of 1944–1945 in Holland was not significantly elevated compared to the general population.[25] Therefore, data from large epidemiological studies suggest that although extreme maternal stress during the second or third trimester of pregnancy may increase the risk factor of developing bipolar disorder, less severe stress does not appear to do so.

Obstetric Complications

Although maternal obstetric complications have been widely regarded as potential environmental risk factors for schizophrenia,[26] obstetric factors may also increase risk for affective disorders. For example, retrospective studies found that patients with bipolar disorder were significantly more likely than their healthy siblings to be exposed to a range of prenatal and perinatal obstetric complications, including maternal anemia, rubella, prematurity, prolonged duration of labor, and neonatal respiratory problems.[27,28] Another study found that low birth weight was associated with mood and non-mood disorders in bipolar offspring even after controlling for family history of unipolar disorder, bipolar disorder, or substance use disorder.[29] However, a fourth study found that patients with bipolar disorder did not experience a greater frequency or severity of labor and delivery complications compared with matched controls, and rates of obstetric adversity were unrelated to the presence or absence of family history of psychiatric disorders.[30] A meta-analysis of 22 studies investigating associations between exposure to obstetric complications and the subsequent development of bipolar disorder did not observe elevated risk (OR: 1.0).[31] Although women with bipolar disorder and their offspring may be at greater risk for obstetric complications,[32–34] extant evidence suggests that maternal obstetric complications do not represent a significant nonheritable risk factor for bipolar disorder.

Urban Birth, Season of Birth, and Birth Order

Evidence regarding season of birth and bipolar disorder is conflicting. At least two studies observed excess winter (December–March) births in patients with bipolar disorder compared with the general population.[35,36] However, a population-based cohort of 2.1 million individuals in the Danish Civil Registration System linked with the Danish Psychiatric Central Register found that season of birth was not associated with increased risk of developing bipolar disorder after adjusting for family history of mental illness.[12] The latter study also did not observe an effect of birth order or being born in an urban area. Taken together, these data suggest that urban birth, season of birth, and birth order are not robust risk factors for bipolar disorder.

Early Parental Loss

In rodents and primates, early maternal separation is associated with a lasting negative impact on healthy brain development and behavior in adulthood.[37] In a population-based cohort of 2.1 million individuals in the Danish Civil Registration System linked with the Danish Psychiatric Central Register, children who experienced parental loss before their fifth birthday had a 4-fold (maternal) or 2-fold (paternal) increased risk of developing bipolar disorder after adjusting for history of mental illness in first-degree relatives.[12] A case-control study similarly found that the rate of early parental loss was increased in bipolar disorder (OR = 2.6).[38] Additionally, suicide of a mother or of a sibling was associated with increased risk of first mania or mixed episode (OR: 5.7), whereas the death of a relative by other causes than suicide was not associated with increased risk.[39] A Japanese study did not find a significant difference in the incidence of paternal or maternal death or separation before age 16 in individuals with bipolar disorder compared with healthy people.[40] These findings suggest that early parental loss may increase the risk for bipolar disorder, and cross-national inconsistencies highlight potential moderating effects of sociocultural factors.

Childhood Trauma and Stressful Life Events

Animal studies have demonstrated the lasting impact of chronic unpredictable stress on behavioral indices of depression.[41] Additionally, a body of evidence suggests that stressful life events and psychosocial stressors frequently precede mood dysregulation in bipolar disorder.[42] Prospective studies have observed a significant association between proximal life events and manic and depressive relapse in patients with bipolar disorder that could not be attributed to medication compliance.[43–45] Moreover, an increase in negative life events during the months and years preceding the initial onset of mood symptoms has been observed in several studies,[46–50] and it may be independent of family history of psychiatric disorders.[51] Interestingly, one study found that prior early adversity was associated with younger age of bipolar disorder onset and a lower threshold for a stress-induced affective episode recurrences.[52] This finding suggests that distal stressful life events can amplify the impact of proximal stressors. Retrospective studies also found that sexual and/or physical abuse is a common distal antecedent of bipolar disorder[53,54] and is associated with a 2-fold increased risk of developing bipolar disorder after adjustment for family psychopathology.[55] Additionally, childhood trauma may result in an earlier age at onset, rapid cycling course, psychotic features, suicidal behavior, and comorbid substance abuse.[53,56,57] These and other findings suggest that early childhood trauma increases the risk for bipolar disorder, perhaps through a sensitizing mechanism that leads to an enduring reduction in the threshold for stress-reactivity.

Antecedent Drug Exposure

In view of cross-national epidemiological evidence that bipolar disorder is more frequently diagnosed in prepubertal children in the United States and rarely in the Netherlands, it was hypothesized that use of psychostimulants and antidepressants may accelerate the onset of bipolar disorder in at-risk children.[58] Indeed, the number of stimulant prescriptions in the United States increased 7-fold over the last decade,[59] and during that period there was a 40-fold increase in the diagnosis of childhood and adolescent bipolar disorder in office-based medical settings.[60] Moreover, counter to treatment guidelines, antidepressants are among the most frequently prescribed class of psychotropics for patients with bipolar disorder in tertiary medical settings.[61] Therefore, developing a more comprehensive understanding of the relationships between psychostimulant and antidepressant medication exposure and the risk for bipolar disorder may have important implications for conventional clinical practice.

Antidepressant Medications

Subsyndromal depression, major depressive disorder, and anxiety frequently precede the initial onset of mania[3,4] and are commonly treated with antidepressant medications regardless of the risk for developing bipolar disorder. An emerging body of evidence suggests that treatment with antidepressants, particularly those with noradrenergic-augmenting effects, may precipitate or exacerbate suicidality and manic symptoms and possibly reduce the age at onset of mania.[62-64] An epidemiological study found that peripubertal children exposed to antidepressants were at highest risk for manic conversion,[65] and a second smaller study found that children who received prior antidepressant treatment had an earlier onset of bipolar disorder than never exposed children.[66] Additionally, several cohort studies of children and adolescents with or at high risk for bipolar disorder have observed a high rate of antidepressant-induced manic symptoms and new-onset suicidal ideation.[68-70] While these data suggest that youth with familial risk for bipolar disorder are vulnerable to antidepressant-induced manic symptoms, it is unclear whether antidepressant medications represent a nonheritable risk factor for bipolar disorder in youth without familial risk.

Psychostimulant Medications

Deficits in concentration and attention also frequently precede the onset of bipolar disorder and are commonly initially treated with psychostimulant medications, including methylphenidate or amphetamine (AMPH) derivatives, regardless of the risk for developing bipolar disorder. While the role of early psychostimulants treatment as a risk factor for bipolar disorder is poorly understood, acute treatment with psychostimulants may produce clinical features that are analogous to idiopathic mania in a subset of individuals.[71] Moreover, the incremental increase in psychomotor responses (e.g., increased eye-blink rate) observed in healthy subjects following repeated AMPH treatment is not exhibited by first-episode manic or psychotic patients,[72] and it may reflect presensitization secondary to prior exposure to psychostimulants and/or stressors. Although controlled trials found that treatment with psychostimulants is effective and safe for treating attention-deficit/hyperactivity disorder (ADHD) in youth with bipolar disorder when administered in conjunction with mood stabilizers,[73-75] it is not clear that they are safe for youth at high risk for developing bipolar disorder in the absence of mood stabilizers. A retrospective study found that adolescents with bipolar disorder and a history of stimulant exposure prior to onset had an earlier age at onset of mania than those without prior stimulant exposure, independent of co-occurring ADHD.[76] In contrast, a 6-year prospective study found that treatment with psychostimulant medications decreased the rate of switching to bipolar disorder in children/adolescents with ADHD.[77] Although controversial and requiring additional investigation to identify vulnerability factors, these data highlight a potential risk associated with early psychostimulant exposure.

Substance Use/Abuse

Substance use and bipolar disorders commonly co-occur, and up to 60% of individuals with bipolar disorder develop substance abuse or dependence at some point during their lives.[78,79] Additionally, substance abuse frequently precedes the initial onset of mania.[80] Moreover, approximately 40% of clinically referred bipolar adolescents have a substance use disorder (SUD), suggesting a 5- to 6-fold increased risk of SUD in adolescents with bipolar disorder compared with adolescents without major psychopathology.[81,82] Although the majority of adolescents with bipolar disorder develop SUD following the onset of bipolar disorder, a substantial portion (approximately one third) will experience bipolar disorder onset following the onset of SUD.[82–84] Additional studies are required to prospectively assess whether substance use and abuse increase risk for developing bipolar disorder independent of familial risk for bipolar disorder.

Medical Conditions
Chronic Infection

Toxoplasma gondii (*T. gondii*) is a common protozoan parasite found in cat urine, and rodent and epidemiological studies suggest that *T. gondii* infection may represent a risk factor for developing mood and psychotic disorders.[85] In a population-based sample of 7,440 respondents from the third National Health and Nutrition Survey, the rate of *T. gondii* infection was greater in respondents with a history of bipolar disorder (OR: 2.4) but not MDD (OR: 0.8) compared with healthy subjects.[86] In a cross-sectional study conducted in France, the prevalence of *T. gondii* infection was greater in patients with bipolar disorder (OR: 2.7) than healthy subjects.[87] Another cross-sectional study found that among patients with bipolar disorder or MDD, suicide attempters had significantly higher *T. gondii* antibody titers than nonattempters independent of diagnosis.[88] Interestingly, mood-stabilizer medications were found to inhibit replication of *T. gondii* in vitro.[89] It may also be relevant that manic symptoms secondary to human immunodeficiency virus (HIV) infection have been documented,[90] and that antiviral therapy was found to be protective against the development of HIV-associated manic symptoms.[91] While these preliminary findings suggest that chronic infection may be associated with bipolar disorder and suicidality, additional research is needed to confirm this suggestion and to rule out the contribution of other risk factors including family history of psychopathology.

Head Injury and Seizures

In a cross-sectional cohort of individuals in the Danish Civil Registration System linked with the Danish Psychiatric Central Register, a history of head injury was associated with an increased risk of bipolar disorder when occurring less than 5 years before the first psychiatric admission (OR: 1.55).[92] However, the latter study did not adjust for other risk factors, including family history of psychopathology or substance abuse. Indeed, a cohort study of 1,275 patients with bipolar disorder and at least two biologically related first-degree relatives with bipolar disorder also observed a higher rate of traumatic head injury patients compared with subjects with no history of mental illness.[93] There is a 3-fold increased risk of developing seizures following mild brain injury and a 5-fold increase following severe brain injury.[94] Bipolar disorder and seizure disorders (i.e., epilepsy) have overlapping clinical features and treatments,[95] and mood disorders are frequently comorbid with epilepsy.[96] In a population-based survey in the United States, symptoms of bipolar disorder were observed in 12% of epilepsy patients, half of whom received a bipolar disorder diagnosis.[97] A population study found that patients with epilepsy had a substantially increased risk for bipolar disorder (OR: 6.3).[98] While these preliminary findings suggest that traumatic head injury and seizures may increase risk for bipolar disorder, additional research is needed to rule out the contribution of family history of psychopathology and reverse causality.

Multiple Sclerosis

Similar to bipolar disorder, multiple sclerosis is a progressive disorder that is often characterized by a relapsing-remitting course, subtotal concordance rates among monozygotic twins, and cross-national variation in lifetime prevalence rates.[99,100] Like multiple sclerosis,[101] bipolar disorder is associated with reduced myelin-associated gene expression[102,103] and myelin staining[104] in postmortem brain, and neuroimaging studies have observed deficits in central white matter structural integrity.[105–107] While depression is the most frequent psychiatric symptom observed in patients with multiple sclerosis,[108–112] a large population study observed a prevalence rate of 2.4% for bipolar disorder among 8,983 patients with multiple sclerosis,[112] a rate that is approximately 2-fold greater than the general population.[113] Early case studies reported "secondary" mania occurring in patients with multiple sclerosis that coincided with neurological manifestations and magnetic resonance imaging (MRI) lesions.[114–116] While these associations suggest that multiple sclerosis and bipolar disorder have overlapping pathoetiological and clinical features, it is not currently clear whether multiple sclerosis is an antecedent of bipolar disorder or visa versa,[117–119] or whether there are common heritable and nonheritable risk factors.

Diet and Nutrition

Although diet and nutrition remain highly neglected variables in investigations of bipolar disorder risk, evidence suggests that patients with bipolar disorder have poor nutritional habits, including diets containing lower amounts of fruits and vegetables, and higher sugar and fat levels.[120-122] Moreover, a large percentage of adults with bipolar disorder are overweight or obese, which may be due in part to poor diet and pharmacological medications,[122-126] though rates of overweight and obesity are also increasing in the general population. Emerging data also suggest that greater consumption of sugary beverages (i.e., soda) is associated with attention problems, hyperactivity, and conduct problems as well as with greater aggression, depression, and suicidality in children and adolescents.[127-129] A meta-analyses additionally suggests that exclusion of artificial food colors from the diet may have clinical benefits in ADHD youth.[130,131] Therefore, poor diet and nutrition may represent a nonheritable risk factor for bipolar symptoms as well as comorbid attention deficits.

Vitamin Deficiencies

Emerging evidence from cross-sectional and preliminary intervention studies suggest that vitamin deficiencies may contribute to the etiology and course of mood disorders.[132,133] Indeed, a large portion of adult patients with mood disorders, including bipolar disorder, were found to consume levels of vitamin B (i.e., thiamine, riboflavin, and folate) that were below the estimated daily requirement,[134] and cross-sectional studies observed lower serum folate levels in patients with unipolar and bipolar depression than the general population.[135] Furthermore, folic acid supplementation reduced the frequency and duration of mood symptoms in a sample of lithium-treated bipolar patients.[136] A preliminary open-label intervention study using a multinutrient supplement (containing 16 minerals, 14 vitamins, 3 amino acids, and 3 antioxidants) observed reductions in depression and mania scores in a small sample of medication-free pediatric patients with bipolar spectrum disorders.[137] Additional controlled trials are needed to determine whether dietary vitamin deficiency represents a nonheritable risk factor for bipolar disorder.

Fatty Acid Deficiencies

Converging evidence also suggests that dietary deficiencies in long-chain omega-3 (LCn-3) fatty acids, found in high concentrations in certain fish, may contribute to the pathophysiology of mood disorders.[138] Cross-national epidemiological studies suggest that greater habitual dietary intake of LCn-3 fatty acid intake from fish/seafood is associated with reduced lifetime prevalence rates for bipolar disorder.[139] Red blood cell (RBC) membrane LCn-3 fatty acid composition is positively correlated with dietary EPA + DHA intake,[140] and case-control studies observed significantly lower RBC LCn-3 fatty acid levels in pediatric and adult patients with bipolar disorder.[141-144] While it not currently known whether LCn-3 fatty acid deficiency observed in bipolar patients is due to dietary insufficiency and/or heritable genetic factors, increasing dietary LCn-3 fatty acid intake is sufficient to normalize RBC LCn-3 fatty acid levels in bipolar patients.[145,146] Independent meta-analyses of controlled trials have observed a significant advantage of LCn-3 fatty acid supplementation over placebo for reducing depression symptom severity in patients with bipolar disorder or MDD.[147–149] A preliminary open-label flexible dosing trial found that LCn-3 fatty acid monotherapy significantly reduced manic symptom severity in pediatric and adolescent bipolar patients.[146] These and other data suggest that dietary LCn-3 fatty acid insufficiency may represent a nonheritable risk factor for bipolar disorder.

Nutrient Sensitivities

Sensitivities to commonly consumed nutrients have also been investigated in the context of bipolar disorder. For example, cross-sectional studies observed increased levels of antibodies to gliadin, which is derived from the wheat protein gluten, in patients with bipolar disorder,[150,151] and adult patients with mood disorders were found to consume higher amounts of whole-grain products compared with Dietary Reference Intakes.[120] It is also notable that *T. gondii* infection significantly increases levels of antigluten antibodies in mice,[152] suggesting a nonheritable etiology. Additionally, a cross-sectional study found significantly higher levels of antibodies to bovine milk casein in patients with bipolar disorder, which were positively associated with manic symptom severity.[153] While these preliminary findings suggest that bipolar disorder may be associated with heightened immunoreactivity to commonly consumed nutrients, it is not currently known whether repeated exposure to these common food components increases risk of developing bipolar disorder independent of genetic risk factors.

Summary and Future Directions

The objective of this chapter was to provide an overview of candidate nonheritable (environmental) risk factors implicated in the etiology of bipolar disorder. Several putative environmental risk factors have been identified that may occur proximal or distal to the initial onset bipolar disorder, involve sensitization mechanisms, and may be tempered by to-be-defined resilience mechanisms (Fig. 6.1). Low-risk factors include maternal infection, obstetric complications, and urban birth, season of birth, and birth order. Intermediate-risk factors include extreme stress during pregnancy and negative life events. High-risk factors include early maternal loss, childhood sexual and/or physical abuse, *T. gondii* infection, head injury, and seizures. Tentative risk factors also include psychostimulant and antidepressant exposure, dietary nutrient sensitivities and deficiencies, and multiple sclerosis. A risk factor, unlike a risk marker, implies a causal link with the illness, correction of which reduces the risk of developing the illness and must satisfy several different criteria, including prediction of illness onset, response to treatment, specificity, and biological plausibility.[17] However, there are limited data available to evaluate fully the validity of these risk factors, methodological limitations including a lack of standard definitions of risk factors and failure to account for gene–environment interactions, and uncertainties regarding whether bipolar symptoms are organic versus idiopathic. Therefore current candidate nonheritable risk factors must be considered tentative pending additional evidence.

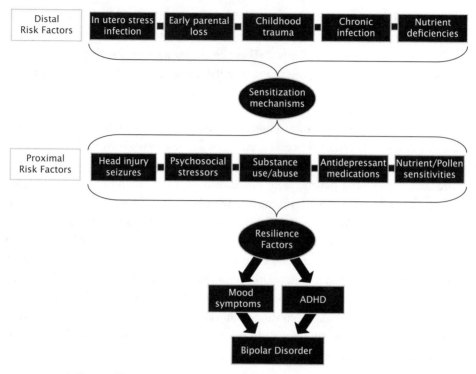

FIGURE 6.1 A diagram illustrating putative distal and proximal nonheritable risk factors for bipolar disorder. Distal risk factors may amplify the impact of proximal risk factors through a sensitization mechanism, and their combined effects may be tempered by resilience factors that could be genetic as well as nongenetic (i.e., nutritional deficiencies). Distal and proximal risk factors may initially lead to the development of prodromal mood (depression) and cognitive (ADHD) symptoms in the years preceding the initial onset of bipolar disorder. ADHD, attention-deficit/hyperactivity disorder.

Regarding the "prediction of illness onset" risk factor criterion, history of extreme stress during pregnancy and distal and/or proximal negative life events, early parental loss, suicide of a mother or of a sibling, childhood sexual and/or physical abuse, *T. gondii* infection, head injury, and antidepressant exposure have been found to precede the onset of bipolar disorder. Because some of the reviewed putative environmental risk factors are more amenable to modification (Table 6.1), it is theoretically possible to investigate whether modification or removal of these risk factors can mitigate the risk of developing bipolar disorder in future prospective longitudinal studies to evaluate the "response to treatment" criterion. While it may be less feasible to modify some candidate environmental risk factors (e.g., *T. gondii* infection, head injury, early parental loss), other risk factors, including antidepressant medication exposure and dietary nutrient sensitivities and deficiencies, are highly amenable to modification.

Regarding the "specificity" risk factor criterion (i.e., the risk factor is specific for bipolar disorder), many of the environmental risk factors reviewed in the context of bipolar disorder have also been implicated as risk factors for schizophrenia and other psychiatric disorders.[26,154,155] It is notable, therefore, that approximately 50% of bipolar

TABLE 6.1 Modifiability of Nonheritable Risk Factors

Lowest	Low	Intermediate	High
Genotype	Stressful life events	Childhood trauma	Diet and nutrition
Parental loss	Multiple sclerosis	Chronic infection	Antidepressants
	Head injury	Maternal stress	Psychostimulants
	Seizures	Obstetric complications	Substance abuse

disorder patients will experience a psychotic episode,[156] and the high rate of comorbid ADHD in pediatric patients with bipolar disorder[5] suggests that there may be common risk factors. For example, preterm birth and low birth weight have been implicated as a risk factor for ADHD[157] and mood disorders, including bipolar disorder.[29] Furthermore, depressive symptoms or MDD frequently may precede the initial onset of mania by several years,[158] and risk factors for MDD may therefore also be relevant to the development of bipolar disorder. For example, cross-national epidemiological studies suggest that greater habitual dietary intake of LCn-3 fatty acid intake is associated with reduced lifetime prevalence rates for both MDD[159,160] and bipolar disorder.[139] These examples suggest that nonheritable risk factors implicated in the etiology of bipolar disorder do not satisfy the "specificity" criterion, and they may instead contribute to pathoetiological and clinical features shared by different psychiatric disorders.

Future investigation of how nonheritable risk factors contribute to quantitative intermediate phenotypes (endophenotypes) associated with bipolar disorder may represent a more sensitive approach over seeking associations with clinical diagnostic features. An endophenotype approach also permits evaluation of the "biological plausibility" risk factor criterion. For example, dysregulation in immune-inflammatory signaling homeostasis, which is mediated in part by circulating peripheral blood mononuclear cells (PBMCs), represents a phenotype relevant to the pathophysiology and treatment of bipolar disorder.[161–163] For example, a case-control study found that lipopolysaccharide-stimulated PBMC cytokine production was elevated in medication-free bipolar patients, and that this elevated response was attenuated in lithium-treated patients.[164] Importantly, concordance rates of elevated markers of immune-inflammatory signaling in circulating PBMC from monozygotic versus dizygotic bipolar twins indicate that nonheritable risk factors are responsible.[165] Candidate nonheritable risk factors that may contribute to elevated PBMC-mediated pro-inflammatory-immune signaling activity in bipolar disorder include LCn-3 fatty acid deficiency,[166] *T. gondii* infection,[87] childhood maltreatment,[167–169] early-life stressors,[170,171] gluten sensitivity,[172] and exposure to seasonal allergens (i.e., pollen)[173–176] (Fig. 6.2). Therefore, PBMC pro-inflammatory-immune signaling may represent a pathophysiologically relevant endophenotype for future studies evaluating risk mechanisms underlying the development of bipolar disorder.

There is also increasing interest in using *central* endophenotypes to identify relevant genetic risk alleles[177] as well as gene–environment interactions.[14] There is growing consensus that disturbances in fronto-limbic structural and functional connectivity

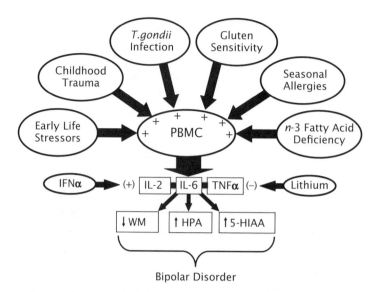

FIGURE 6.2 A diagram illustrating the impact of putative nonheritable risk factors for bipolar disorder on a candidate endophenotype, pro-inflammatory cytokine (IL-2, IL-6, TNFα) production by circulating peripheral blood mononuclear cells (PBMC). Similarly, interferon-alpha (INFα) increases PBMC pro-inflammatory cytokine production and is associated with manic and depressive symptoms in a subset of individuals, whereas the mood-stabilizer lithium decreases PBMC pro-inflammatory cytokine production. Pro-inflammatory cytokines may have detrimental downstream effects on central white matter (WM) integrity, hypothalamic-pituitary-adrenal axis (HPA) activity, and central serotonin turnover (5-HIAA), which in turn lead to fronto-limbic connectivity deficits, stress-axis hyperactivity, and mood features that characterize bipolar disorder.

may represent an endophenotype relevant to the pathoetiology of bipolar disorder.[178] Although not traditionally thought of as a neurodevelopmental disorder, the initial onset of mania frequently occurs during childhood and adolescence, a period associated with maturational changes in fronto-limbic circuits.[179] Indeed, longitudinal and cross-sectional neuroimaging evidence suggests that fronto-limbic connectivity deficits, reductions in amygdala volume, and frontal white matter structural pathology are evident early in the course of the disorder.[180–182] Candidate nonheritable risk factors that may contribute to reductions in amygdala volume include perinatal asphyxia[183] and *T. gondii* infection,[184] and nonheritable risk factors that may contribute to white matter structural pathology include elevated immune-inflammatory signaling[185] and chronic psychostimulant exposure.[186–188]

Because evidence from family and twin studies indicating that the risk of developing bipolar disorder is mediated by both environmental and genetic factors, a more integrated approach will be required to elucidate risk and resilience mechanisms. There is increasing theoretical and experimental interest in using a "gene–environment interaction" approach, which posits that environmental factors cause the disorder and that genotype determines either vulnerability or resilience to an environmental insult.[14] For example, a prospective-longitudinal study found that maltreated children possessing a polymorphism associated with lower monoamine oxidase A (MAOA) activity were more likely to develop conduct disorder, antisocial personality, and adult violent crime than maltreated children with a high-activity genotype.[189] A second study found that individuals with one or two copies of the short allele in the promoter region of the serotonin transporter exhibited more depressive symptoms and suicidality following stressful life events than individuals with two copies of the long allele.[190] A third study found that the precipitation of manic symptoms (anger/irritability) in hepatitis C patients following interferon-alpha treatment occurred only in carriers of the tumor necrosis factor-alpha promoter polymorphism with lower LCn-3 fatty acid levels.[191] These examples highlight the importance of evaluating interactions between candidate genetic and environmental risk factors in future studies investigating risk mechanisms associated with the development of bipolar disorder.

Because some of the nonheritable risk factors are highly amenable to modification, additional prospective longitudinal studies are needed to determine whether their manipulation can mitigate the risk of developing bipolar disorder. Indeed, there is growing interest in identifying individuals that are at ultra-high risk for developing bipolar disorder,[67] and developing safe and feasible intervention strategies to delay or prevent the initial onset of bipolar disorder.[192] Because there is strong evidence for familial transmission of bipolar disorder, offspring of bipolar parents may be ideally suited to evaluate the protective effects of early interventions, as well as for elucidating gene–environment interactions, relevant central and peripheral endophenotypes, and optimal developmental windows for interventions. As proof of principle, a prospective intervention trial found that dietary LCn-3 fatty acid supplementation was more efficacious than placebo for preventing or delaying the initial onset of psychosis in adolescents meeting ultra-high-risk criteria.[193] Analogous primary prevention trials that manipulate modifiable risk factors in adolescents meeting ultra-high-risk criteria for developing mania are currently feasible and warranted.

In conclusion, subtotal heritability estimates based on family and twin studies indicate that the risk for developing bipolar disorder is mediated by both genetic and nonheritable risk factors. Because nonheritable risk factors may be amenable to modification, elucidating their role in the etiology of bipolar disorder will be necessary to inform early intervention and prevention strategies.

Author Disclosures

Dr. McNamara was a member of the scientific advisory board for the Inflammation Research Foundation. He has received grant support from Martek Biosciences Inc, Inflammation Research Foundation, Ortho-McNeil Janssen, NARSAD, and the National Institutes of Health.

Dr. Strawn has received grant support from Eli Lilly, Shire, Forest Research Laboratories, Lundbeck, and the American Academy of Child and Adolescent Psychiatry.

This work was supported in part by National Institute of Health grants MH083924 and AG03617, and a NARSAD Independent Investigator Award to R.K.M. R.K.M. has received research support from Martek Biosciences Inc, Inflammation Research Foundation (IRF), Ortho-McNeil Janssen, AstraZeneca, Eli Lilly. R.K.M. has served as a member of the IRF scientific advisory board. J.R.S. has received research support from Eli Lilly, Shire and from the American Academy of Child and Adolescent Psychiatry.

References

1. Goodwin FK, Jamison KR. *Manic-Depressive Illness: Bipolar Disorders and Recurrent Depression.* 2nd ed. New York, NY: Oxford University Press; 2007.
2. Perlis RH, Dennehy EB, Miklowitz DJ, et al. Retrospective age at onset of bipolar disorder and outcome during two-year follow-up: results from the STEP-BD study. *Bipolar Disord.* 2009;11:391–400.
3. Berk M, Conus P, Lucas N, et al. Setting the stage: from prodrome to treatment resistance in bipolar disorder. *Bipolar Disord.* 2007;9:671–8.
4. Conus P, Ward J, Hallam KT, et al. The proximal prodrome to first episode mania—a new target for early intervention. *Bipolar Disord.* 2008;10:555–65.
5. Singh MK, DelBello MP, Kowatch RA, Strakowski SM. Co-occurrence of bipolar and attention-deficit hyperactivity disorders in children. *Bipolar Disord.* 2006;8:710–20.
6. Angst F, Stassen HH, Clayton PJ, Angst J. Mortality of patients with mood disorders: follow-up over 34–38 years. *J Affect Disord.* 2002;68:167–81.
7. Osby U, Brandt L, Correia N, Ekbom A, Sparén P. Excess mortality in bipolar and unipolar disorder in Sweden. *Arch Gen Psychiatry.* 2001;58:844–50.
8. Begley CE, Annegers JF, Swann AC, et al. The lifetime cost of bipolar disorder in the US: an estimate for new cases in 1998. *Pharmacoeconomics.* 2001;19:483–95.
9. Kleinman L, Lowin A, Flood E, Gandhi G, Edgell E, Revicki D. Costs of bipolar disorder. *Pharmacoeconomics.* 2003;21:601–22.
10. Smoller JW, Finn CT. Family, twin, and adoption studies of bipolar disorder. *Am J Med Genet C Semin Med Genet.* 2003;123C:48–58.
11. Seifuddin F, Mahon PB, Judy J, et al. Meta-analysis of genetic association studies on bipolar disorder. *Am J Med Genet B Neuropsychiatr Genet.* 2012;159:508–18.
12. Mortensen PB, Pedersen CB, Melbye M, Mors O, Ewald H. Individual and familial risk factors for bipolar affective disorders in Denmark. *Arch Gen Psychiatry.* 2003;60:1209–15.
13. Weissman MM, Bland RC, Canino GJ, et al. Cross-national epidemiology of major depression and bipolar disorder. *JAMA* 1996;276:293–9.
14. Caspi A, Moffitt TE. Gene-environment interactions in psychiatry: joining forces with neuroscience. *Nat Rev Neurosci.* 2006;7:583–90.
15. Perroud N, Dayer A, Piguet C, et al. Childhood maltreatment and methylation of the glucocorticoid receptor gene NR3C1 in bipolar disorder. *Br J Psychiatry.* 2014;204(1):30–5.
16. Zhang TY, Labonté B, Wen XL, Turecki G, Meaney MJ. Epigenetic mechanisms for the early environmental regulation of hippocampal glucocorticoid receptor gene expression in rodents and humans. *Neuropsychopharmacology.* 2013;38:111–23.
17. Hill, AB. The environment and disease: association or causation? *Proc R Soc Med.* 1965; 58:295–300.
18. Boksa P. Effects of prenatal infection on brain development and behavior: a review of findings from animal models. *Brain Behav Immun.* 2010;24:881–97.
19. Kofman O. The role of prenatal stress in the etiology of developmental behavioural disorders. *Neurosci Biobehav Rev.* 2002;26:457–70.
20. Machón RA, Mednick SA, Huttunen MO. Adult major affective disorder after prenatal exposure to an influenza epidemic. *Arch Gen Psychiatry.* 1997;54:322–8.

21. Cannon M, Cotter D, Coffey VP, et al. Prenatal exposure to the 1957 influenza epidemic and adult schizophrenia: a follow-up study. *Br J Psychiatry*. 1996;168:368–71.

22. Morgan V, Castle D, Page A, et al. Influenza epidemics and incidence of schizophrenia, affective disorders and mental retardation in Western Australia: no evidence of a major effect. *Schizophr Res*. 1997;26:25–39.

23. Class QA, Abel KM, Khashan AS, et al. Offspring psychopathology following preconception, prenatal and postnatal maternal bereavement stress. *Psychol Med*. 2014;44(1):71–84.

24. Kleinhaus K, Harlap S, Perrin M, et al. Prenatal stress and affective disorders in a population birth cohort. *Bipolar Disord*. 2013;15:92–9.

25. Brown AS, van Os J, Driessens C, Hoek HW, Susser ES. Further evidence of relation between prenatal famine and major affective disorder. *Am J Psychiatry*. 2000;157:190–5.

26. Brown AS. The environment and susceptibility to schizophrenia. *Prog Neurobiol*. 2011;93:23–58.

27. Kinney DK, Yurgelun-Todd DA, Levy DL, Medoff D, Lajonchere CM, Radford-Paregol M. Obstetrical complications in patients with bipolar disorder and their siblings. *Psychiatry Res*. 1993;48:47–56.

28. Kinney DK, Yurgelun-Todd DA, Tohen M, Tramer S. Pre- and perinatal complications and risk for bipolar disorder: a retrospective study. *J Affect Disord*. 1998;50:117–24.

29. Wals M, Reichart CG, Hillegers MH, et al. Impact of birth weight and genetic liability on psychopathology in children of bipolar parents. *J Am Acad Child Adolesc Psychiatry*. 2003;42:1116–21.

30. Browne R, Byrne M, Mulryan N, et al. Labour and delivery complications at birth and later mania. An Irish case register study. *Br J Psychiatry*. 2000;176:369–72.

31. Scott J, McNeill Y, Cavanagh J, Cannon M, Murray R. Exposure to obstetric complications and subsequent development of bipolar disorder: systematic review. *Br J Psychiatry*. 2006;189:3–11.

32. Jablensky AV, Morgan V, Zubrick SR, Bower C, Yellachich LA. Pregnancy, delivery, and neonatal complications in a population cohort of women with schizophrenia and major affective disorders. *Am J Psychiatry*. 2005;162:79–91.

33. Lee HC, Lin HC. Maternal bipolar disorder increased low birthweight and preterm births: a nationwide population-based study. *J Affect Disord*. 2010;121:100–5.

34. Singh MK, DelBello MP, Soutullo C, Stanford KE, McDonough-Ryan P, Strakowski SM. Obstetrical complications in children at high risk for bipolar disorder. *J Psychiatr Res*. 2007;41:680–5.

35. Mino Y, Oshima I, Okagami K. Seasonality of birth in patients with mood disorders in Japan. *J Affect Disord*. 2000;59:41–6.

36. Torrey EF, Rawlings RR, Ennis JM, Merrill DD, Flores DS. Birth seasonality in bipolar disorder, schizophrenia, schizoaffective disorder and stillbirths. *Schizophr Res*. 1996;21:141–9.

37. Sánchez MM, Ladd CO, Plotsky PM. Early adverse experience as a developmental risk factor for later psychopathology: evidence from rodent and primate models. *Dev Psychopathol*. 2001;13:419–49.

38. Agid O, Shapira B, Zislin J, et al. Environment and vulnerability to major psychiatric illness: a case control study of early parental loss in major depression, bipolar disorder and schizophrenia. *Mol Psychiatry*. 1999;4:163–72.

39. Kessing LV, Agerbo E, Mortensen PB. Major stressful life events and other risk factors for first admission with mania. *Bipolar Disord*. 2004;6:122–29.

40. Furukawa TA, Ogura A, Hirai T, Fujihara S, Kitamura T, Takahashi K. Early parental separation experiences among patients with bipolar disorder and major depression: a case-control study. *J Affect Disord*. 1999;52:85–91.

41. Hill MN, Hellemans KG, Verma P, Gorzalka BB, Weinberg J. Neurobiology of chronic mild stress: parallels to major depression. *Neurosci Biobehav Rev*. 2012;36:2085–117.

42. Post RM, Leverich GS. The role of psychosocial stress in the onset and progression of bipolar disorder and its comorbidities: the need for earlier and alternative modes of therapeutic intervention. *Dev Psychopathol*. 2006;18:1181–211.

43. Christensen EM, Gjerris A, Larsen JK, et al. Life events and onset of a new phase in bipolar affective disorder. *Bipolar Disord*. 2003;5:356–61.

44. Ellicott A, Hammen C, Gitlin M, Brown G, Jamison K. Life events and the course of bipolar disorder. *Am J Psychiatry*. 1990;147:1194–8.

45. Hunt N, Bruce-Jones W, Silverstone T. Life events and relapse in bipolar affective disorder. *J Affect Disord*. 1992;25:13–20.

46. Horesh N, Apter A, Zalsman G. Timing, quantity and quality of stressful life events in childhood and preceding the first episode of bipolar disorder. *J Affect Disord*. 2011;134:434–7.

47. Horesh N, Iancu I. A comparison of life events in patients with unipolar disorder or bipolar disorder and controls. *Compr Psychiatry*. 2010;51:157–64.

48. Kennedy S, Thompson R, Stancer HC, Roy A, Persad E. Life events precipitating mania. *Br J Psychiatry*. 1983;142:398–403.

49. Mathew MR, Chandrasekaran R, Sivakumar V. A study of life events in mania. *J Affect Disord*. 1994;32:157–161.

50. Sclare P, Creed F. Life events and the onset of mania. *Br J Psychiatry*. 1990;156:508–14.

51. Hillegers MH, Burger H, Wals M, et al. Impact of stressful life events, familial loading and their interaction on the onset of mood disorders: study in a high-risk cohort of adolescent offspring of parents with bipolar disorder. *Br J Psychiatry*. 2004;185:97–101.

52. Dienes KA, Hammen C, Henry RM, Cohen AN, Daley SE. The stress sensitization hypothesis: understanding the course of bipolar disorder. *J Affect Disord*. 2006;95:43–9.

53. Garno JL, Goldberg JF, Ramirez PM, Ritzler BA. Impact of childhood abuse on the clinical course of bipolar disorder. *Br J Psychiatry*. 2005;186:121–5.

54. Romero S, Birmaher B, Axelson D, et al. Prevalence and correlates of physical and sexual abuse in children and adolescents with bipolar disorder. *J Affect Disord*. 2009;112:144–50.

55. Sugaya L, Hasin DS, Olfson M, Lin KH, Grant BF, Blanco C. Child physical abuse and adult mental health: a national study. *J Trauma Stress*. 2012;25:384–92.

56. Hammersley P, Dias A, Todd G, Bowen-Jones K, Reilly B, Bentall RP. Childhood trauma and hallucinations in bipolar affective disorder: preliminary investigation. *Br J Psychiatry* 2003;182:543–7.

57. Leverich GS, Post RM. Course of bipolar illness after history of childhood trauma. *Lancet*. 2006;367:1040–2.

58. Reichart CG, Nolen WA. Earlier onset of bipolar disorder in children by antidepressants or stimulants? An hypothesis. *J Affect Disord*. 2004;78:81–4.

59. Mayes R, Bagwell C, Erkulwater J. ADHD and the rise in stimulant use among children. *Harv Rev Psychiatry*. 2008;16:151–66.

60. Moreno C, Laje G, Blanco C, Jiang H, Schmidt AB, Olfson M. National trends in the outpatient diagnosis and treatment of bipolar disorder in youth. *Arch Gen Psychiatry*. 2007 64:1032–9.

61. Paterniti S, Bisserbe JC. Pharmacotherapy for bipolar disorder and concordance with treatment guidelines: survey of a general population sample referred to a tertiary care service. *BMC Psychiatry*. 2013;13:211.

62. Goldsmith M, Singh M, Chang K. Antidepressants and psychostimulants in pediatric populations. Is there an association with mania? *Pediatric Drugs*. 2011;13:225–39.

63. Post RM, Altshuler LL, Leverich GS, et al. Mood switch in bipolar depression: comparison of adjunctive venlafaxine, bupropion and sertraline. *Br J Psychiatry*. 2006;189:124–31.

64. Yerevanian BI, Koek RJ, Mintz J, Akiskal HS. Bipolar pharmacotherapy and suicidal behavior Part 2. The impact of antidepressants. *J Affect Disord*. 2007;103:13–21.

65. Martin A, Young C, Leckman JF, Mukonoweshuro C, Rosenheck R, Leslie D. Age effects on antidepressant-induced manic conversion. *Arch Pediatr Adolesc Med*. 2004;158:773–80.

66. Cicero D, El-Mallakh RS, Holman J, Robertson J. Antidepressant exposure in bipolar children. *Psychiatry*. 2003;66:317–22.

67. Bechdolf A, Nelson B, Cotton SM, et al. A preliminary evaluation of the validity of at-risk criteria for bipolar disorders in help-seeking adolescents and young adults. *J Affect Disord*. 2010;127:316–20.

68. Baumer FM, Howe M, Gallelli K, Simeonova DI, Hallmayer J, Chang KD. A pilot study of antidepressant-induced mania in pediatric bipolar disorder: characteristics, risk factors, and the serotonin transporter gene. *Biol Psychiatry*. 2006;60:1005–12.

69. Findling RL, Lingler J, Rowles BM, McNamara NK, Calabrese JR. A pilot pharmacotherapy trial for depressed youths at high genetic risk for bipolarity. *J Child Adolesc Psychopharmacol*. 2008;18:615–21.

70. Strawn JR, Adler, CM, McNamara RK, et al. Antidepressant tolerability in anxious and depressed youth at high-risk for bipolar disorder: a prospective naturalistic treatment study. *Bipolar Disord*. 2013. Epub ahead of print; doi: 10.1111/bdi.12113

71. Van Kammen DP, Murphy DL. Attenuation of the euphoriant and activating effects of d- and l-amphetamine by lithium carbonate treatment. *Psychopharmacologia*. 1975;44:215–24.

72. Strakowski SM, Sax KW, Setters MJ, Stanton SP, Keck PE Jr. Lack of enhanced response to repeated d-amphetamine challenge in first-episode psychosis: implications for a sensitization model of psychosis in humans. *Biol Psychiatry*. 1997;42:749–55.

73. Findling RL, Short EJ, McNamara NK, et al. Methylphenidate in the treatment of children and adolescents with bipolar disorder and attention-deficit/hyperactivity disorder. *J Am Acad Child Adolesc Psychiatry*. 2007;46:1445–53.

74. Kowatch RA, Sethuraman G, Hume JH, Kromelis M, Weinberg WA. Combination pharmacotherapy in children and adolescents with bipolar disorder. *Biol Psychiatry*. 2003;53:978–84.

75. Scheffer RE, Kowatch RA, Carmody T, Rush AJ. Randomized, placebo-controlled trial of mixed amphetamine salts for symptoms of comorbid ADHD in pediatric bipolar disorder after mood stabilization with divalproex sodium. *Am J Psychiatry*. 2005;162:58–64.

76. DelBello MP, Soutullo CA, Hendricks W, Niemeier RT, McElroy SL, Strakowski SM. Prior stimulant treatment in adolescents with bipolar disorder: association with age at onset. *Bipolar Disord*. 2001;3:53–7.

77. Tillman R, Geller B. Controlled study of switching from attention-deficit/hyperactivity disorder to a prepubertal and early adolescent bipolar I disorder phenotype during 6-year prospective follow-up: rate, risk, and predictors. *Dev Psychopathol*. 2006;18:1037–53.

78. Kessler RC, Crum RM, Warner LA, Nelson CB, Schulenberg J, Anthony JC. Lifetime co-occurrence of DSM-III-R alcohol abuse dependence with other psychiatry disorders in the National Comorbidity Survey. *Arch Gen Psychiatry*. 1997;54:313–21.

79. Regier DA, Farmer ME, Rae DS, et al. Comorbidity of mental disorders with alcohol and other drug abuse: results from the Epidemiologic Catchment Area ECA Study. *JAMA*. 1990;264:2511–8.

80. Azorin JM, Kaladjian A, Adida M, Fakra E, Hantouche E, Lancrenon S. Correlates of first-episode polarity in a French cohort of 1089 bipolar I disorder patients: role of temperaments and triggering events. *J Affect Disord*. 2011;129:39–46.

81. West SA, Strakowski SM, Sax KW, McElroy SL, Keck PE Jr, McConville BJ. Phenomenology and comorbidity of adolescents hospitalized for the treatment of acute mania. *Biol Psychiatry*. 1996;39:458–60.

82. Wilens TE, Biederman J, Abrantes AM, Spencer TJ. Clinical characteristics of psychiatrically referred adolescent outpatients with substance use disorder. *J Am Acad Child Adolesc Psychiatry*. 1997;36:941–7.

83. Goldstein BI, Strober MA, Birmaher B, et al. Substance use disorders among adolescents with bipolar spectrum disorders. *Bipolar Disord*. 2008;10:469–78.

84. Goldstein BI, Bukstein OG. Comorbid substance use disorders among youth with bipolar disorder: opportunities for early identification and prevention. *J Clin Psychiatry*. 2010;71:348–58.

85. Fond G, Capdevielle D, Macgregor A, et al. Toxoplasma gondii: a potential role in the genesis of psychiatric disorders. *Encephale*. 2013;39:38–43.

86. Pearce BD, Kruszon-Moran D, Jones JL. The relationship between Toxoplasma gondii infection and mood disorders in the Third National Health and Nutrition Survey. *Biol Psychiatry*. 2012;72:290–5.

87. Hamdani N, Daban-Huard C, Lajnef M, et al. Relationship between Toxoplasma gondii infection and bipolar disorder in a French sample. *J Affect Disord*. 2013;148:444–8.

88. Arling TA, Yolken RH, Lapidus M, et al. Toxoplasma gondii antibody titers and history of suicide attempts in patients with recurrent mood disorders. *J Nerv Ment Dis*. 2009;197:905–8.

89. Jones-Brando L, Torrey EF, Yolken R. Drugs used in the treatment of schizophrenia and bipolar disorder inhibit the replication of Toxoplasma gondii. *Schizophr Res*. 2003;62:237–44.

90. Ellen SR, Judd FK, Mijch AM, Cockram A. Secondary mania in patients with HIV infection. *Aust NZ J Psychiatry*. 1999;33:353–60.

91. Mijch AM, Judd FK, Lyketsos CG, Ellen S, Cockram A. Secondary mania in patients with HIV infection: are antiretrovirals protective? *J Neuropsychiatry Clin Neurosci*. 1999;11:475–80.

92. Mortensen PB, Mors O, Frydenberg M, Ewald H. Head injury as a risk factor for bipolar affective disorder. *J Affect Disord*. 2003;76:79–83.

93. Malaspina D, Goetz RR, Friedman JH, et al. Traumatic brain injury and schizophrenia in members of schizophrenia and bipolar disorder pedigrees. *Am J Psychiatry*. 2001;158:440–6.

94. Yeh CC, Chen TL, Hu CJ, Chiu WT, Liao CC. Risk of epilepsy after traumatic brain injury: a retrospective population-based cohort study. *J Neurol Neurosurg Psychiatry*. 2013;84:441–5.

95. Amann B, Grunze H. Neurochemical underpinnings in bipolar disorder and epilepsy. *Epilepsia*. 2005;46(Suppl. 4):26–30.

96. Mula M, Marotta AE, Monaco F. Epilepsy and bipolar disorders. *Expert Rev Neurother*. 2010;10:13–23.

97. Ettinger AB, Reed ML, Goldberg JF, Hirschfeld RM. Prevalence of bipolar symptoms in epilepsy vs other chronic health disorders. *Neurology*. 2005;65:535–40.

98. Clarke MC, Tanskanen A, Huttunen MO, Clancy M, Cotter DR, Cannon M. Evidence for shared susceptibility to epilepsy and psychosis: a population-based family study. *Biol Psychiatry*. 2012;71:836–9.

99. Kuusisto H, Kaprio J, Kinnunen E, Luukkaala T, Koskenvuo M, Elovaara I. Concordance and heritability of multiple sclerosis in Finland: study on a nationwide series of twins. *Eur J Neurol*. 2008;15:1106–10.

100. Weinshenker BG. Epidemiology of multiple sclerosis. *Neurol Clin*. 1996;14:291–308.

101. Reynolds R, Roncaroli F, Nicholas R, Radotra B, Gveric D, Howell O. The neuropathological basis of clinical progression in multiple sclerosis. *Acta Neuropathol*. 2011;122:155–70.

102. Aston C, Jiang L, Sokolov BP. Transcriptional profiling reveals evidence for signaling and oligodendroglial abnormalities in the temporal cortex from patients with major depressive disorder. *Mol Psychiatry*. 2005;10:309–22.

103. Tkachev D, Mimmack ML, Ryan MM, et al. Oligodendrocyte dysfunction in schizophrenia and bipolar disorder. *Lancet*. 2003;362:798–805.

104. Regenold WT, Phatak P, Marano CM, Gearhart L, Viens CH, Hisley KC. Myelin staining of deep white matter in the dorsolateral prefrontal cortex in schizophrenia, bipolar disorder, and unipolar major depression. *Psychiatry Res*. 2007;151:179–88.

105. Adler CM, Holland SK, Schmithorst V, et al. Abnormal frontal white matter tracts in bipolar disorder: a diffusion tensor imaging study. *Bipolar Disord*. 2004;6:197–203.

106. Benedetti F, Absinta M, Rocca MA, et al. Tract-specific white matter structural disruption in patients with bipolar disorder. *Bipolar Disord*. 2011;13:414–24.

107. Heng S, Song AW, Sim K. White matter abnormalities in bipolar disorder: insights from diffusion tensor imaging studies. *J Neural Transm*. 2010;117:639–54.

108. Bamer AM, Cetin K, Johnson KL, Gibbons LE, Ehde DM. Validation study of prevalence and correlates of depressive symptomatology in multiple sclerosis. *Gen Hosp Psychiatry*. 2008;30:311–7.

109. Patten SB, Beck CA, Williams JV, Barbui C, Metz LM. Major depression in multiple sclerosis. A population-based perspective. *Neurology*. 2003;61:1524–7.

110. Chwastiak L, Ehde DM, Gibbons LE, Sullivan M, Bowen JD, Kraft GH. Depressive symptoms and severity of illness in multiple sclerosis: epidemiologic study of a large community sample. *Am J Psychiatry*. 2002;159:1862–8.

111. Fisk JD, Morehouse SA, Brown MG, Skedgel C, Murray TJ. Hospital-based psychiatric service utilization and morbidity in multiple sclerosis. *Can J Neurol Sci*. 1998;25:230–5.

112. Marrie RA, Horwitz R, Cutter G, Tyry T, Campagnolo D, Vollmer T. The burden of medical comorbidity in multiple sclerosis: frequent, underdiagnosed and undertreated. *Mult Scler*. 2009; 15:385–92.

113. Kessler RC, Merikangas KR, Wang PS. Prevalence, comorbidity, and service utilization for mood disorders in the United States at the beginning of the twenty-first century. *Annu Rev Clin Psychol*. 2007;3:137–58.

114. Heilä H, Turpeinen P, Erkinjuntti T. Case study: mania associated with multiple sclerosis. *J Am Acad Child Adolesc Psychiatry*. 1995;34:1591–5.

115. Mapelli G, Ramelli E. Manic syndrome associated with multiple sclerosis: secondary mania? *Acta Psychiatr Belg*. 1981;81:337–49.

116. Ron MA, Logsdail SJ. Psychiatric morbidity in multiple sclerosis: a clinical and MRI study. *Psychol Med*. 1989;19:887–95.

117. Hutchinson M, Stack J, Buckley P. Bipolar affective disorder prior to the onset of multiple sclerosis. *Acta Neurol Scand*. 1993;88:388–93.

118. Joffe RT, Lippert GP, Gray TA, Sawa G, Horvath Z. Mood disorder and multiple sclerosis. *Arch Neurol*. 1987;44:376–8.

119. Pine DS, Douglas CJ, Charles E, Davies M, Kahn D. Patients with multiple sclerosis presenting to psychiatric hospitals. *J Clin Psychiatry*. 1995;56:297–306.

120. Davison KM, Kaplan BJ. Food intake and blood cholesterol levels of community-based adults with mood disorders. *BMC Psychiatry*. 2012;12:10.
121. Jacka FN, Pasco JA, Mykletun A, et al. Diet quality in bipolar disorder in a population based sample of women. *J Affect Disord*. 2011;129:332–7.
122. Kilbourne AM, Rofey DL, McCarthy JF, Post EP, Welsh D, Blow FC. Nutrition and exercise behavior among patients with bipolar disorder. *Bipolar Disord*. 2007;9:443–52.
123. Fagiolini A, Frank E, Houck PR, et al. Prevalence of obesity and weight change during treatment in patients with bipolar I disorder. *J Clin Psychiatry*. 2002;63:528–33.
124. Fiedorowicz JG, Palagummi NM, Forman-Hoffman VL, Miller DD, Haynes WG. Elevated prevalence of obesity, metabolic syndrome, and cardiovascular risk factors in bipolar disorder. *Ann Clin Psychiatry*. 2008;20:131–7.
125. McElroy SL, Frye MA, Suppes T, et al. Correlates of overweight and obesity in 644 patients with bipolar disorder. *J Clin Psychiatry*. 2002;63:207–13.
126. Wang PW, Sachs GS, Zarate CA, et al. Overweight and obesity in bipolar disorders. *J Psychiatr Res*. 2006;40:762–4.
127. Lien L, Lien N, Heyerdahl S, Thoresen M, Bjertness E. Consumption of soft drinks and hyperactivity, mental distress, and conduct problems among adolescents in Oslo, Norway. *Am J Public Health*. 2006;96:1815–20.
128. Solnick SJ, Hemenway D. Soft drinks, aggression and suicidal behaviour in US high school students. *Int J Inj Contr Saf Promot*. 2013. Epub ahead of print.
129. Suglia SF, Solnick S, Hemenway D. Soft drink consumption is associated with behavior problems in 5-year-olds. *J Pediatr*. 2013;163(5):1323–8.
130. Nigg JT, Lewis K, Edinger T, Falk M. Meta-analysis of attention-deficit/hyperactivity disorder or attention-deficit/hyperactivity disorder symptoms, restriction diet, and synthetic food color additives. *J Am Acad Child Adolesc Psychiatry*. 2012;51:86–97.
131. Sonuga-Barke EJ, Brandeis D, Cortese S, et al. Nonpharmacological interventions for ADHD: systematic review and meta-analyses of randomized controlled trials of dietary and psychological treatments. *Am J Psychiatry*. 2013;170:275–89.
132. Folstein M, Liu T, Peter I, Buell J, Arsenault L, Scott T, Qiu WW. The homocysteine hypothesis of depression. *Am J Psychiatry*. 2007;164:861–7.
133. Morris DW, Trivedi MH, Rush AJ. Folate and unipolar depression. *J Altern Complement Med*. 2008;14:277–85.
134. Davison KM, Kaplan BJ. Vitamin and mineral intakes in adults with mood disorders: comparisons to nutrition standards and associations with sociodemographic and clinical variables. *J Am Coll Nutr*. 2011;30:547–8.
135. Morris MS, Fava M, Jacques PF, Selhub J, Rosenberg IH. Depression and folate status in the US Population. *Psychother Psychosom*. 2003;72:80–7.
136. Coppen A, Chaudhry S, Swade C. Folic acid enhances lithium prophylaxis. *J Affect Disord*. 1986;10:9–13.
137. Frazier EA, Fristad MA, Arnold LE. Feasibility of a nutritional supplement as treatment for pediatric bipolar spectrum disorders. *J Altern Complement Med*. 2012;18:678–85.
138. McNamara RK. Long-chain omega-3 fatty acid deficiency in mood disorders: Rationale for treatment and prevention. *Curr Drug Discov Technol*. 2013;10:233–44.
139. Noaghiul S, Hibbeln JR. Cross-national comparisons of seafood consumption and rates of bipolar disorders. *Am J Psychiatry*. 2003;160:2222–7.
140. Cao J, Schwichtenberg KA, Hanson NQ, Tsai MY. Incorporation and clearance of omega-3 fatty acids in erythrocyte membranes and plasma phospholipids. *Clin Chem*. 2006;52:2265–72.
141. Chiu CC, Huang SY, Su KP, et al. Polyunsaturated fatty acid deficit in patients with bipolar mania. *Eur Neuropsychopharmacol*. 2003;13:99–103.
142. Clayton EH, Hanstock TL, Hirneth SJ, Kable CJ, Garg ML, Hazell PL. Long-chain omega-3 polyunsaturated fatty acids in the blood of children and adolescents with juvenile bipolar disorder compared to healthy controls. *Lipids*. 2008;43:1031–8.

143. McNamara RK, Jandacek R, Rider T, Tso P, Dwivedi Y, Pandey GN. Selective deficits in erythrocyte docosahexaenoic acid composition in adult patients with bipolar disorder and major depressive disorder. *J Affect Disord.* 2010;126:303–11.

144. Ranjekar PK, Hinge A, Hegde MV, et al. Decreased antioxidant enzymes and membrane essential polyunsaturated fatty acids in schizophrenic and bipolar mood disorder patients. *Psychiatry Res.* 2003;121:109–122.

145. Clayton EH, Hanstock TL, Hirneth SJ, Kable CJ, Garg ML, Hazell PL. Reduced mania and depression in juvenile bipolar disorder associated with long-chain omega-3 polyunsaturated fatty acid supplementation. *Eur J Clin Nutr.* 2009;63:1037–40.

146. Wozniak J, Biederman J, Mick E, et al. Omega-3 fatty acid monotherapy for pediatric bipolar disorder: a prospective open-label trial. *Eur Neuropsychopharmacol.* 2007;17:440–7.

147. Freeman MP, Hibbeln JR, Wisner KL, et al. Omega-3 fatty acids: evidence basis for treatment and future research in psychiatry. *J Clin Psychiatry.* 2006;67:1954–67.

148. Lin PY, Su KP. A meta-analytic review of double-blind, placebo-controlled trials of antidepressant efficacy of omega-3 fatty acids. *J Clin Psychiatry.* 2007;68:1056–61.

149. Sarris J, Mischoulon D, Schweitzer I. Omega-3 for bipolar disorder: meta-analyses of use in mania and bipolar depression. *J Clin Psychiat.* 2012;73:81–6.

150. Dickerson F, Stallings C, Origoni A, et al. Markers of gluten sensitivity and celiac disease in bipolar disorder. *Bipolar Disord.* 2011;13:52–8.

151. Dickerson F, Stallings C, Origoni A, Vaughan C, Khushalani S, Yolken R. Markers of gluten sensitivity in acute mania: a longitudinal study. *Psychiatry Res.* 2012;196:68–71.

152. Severance EG, Kannan G, Gressitt KL, et al. Anti-gluten immune response following Toxoplasma gondii infection in mice. *PLoS One.* 2012;7:e50991.

153. Severance EG, Dupont D, Dickerson FB, et al. Immune activation by casein dietary antigens in bipolar disorder. *Bipolar Disord* 2010;12:834–42.

154. Banerjee TD, Middleton F, Faraone SV. Environmental risk factors for attention-deficit hyperactivity disorder. *Acta Paediatr.* 2007;96:1269–74.

155. Torrey EF, Bartko JJ, Yolken RH. Toxoplasma gondii and other risk factors for schizophrenia: an update. *Schizophr Bull.* 2012;38:642–7.

156. Dunayevich E, Keck PE Jr. Prevalence and description of psychotic features in bipolar mania. *Curr Psychiatry Rep.* 2000;2:286–90.

157. Bhutta AT, Cleves MA, Casey PH, Cradock MM, Anand KJ. Cognitive and behavioral outcomes of school-aged children who were born preterm: a meta-analysis. *JAMA.* 2002;288:728–37.

158. Egeland JA, Hostetter AM, Pauls DL, Sussex JN. Prodromal symptoms before onset of manic-depressive disorder suggested by first hospital admission histories. *J Am Acad Child Adolesc Psychiatry.* 2000;39:1245–52.

159. Hibbeln JR. Fish consumption and major depression. *Lancet.* 1998;351(9110):1213.

160. Peet M. International variations in the outcome of schizophrenia and the prevalence of depression in relation to national dietary practices: an ecological analysis. *Br J Psychiatry.* 2004;184:404–8.

161. Goldstein BI, Kemp DE, Soczynska JK, McIntyre RS. Inflammation and the phenomenology, pathophysiology, comorbidity, and treatment of bipolar disorder: a systematic review of the literature. *J Clin Psychiatry.* 2009;70:1078–90.

162. McNamara RK, Lotrich FE. Elevated immune-inflammatory signaling in mood disorders: a new therapeutic target? *Expert Rev Neurother.* 2012;12:1143–61.

163. Rapoport SI, Basselin M, Kim HW, Rao JS. Bipolar disorder and mechanisms of action of mood stabilizers. *Brain Res Rev.* 2009;61:185–209.

164. Knijff EM, Breunis MN, Kupka RW, et al. An imbalance in the production of IL-1beta and IL-6 by monocytes of bipolar patients: restoration by lithium treatment. *Bipolar Disord.* 2007;9:743–53.

165. Padmos RC, Van Baal GC, Vonk R, et al. Genetic and environmental influences on pro-inflammatory monocytes in bipolar disorder: a twin study. *Arch Gen Psychiatry.* 2009;66:957–65.

166. Calder PC. The relationship between the fatty acid composition of immune cells and their function. *Prostaglandins Leukot Essent Fatty Acids.* 2008;79:101–8.

167. Danese A, Pariante CM, Caspi A, Taylor A, Poulton R. Childhood maltreatment predicts adult inflammation in a life-course study. *Proc Natl Acad Sci USA*. 2007;104:1319–24.
168. Danese A, Moffitt TE, Pariante CM, Ambler A, Poulton R, Caspi A. Elevated inflammation levels in depressed adults with a history of childhood maltreatment. *Arch Gen Psychiatry*. 2008;65:409–15.
169. McDade TW, Hawkley LC, Cacioppo JT. Psychosocial and behavioral predictors of inflammation in middle-aged and older adults: the Chicago health, aging, and social relations study. *Psychosom Med*. 2006;68;376–81.
170. Miller GE, Rohleder N, Cole SW. Chronic interpersonal stress predicts activation of pro- and anti-inflammatory signaling pathways 6 months later. *Psychosom Med*. 2009;71;57–62.
171. Pace TW, Mletzko TC, Alagbe O, et al. Increased stress-induced inflammatory responses in male patients with major depression and increased early life stress. *Am J Psychiatry*. 2006;163;1630–3.
172. Romaldini CC, Barbieri D, Okay TS, Raiz R Jr, Cançado EL. Serum soluble interleukin-2 receptor, interleukin-6, and tumor necrosis factor-alpha levels in children with celiac disease: response to treatment. *J Pediatr Gastroenterol Nutr*. 2002;35:513–7.
173. Manalai P, Hamilton RG, Langenberg P, et al. Pollen-specific immunoglobulin E positivity is associated with worsening of depression scores in bipolar disorder patients during high pollen season. *Bipolar Disord*. 2012;14:90–8.
174. Lee HC, Tsai SY, Lin HC. Seasonal variations in bipolar disorder admissions and the association with climate: a population-based study. *J Affect Disord*. 2007;97:61–9.
175. Cassidy F, Carroll BJ. Seasonal variation of mixed and pure episodes of bipolar disorder. *J Affect Disord*. 2002;68:25–31.
176. Sim TC, Grant JA, Hilsmeier KA, Fukuda Y, Alam R. Proinflammatory cytokines in nasal secretions of allergic subjects after antigen challenge. *Am J Respir Crit Care Med*. 1994;149:339–44.
177. Sprooten E, Fleming KM, Thomson PA, et al. White matter integrity as an intermediate phenotype: exploratory genome-wide association analysis in individuals at high risk of bipolar disorder. *Psychiatry Res*. 2013;206:223–31.
178. Strakowski SM, Adler CM, Almeida J, et al. The functional neuroanatomy of bipolar disorder: a consensus model. *Bipolar Disord*. 2012;14:313–25.
179. Giedd JN, Lalonde FM, Celano MJ, et al. Anatomical brain magnetic resonance imaging of typically developing children and adolescents. *J Am Acad Child Adolesc Psychiatry*. 2009;48:465–70.
180. Pfeifer JC, Welge J, Strakowski SM, Adler CM, DelBello MP. Meta-analysis of amygdala volumes in children and adolescents with bipolar disorder. *J Am Acad Child Adolesc Psychiatry*. 2008;47:1289–98.
181. Nortje G, Stein DJ, Radua J, Mataix-Cols D, Horn N. Systematic review and voxel-based meta-analysis of diffusion tensor imaging studies in bipolar disorder. *J Affect Disord*. 2013;150:192–200.
182. Schneider RM, DelBello MP, McNamara RK, Strakowski SM, Adler CM. Neuroprogression of bipolar disorder. *Bipolar Disord*. 2012;14:356–74.
183. Haukvik UK, McNeil T, Lange EH, et al. Pre- and perinatal hypoxia associated with hippocampus/amygdala volume in bipolar disorder. *Psychol Med*. 2013 Jun 27:1–11. Epub ahead of print.
184. Mitra R, Sapolsky RM, Vyas A. Toxoplasma gondii infection induces dendritic retraction in basolateral amygdala accompanied by reduced corticosterone secretion. *Dis Model Mech*. 2013;6:516–20.
185. Stolp HB, Dziegielewska KM, Ek CJ, Potter AM, Saunders NR. Long-term changes in blood-brain barrier permeability and white matter following prolonged systemic inflammation in early development in the rat. *Eur J Neurosci*. 2005;22:2805–16.
186. Alicata D, Chang L, Cloak C, Abe K, Ernst T. Higher diffusion in striatum and lower fractional anisotropy in white matter of methamphetamine users. *Psychiatry Res*. 2009;174:1–8.
187. Lim KO, Choi SJ, Pomara N, Wolkin A, Rotrosen JP. Reduced frontal white matter integrity in cocaine dependence: a controlled diffusion tensor imaging study. *Biol Psychiatry*. 2002;51:890–5.
188. Romero MJ, Asensio S, Palau C, Sanchez A, Romero FJ. Cocaine addiction: diffusion tensor imaging study of the inferior frontal and anterior cingulate white matter. *Psychiatry Res*. 2010;181:57–63.
189. Caspi A, McClay J, Moffitt TE, et al. Role of genotype in the cycle of violence in maltreated children. *Science*. 2002;297:851–4.

190. Caspi A, Sugden K, Moffitt TE, et al. Influence of life stress on depression: moderation by a polymorphism in the 5-HTT gene. *Science*. 2003;301:386–9.

191. Lotrich FE, Sears B, McNamara RK. Anger induced by interferon-alpha treatment is moderated by the ratio of arachidonic acid to omega-3 fatty acids. *J Psychosom Res*. 2013;75(5):475–83.

192. McNamara RK, Strawn JR, Chang KD, DelBello MP. Interventions for youth at high risk for bipolar disorder and schizophrenia. *Child Adolesc Psychiatric Clin N Am*. 2012;21:739–51.

193. Amminger GP, Schäfer MR, Papageorgiou K, et al. Long-chain omega-3 fatty acids for indicated prevention of psychotic disorders: a randomized, placebo-controlled trial. *Arch Gen Psychiatry*. 2010;67:146–54.

Treatment of Bipolar Disorder in Youth

Section Editor: Melissa P. DelBello

Ethical Consideration for Treating At-Risk Populations

Aswin Ratheesh, Michael Berk,
and Patrick D. McGorry

Introduction

Bipolar disorder (BD) in its more severe forms can be a debilitating and recurrent illness, and it has been ranked the eighth leading cause of medical disability in the world. The recurrent episodes often lead to a high level of physical and vocational disability, contributing to a substantial economic burden, as well as social and family dysfunction.[1] The universal prevalence and the peak age of onset in the most productive and developmentally significant life years contribute to the magnitude of this disability. Early intervention (EI) in BD, specifically targeting at-risk groups, may help achieve better outcomes, limit comorbidity, and improve functional outcome, as it has for persons with psychotic disorders.[2] However, two decades of EI efforts in psychosis and of high-risk family studies in BD have revealed ethical and moral challenges that clinicians and researchers face while providing EI efforts for at-risk individuals. We will attempt to explore these challenges in the context of the current data on EI and at-risk research in BD and address the ethical dilemmas associated with such efforts against the background of currently accepted ethical frameworks in medicine and psychiatry.

Interventions in At-Risk Mental Health Populations

The psychotic and serious mood disorders contribute to substantial economic and emotional burden in the wider population.[3,4] This is largely due to their onset in the most productive and developmentally significant years of life, with nearly 75% of new onsets being before the age of 25. In the past, the dysfunction and disability associated with these ill-nesses maintained the pessimism and stigma surrounding them, which has only recently begun to lift across many parts of the world. EI is an idea that has helped change this landscape over the last few decades, and it is now a well-established concept for psychotic illnesses. With an explosion of research in the field demonstrating the effectiveness of such EI efforts, EI services have mushroomed across many parts of the world.[5] Consistent with the approach to other conditions of global impact in medicine, such as cancer and coronary artery disease, and following the description of various high-risk (HR) states for psychosis, EI has given way to earlier or preemptive interventions.[6] This is also linked to the observation that the need for care begins well before the development of fully formed and threshold psychotic or mood disorder diagnoses. Attention to potentially modifiable risk factors has been extended to a preventive focus.[7] An extrapolation of this approach suggests that universal or primary prevention may be the ultimate aim for serious mental disorders across the life span, thereby reducing the incidence of risk states and thus the need for care for mental disorders. However, an examination of the statistical power nec-essary for studies on universal prevention of mental disorders indicates that the feasibility of this approach may be limited.[8]

With the burgeoning research on at-risk states for psychosis, clinicians and researchers have debated various ethical challenges in this area.[9,10] The primary issue with at-risk samples has been one of false positives. As noted very early in the field of at-risk research in psychosis, the term *prodrome* is ethically complicated as this seemed to indicate an inevitability in the transition to psychosis or schizophrenia.[11] However, as a recent meta-analysis[6] indicates, a majority of help-seeking clients—approximately 64%—who fulfil one of the many criteria for the HR state for psychosis do not develop a psychotic illness, even at 3 years after identification, and are thus "false positives" in the screening strategy for psychosis. However, people exhibiting emerging distress may be at risk for developing other nonpsychotic disorders. These individuals, by their association with the "converters," may be at risk of labeling and its potential negative effects and that of side effects of interventions aimed at reducing the transition to psychosis. Though the concern about labeling and stigma associated with psychosis is genuine, EI services have attempted to alleviate this in some centers by providing education about the relatively low probability of developing psychosis, by emphasizing the fact that psychosis is highly treatable even if it initially worsens and is sustained, and by avoiding the term *psychosis* in the name of the service.[12] Making the culture of services youth friendly and optimistic also deals effectively with the theoretical risks of labeling and stigma. However, providing early intervention in traditional psychiatric settings in which disabled and marginalized older patients dominate clearly poses risks. The risk of antipsychotic exposure may be a more serious problem in this particular population; however, this may be especially so in the hands of primary care physicians and private psychiatric practice, and specialist early intervention services provide protection against this premature use of antipsychotic medications through ensuring adherence to clinical practice guidelines. Though early studies of risperidone[13] and olanzapine[14] were shown to be more effective than placebo, antipsychotics are currently thought to be "overtreatment" for at-risk states for psychosis.[15] In routine clinical care for young people experiencing at-risk symptoms in general psychiatric care or in general medical practice, the prescription of antipsychotic medications, combined with a relative lack of appreciation of the risks of these medications, may lead to poorer outcomes for some young people. Instead, low-risk interventions such as cognitive-behavioral strategies and omega-3 fatty acids present a better risk-benefit profile as first-line treatment for subthreshold psychotic illnesses. Education and dissemination of evidence-based recommendations for interventions in at-risk youth may help bridge the gap between research and clinical practice, especially in primary care settings.

Even if safer interventions were to be used initially, another ethical challenge has been that of intervention cessation for apparently successful at-risk participants, or the so-called exit question. Among these at-risk individuals, the concern is that of withdrawal of interventions and the potential for clinical worsening or functional deterioration. However, it could be argued that this deterioration may have occurred in any case, and that prepsychotic intervention may have simply delayed this inevitable deterioration and thus may have provided overall benefit. The duration of care necessary is far from clear in the evidence base and may vary from case to case; thus, further research is urgently needed. Often due to pressure for resources, particularly in managed care settings, the ability to provide prepsychotic intervention may be time limited. In such a scenario, if an at-risk young person continues to experience symptoms at a level where ongoing care is indicated, but not at a level where a psychotic illness can be diagnosed, care may need to be ceased, which may leave the young person vulnerable. It is also the case that patients who have been successfully treated for first-episode psychosis for 2 years and then discharged to standard care also suffer deterioration due to the reduction in quality of care. This is obviously an argument for sustaining the quality and tenure of the early intervention approach, not for suggesting that the initial benefits were somehow illusory or not worthwhile. If a remission is achieved in cancer, every effort is made to sustain it with appropriate maintenance therapy. The same should be offered in psychiatric illness. Furthermore, it has been shown that young people with HR states, but who have nonpsychotic outcomes, have significant dysfunction and impairment[16,17] on follow-up. However, it is hoped that with youth-friendly, evidence-based, staged EI services that are well linked with local general practice systems, these disruptions of care may be minimized. Such systems are already operational in countries like Australia, Ireland, and the United Kingdom.[5]

A further ethical issue is raised by the neuroprogression hypothesis,[18] which posits that there is an active process of illness progression, most marked at the earliest stages, which may be amenable to therapeutic intervention with agents, including conventional agents such as lithium, which may be neuroprotective.[19]

Another question in prepsychotic interventions has been the ability of those at risk to be able to give informed consent for research or clinical interventions.[20] Since even a proportion of nonpsychiatric patients or members of the general population have demonstrable difficulties with informed consent,[10] it may be possible that some of these individuals are unable to provide full informed consent for interventions. It is possible that psychotic symptoms could interfere with the ability to give consent, even though the psychosis is not "full threshold." This particular difficulty is managed relatively well by institutional review boards (IRBs), with the requirement for signed written informed consent forms for research. These ethical challenges in psychosis, many of which have been successfully resolved, have set the scene for clinicians and researchers in our evolving understanding of at-risk states and in the efforts for EI for BD.

Early Intervention in Bipolar Disorder

In the case of BD, prevention means the detection and targeting of early-life risk factors that have been linked to the development of subsequent illness and the provision of targeted interventions to reduce the impact of these risk factors. Due to the high relative contribution of genetic factors in the development of BD, early identification efforts have focused on familial HR groups.[21] Many of the other early risk factors for BD, as for other psychiatric disorders, are often ill defined and nonspecific, meaning that primary prevention efforts must be transdiagnostic and measure multiple outcomes. EI, in contrast, means identifying the early clinical phenotypes or stages and providing specific or nonspecific interventions to reduce the risk of progression to full-threshold illness or the morbidity and functional impairment associated with the illness, or both. Recent retrospective[22] and prospective studies (Bechdolf et al., 2014)[23] indicate that some of the subthreshold stages or early clinical phenotypes (which may be referred to as the "prodrome") may be able to be identified, though this is more challenging than with the psychotic disorders.

The observation that BD is a progressive illness, at least in a majority of patients, and has at least a partially predictable trajectory is central to the idea of EI. Due to this identifiable and typically recurrent or progressive course, the illness may be conceptualized to progress across multiple stages. According to this proposal,[24] at least a proportion of patients with BD progress from an asymptomatic at-risk stage to the emergence of prodromal symptoms, a first episode of illness, recurrence, and some eventually to a chronic and treatment-refractory stage. The asymptomatic at-risk stage (Stage 0) includes individuals at risk of developing BD by virtue of familial, physiological, or psychosocial risk. Familial or genetic risk is one the strongest risk factors associated with development of BD. Physical or sexual abuse, substance use, and life events are evidence-based psychosocial risk factors reported in the early lives of patients with BD. Stage 1 is the prodromal or subthreshold stage, which comprises Stage 1a, characterized by mild and nonspecific symptoms; and Stage 1b, with identifiable and relatively more specific subthreshold and potentially prodromal symptoms. Currently, it is not clear that the course of the illness can be predicted with substantial accuracy or whether there is a more common or "pluripotential" first stage, though it is hoped that the ability to predict outcomes will improve with further research. As this subthreshold stage involves clinical symptoms of low specificity, especially in young people, therapeutic interventions need to be broad spectrum, including cognitive-behavioral therapy and family interventions. There may be a role for neuroprotective and other safe biotherapies that may reduce risks, not only for BD but also for other potentially serious and enduring mental disorders. Single or recurrent hypomanic episodes without severe depressive episodes may be conceptualized to be in Stage 1b, as hypomania is considered by many to not mark the onset of severe mood disorders.[25] Stage 2 is defined as the first episode of full-threshold mood disorder, which conceptually may include mania or severe depression. However, since depressive episodes often precede manic episodes and since a manic or hypomanic episode is required for *ICD-10* or *DSM-5* criteria for BD, this stage may sometimes have to be defined in retrospect. Stage 3 is one of recurrence of depression and/or mania, and unfortunately, it is at this stage that many patients are correctly identified and specific treatment is instituted. When repeated and unremitting illness episodes occur, the illness is conceptualized to be in Stage 4.

According to this staging model, the main goals of EI would be to bring forward clinical diagnosis and treatment to an earlier stage. The imperative for this is driven by studies indicating that delays in correct diagnosis of BD are associated with poorer outcomes in adulthood.[26] Studies examining the efficacy of antipsychotics and mood stabilizers among participants with BD have also demonstrated that fewer episodes are associated with better treatment response.[27,28] However, it should also be borne in mind that this heuristic model is probabilistic rather than deterministic, as some patients are likely to have a different course. The current progress on at-risk interventions in BD will be considered in the context of these stages.

Stage 0: Genetic Risk for Bipolar Disorder: High-Risk Offspring as a Target for Early Intervention

Based on family, twin, and adoption studies, BD has been found to be one of the most heritable conditions in psychiatry.[29] A family history of BD is one of the most robust predictive risk factors for this disorder,[30] with the risk increasing 10-fold up to the age of 52 in individuals with a family member with BD. These factors inevitably point to the offspring of probands with BD as the targets of EI.

In the last three decades, there have been a number of cross-sectional and longitudinal studies that suggested a higher prevalence of mood, anxiety, and disruptive behavioral disorders in children with at least one parent with BD.[31] The longitudinal studies have clarified the evolution of these symptoms from broad nonspecific clusters in childhood to depressive disorders in early adolescence and bipolar spectrum disorders in later adolescence and early adulthood.[32] An early 3-year follow-up study indicated that depressive and anxiety symptoms predominated in the early childhood years, while full-threshold hypomania or mania was not observed until the age of 13 years.[33] In a Dutch longitudinal study of children (aged 12–21 years) of bipolar parents,[34] 13 met lifetime criteria for BD. Among these young people, the first mood episode was of depressive polarity in 12 subjects, and the average age of onset was 13 years (range 9–22 years). The average latency between the first depressive episode and the first activated episode (hypomania or mania) was 4.9 years (SD 3.4 years). None of the offspring met full-blown criteria for mania, hypomania, or cyclothymia before the age of 12 years. A Canadian longitudinal study identified a higher rate of childhood sleep and anxiety disorders among offspring of parents with a lithium-responsive form of BD.[35] In addition to sleep and anxiety disorders, the study also identified a higher rate of attention difficulties, learning disabilities, and Cluster A traits in children of parents with a lithium nonresponsive form of BD. A cohort of children with at least one bipolar parent from the Amish community in the United States were identified to have depressive and anxiety symptoms in childhood over a 10-year follow-up period,[36] and eight of these participants had developed BD type I at 16-year follow-up. The age of onset of mania varied from 13 to 29 years and episodicity of mood symptoms was characteristic in later childhood[37] among these participants. In these studies, prepubertal full-threshold hypomanic or manic syndromes have only rarely been identified as preceding manic illnesses in adulthood.

Within this group of HR offspring, Duffy and colleagues argue for a number of syndromes across the developmental period[31] to constitute stages in the development of BD. In childhood, three separate, but overlapping, clusters of anxiety, sleep disorders, and externalizing disorders were observed, while in adolescence, minor mood episodes occurred initially, while threshold depressive episodes in later adolescence preceded the onset of mania in a subset of these offspring. This may be consistent with the Stages 1a and 1b of nonspecific and specific syndromes, respectively, as discussed by Berk et al. 2007.[24]

However, nongenetic determinants of BD seem to exist, given that even among identical twins the concordance rate is less than 100%.[38] Nongenetic risk factors for BD may include substance use disorders; physical or sexual abuse and other psychosocial stressors; stimulant and antidepressant medication exposure; and omega-3 fatty acid or vitamin deficiencies.[39] Given that a number of different risk factors may operate to create the same phenotypic outcome (equifinality), approaches that are more pragmatic than risk factor research have attempted to identify a prodromal stage of BD.

Stage 1: Risk States for Bipolar Disorder: Is There an Identifiable Prodrome for Bipolar Disorder?

One of the challenges in EI for BD has been the lack of well-described risk groups who could be referred to as being in the "prodrome" of BD—itself a retrospective term that can only be defined with the clear onset of the illness. However, in the last decade, multiple approaches indicate the presence of such a proximal at-risk stage for BD.

One approach has been to describe retrospectively symptoms or experiences that immediately predate the onset of first manic episodes. Twelve such studies have described a range of symptoms, including depressed mood, mood swings, anxiety, irritability, and sleep disturbances among participants prior to manic episodes. Recall bias and reliability issues have been partially addressed in some of these studies by using multiple informants, and with assessments at different time points. A recent development has been the use of systematic examination of state and trait markers of risk for BD using specific instruments devised for this purpose.[22,40] However, these studies have focused on BD participants with psychosis, or participants who were identified as being at ultra-high risk of psychosis and who later developed BD. It should be noted that such samples are not representative of the larger group of persons who are in the preillness stages of BD.

Prospective studies represent the most methodologically rigorous way to assess phenomenological characteristics of at-risk subjects prior to the onset of the first manic episode. A 10-year follow-up of a subset of a community sample of teens from the Oregon Adolescent Development project identified two participants who developed BD type I and 16 others who developed BD type II or cyclothymia.[41] From the Dunedin birth cohort, which was assessed at age 3 and then reassessed at age 26, 93% of participants who developed mania had an antecedent adolescent diagnosis of depression or conduct disorders.[42] In both of these studies, the participants who developed BD in young adulthood had threshold or subthreshold depressive or conduct disorders in earlier adolescence.[42,43] In a population sample of 1,902 adolescents and young adults living in the Munich area (Germany), aged 14–24 years at baseline, 21 developed BD within a mean follow-up of 8.3 years and most of these converters presented with hypomanic symptoms and/or depressive symptoms prior to conversion, compared to the nonconverters.[44] A review of high-risk prospective studies[45] indicated that symptoms of inattention may be present early in the course of young persons who later develop BD, suggesting that attentional difficulties may also be a marker of higher risk. However, another review of prospective studies that examined children and young people prior to the onset of BD concluded that syndromal attention-deficit/hyperactivity disorder (ADHD) may not precede the onset of classical *DSM-IV* or *DSM-5* forms of BD (types I and II).[46] Phenomenological overlap between BD and ADHD, especially in the behavioral domains also contributes to the difficulty in parsing out these syndromes in the earlier stages of the evolution of the illness.

Another strategy combining multiple risk factors has been described by Bechdolf et al.[47] The authors described a set of bipolar at-risk (BAR) criteria, including the age group (15–25 years) that has the highest risk of onset for psychosis and mania; subthreshold depressive symptoms, which are commonly reported by participants in the 12 months prior to manic episodes; family history of BD in a first-degree relative; cyclothymic temperament, which serves as a marker of longer term cyclical mood dysregulation; and subthreshold manic symptoms, which are common in participants in the immediate period prior to a manic episode. A retrospective chart review of 173 patients treated at Orygen Youth Health, Melbourne, Australia, suggested that 22 (12.7%) of these young people fit the BAR criteria and 5 out of these converted to BD over a follow-up period of 265 days, compared with one young person in the group that did not fit the BAR criteria. Recently, it has been suggested that a third risk group of HR biomarkers could be added to genetic and environmental risk groups.[48] This biomarker profile may include markers of neuro-plasticity, such as BDNF; pro-inflammatory agents, including TNF-α, IL-6, and IL-8; and markers of oxidative stress, including superoxide dismutase (SOD); catalase; and markers of lipid peroxidation.[49] Neurocognitive and neuroimaging markers have been observed in participants prior to their onset of first episode of mania, but they have been shown to be relatively nonspecific.[50,51]

Interventions in At-Risk Stages (Stages 0 and 1)

As the description of the prodromal period of BD is a relatively recent development, intervention studies are limited and have been largely confined to HR offspring of BD probands. In double-blind placebo-controlled studies, lithium[52] and divalproex[53] have been found to be ineffective for alleviating depression and manic symptoms, respectively, among symptomatic HR offspring groups. A single-blind trial of 300–600 mg of quetiapine was demonstrated to be significantly better than placebo for improving manic, depressive, and overall clinical severity ratings in 20 adolescents presenting with mood disorders other than mania, but with a first-degree relative with mania.[54] However, 55% of these adolescents experienced somnolence during the trial, and there was a statistically significant increase in body mass index over the 12-week period in the intervention arm. Given the risks of medication use, psychological interventions may be safer and equally effective in reducing distress, improving functional outcomes, and possibly preventing or delaying the transition to full-threshold disorder. A 1-year open trial of family-focused therapy with 13 children who had a parent with BP resulted in significant improvements in depression, hypomania, and psychosocial functioning scores in this sample.[55] Among adolescent subjects with major depression or manic symptoms, long chain omega-3 fatty acid supplementation was associated with a reduction in these symptoms in preliminary studies.[56,57] Given its role as a nutritional agent and its high tolerability, omega-3 fatty acids may represent a low-risk strategy for intervention in at-risk youth. Such an evaluation of risks and benefits forms the core of the ethical considerations in at-risk states, mental illness, and medical practice in general.

Ethical Frameworks for Early Intervention

A number of ethical principles have evolved over the last two centuries that allow physicians to rationalize moral rules and thus decide the right course of action in clinical settings. Classical utilitarian and Kantian theories have been modified and incorporated into the set of four principles suggested by Beauchamp and Childress[58] that is currently widely accepted in biomedical literature, and elements of which are included in the Declaration of Helsinki. These principles of (a) respect for autonomy, (b) nonmaleficence, (c) beneficence, and (d) justice will provide a heuristic framework for the following discussion on the ethical dilemmas in EI. According to Beauchamp and Childress,[56] respect for autonomy is one of the primary principles and is rooted in the liberal moral and political tradition of the importance of individual freedom and choice. Autonomy indicates freedom from external constraint and the presence of critical mental capacities such as understanding, intending, and voluntary decision-making capacity.[59] Respect for autonomy is enshrined in the necessity for informed consent in psychiatric research and shared decision making in the treatment of mental illnesses, especially in EI or in working with young people. Nonmaleficence, embodied in the maxim "*primum non nocere*," refers to the simple idea of abstaining from harm. However, this can be a far from simple notion in modern clinical practice, where almost all aspects of care, including psychotherapy, have attendant risks. Hence, all harms must be balanced against the benefits of interventions or beneficence. The principle of beneficence requires clinicians to help others further their important and legitimate interests, often by preventing or removing possible harms. Though the principle of nonmaleficence may intuitively be seen to be more important than the duty of beneficence, this hierarchical ordering is not supported by ethical theory or morality. A harm inflicted may be negligible or trivial, while a harm to be prevented may be substantial. Lastly, the distribution of limited resources for the medical care of the mentally ill or for prevention of mental ill health is significant in most modern societies and requires a close consideration of the principle of justice. Egalitarian theories of justice emphasize equal access to primary goods; libertarian theories emphasize rights to social and economic liberties; and utilitarian theories emphasize a mixed use of such criteria so that public and private utility are maximized. In the days of mental health care provision that is often "managed" by private health management organizations (HMOs) or public bodies in more universalized health systems, the limits of coverage for mental suffering has a particular significance in the area of EI. Ensuring parity for mental health with investment in other areas of health care should aid the cause of EI. Principles of justice may have a role in determining such limits. Strategies that can be demonstrated to do more good for a larger proportion of the population may be preferred over those that are less efficient using such principles.

These four principles often operate together, and sometimes in opposition, in various situations in clinical practice. One or more of these principles may be overridden by others when they exist in conflict. Thus, one's actual duty may be determined by the relative weights of competing duties in particular situations. The restrictions and liberties that different societies value may vary, and this will lead to slightly different interpretations across the world. When these moral principles are in conflict, especially in legal situations, practices such as casuistry where previous judgments direct future ones, may have a role in their resolution.

Ethical Issues in Treating At-Risk Populations

The ethical considerations in dealing with young or at-risk populations will be considered along the lines of the aforementioned principles for the two groups of EI targets for BD, namely familial HR subjects (Stage 0) and clinical HR or subjects with subthreshold mood symptoms (Stage 1).

Benefits of Early Intervention

A substantial minority of adults with BD have reported long delays of over 10–12 years before receiving a correct diagnosis.[60,61] This may partly be due to the onset of depressive episodes or other externalizing disorders well before the onset of full-blown manic episodes in most patients. However, in a number of patients, the diagnosis may be missed in the absence of a carefully taken history or corroborating information.[60] Though there may be confounders in the research indicating this diagnostic delay, any delay in receiving appropriate treatment may have significant consequences for those with BD.

In a 4-year follow-up of adult outpatients with BD, length of delay to first treatment was associated with spending more time depressed, greater severity of depression, greater number of episodes, more days of ultradian cycling, and fewer euthymic days.[26] Though the delay in first treatment was associated with the age of onset in two studies,[26,62] in the study by Post et al.[26] the delay in treatment was independently associated with poor outcomes. In the latter study,[62] the immediate pretreatment morbidity was similar in the individuals with longest and the shortest treatment delay. This may indicate some of the difficulties with the concept of duration of untreated/incorrectly treated illness, where acute onset of severe symptoms in a subset of participants led to emergency access to care. This also highlights the heterogeneity inherent in BD, where the number of episodes may be a better indicator of illness load.[63]

There is substantial evidence to suggest that a greater number of prior episodes or duration of illness is associated with higher cognitive dysfunction, treatment resistance, greater medical comorbidity, and more neurobiological abnormalities in recurrent unipolar and BD.[64] Though the evidence from imaging is equivocal,[65] an examination of cognition in BD suggests that cognitive functions may be preserved prior to illness onset, with deterioration occurring after.[66] However, longitudinal studies examining brain imaging and cognition from before illness onset to later outcomes may help clarify the question of neuroprogression.[65,67] A larger number of episodes has been associated with a poorer treatment response in the acute and maintenance phases[27] and with poorer cross-sectional and longitudinal symptomatic and functional outcome in persons with BD.[68] The response to lithium[69,70] and psychological interventions[28,71] has also been found to be better in persons with earlier initiation of treatment or fewer episodes.

Taken together, these findings strongly point to the benefits of earlier intervention in BD. However, the strongest evidence for the benefit of intervention in at-risk groups in the preillness stage (Stage 0 or 1) may be the improvement seen with therapeutic measures (quetiapine or family-focused therapy) in symptomatic familial at-risk participants, as described earlier. In addition, the finding of normal cognitive function prior to the first manic episode with deterioration later in the course of illness points to the need for intervention prior to the first episode of mania.

Risks of Treating At-Risk Groups

As familial HR groups of children, adolescents, and young adults are better studied to monitor the onset of early symptoms and family difficulties, the potential problems of such approaches are also becoming apparent. Family history–based risk may be an emotionally difficult concept for many families, especially when the risk for bipolar outcomes among offspring of one bipolar parent is quite low. In one of the few studies that have examined this risk covering most of the age of risk (up to the age of 52), the prevalence of BD among offspring of one parent with BD was only 4.4%.[30] Another review of this risk concluded that the weighted summary estimate of the risk of developing the classical forms of BD among offspring of BD parents was 8.7%.[29] These findings suggest that 91%–95% of offspring of BD probands do not develop BD, although a substantial proportion is at increased risk of other problems, including substance abuse and unipolar depression. This, in turn, raises the concern that most of the young people deemed to be at risk for BD in fact may not be and are thus "false positives" in the screening strategy for BD. The potential harms of falsely identifying children and adolescents as being at risk of BD may be many. Young persons may be particularly vulnerable to being labeled as being at risk of BD and may not be able to appreciate the probability of such risk. Literature on the attitudes of children or young persons to risk for BD is limited. In an exploratory study of attitudes to genetic testing among HR adult family members with BD, most participants said that they would chose to take a predictive test for BD if the test answer was definitive, but most would prefer not to if the answer was only probable.[72] Given the very low positive predictive value of a positive family history and these attitudes to genetic testing, it is not clear that HR children or adolescents would willingly choose to be identified as being at risk of BD. Among young persons, concerns about lack of medical insurance coverage when identified to be at genetic HR may also be a negative consequence in some countries. Approximately 63% of a subgroup of participants with BD in the US Bipolar Genome study expressed this worry when asked about their concerns about genetic testing for BD.[73]

Thus, the benefits of EI may have to be weighed against the risks of harm in genetic at-risk populations. Even considering that the seriousness of such harms may be limited and the benefits considerable, the probability of such harm may be high and the probability of the benefits low because of the very high false-positive risk. Given this balance of risks and benefits, special consideration must be taken in identifying at-risk children under the age of consent, to prevent potential negative implications of labeling. These may include the use of developmentally appropriate psychotherapeutic approaches that may help reduce stigma among such young persons. Less specific interventions with multiple diagnostic and psychosocial functioning outcome targets are less contentious from a labeling perspective and may diffuse the "false-positive" problem. This risk-benefit balance may also be altered where interventions are offered to young people only when the young person themselves or their family members have sought help for treatment for symptomatic conditions, including major depression, BD NOS or other nonbipolar psychiatric diagnoses. It is heartening that the pharmacological and psychotherapeutic interventions reported to date among genetic at-risk BD groups have been limited to such symptomatic or help-seeking participants. In these participants, the benefits of potential improvement with these interventions and the preserved autonomy inherent in help seeking may balance the risks of labeling and stigma.

Even among help-seeking groups of young persons, the potential harms from HR interventions such as antipsychotics or mood stabilizers may be considerable. In the previously mentioned single-blind study of quetiapine for nonbipolar mood disorders among familial HR youth, 55% of the participants experienced somnolence, and there was a statistically significant increase in body mass index during the course of this 12-week study.[54] Psychosocial treatments such as family-focused therapy (FFT)[55] and/or nutritional supplements such as omega-3 fatty acids may have a much lower risk as first-line approaches and thus a better risk-benefit ratio than traditional antimanic agents. Furthermore, the impact of such agents needs further study, given the rapid cortical maturational changes in adolescence, including myelination and pruning, and animal studies indicating risks associated with antidepressants[74] and lithium[75] during neurodevelopment.

There may be additional concerns about the assessment of manic-like symptoms in research and clinical practice in at-risk youth. The assessment of psychopathology is often reliant on multiple informants, particularly in children. The agreement between children and parents[76] or teachers and parents[77] has been found to be limited in studies aiming to assess manic symptoms in children. This raises concerns about single-informant research or clinical practice, and the difficulties in achieving agreement in multi-informant research in the examination of manic symptoms among children. Duffy and Carlson[78] also raise concerns about the developmental difficulties in the downward extrapolation of "euphoria" and "irritability," the cardinal symptoms of mania, to children. When parents have described children to be "euphoric" as evidenced by silly and giddy behavior, children have been able to provide a reasonable, developmentally appropriate explanation[79] for these descriptions. The authors also question the ability of children to consistently and easily understand the cognitively complicated notion of euphoria, especially when suffering from comorbid attentional difficulties. Grandiosity is another symptom that is potentially misleading in children, where bragging about their abilities or having an unrealistic positive view of their popularity may in fact be associated with difficulties in learning, attention, or social cognition. Primarily, these diagnostic dilemmas raise questions about the identification of subthreshold mania in children. In addition, these concerns about identification of manic symptoms question the weight of the principle of autonomy over the risks of harm or nonmaleficence. If the interpretation of the parent's report of his or her child's symptoms is potentially erroneous, the help seeking may not be for manic symptoms, and then the concern for potential harm could outweigh the autonomy of the guardian inherent in help seeking.

The other major research strategy in the quest for defining at-risk states for BD has explored subthreshold manic symptoms as a "state marker" for the preillness stage. Retrospective and prospective studies have described a set of putative prodromal criteria that have sought to identify risk groups that may transition to full-threshold BD. One of the main ethical challenges with this approach is the risk of "medicalizing" symptoms that may be seen to be an extension of human emotions such as joy and suffering, or which may be part of personality dysfunction where mood dysregulation is a feature. This may have grave consequences if treatments that are effective in BD (lithium, antipsychotics) are injudiciously administered to this subthreshold group. In such a situation, the risk of maleficence to a subset of the population may override the possibility of beneficence to a similar subgroup that may benefit from such EIs. Indeed, a community-based stratified epidemiological sample of young adults identified 23 individuals with "pure hypomania," where there were periods of hypomania in the absence of depressive episodes.[80] These individuals had higher monthly incomes, were married more often than controls, had little distress about their hypomanic symptoms, and had comparable quality of life to control subjects. This raises the potential that in a small minority of subthreshold hypomanic subjects, interventions may not be necessary, or potentially even harmful. Hence, mild hypomania unless and until it evolves into a full manic or depressive phase may not constitute a disorder in many or most people. So optimal timing of intervention may be critical and quite a different scenario than in subthreshold depression or psychosis.

One of the approaches to improving the positive predictive value of these criteria has been to include major or minor depressive episodes to subthreshold manic symptoms.[47] In general population samples[81] and clinically help-seeking primary care patients,[82] roughly a third (31%–40%) of depressed participants had hypomanic symptoms. This population with both depressive and hypomanic symptoms may be more vulnerable to developing full-threshold BD and have a higher need for care than the previously described "pure hypomanics." In addition, research attempts are being made to understand the clinical validity of these subthreshold groups in a prospective manner [83] before interventions are considered. It should also be considered that population-based studies in the United States[84] and across the world[85] using structured instruments have determined the prevalence of subthreshold BD, as defined by hypomanic symptoms that do not meet the full-threshold *DSM-IV* criteria, to be around 2.4%. As demonstrated by these studies, when such criteria are used carefully and in a rigorous manner, a smaller subset of at-risk participants may be identified that may reduce the false positives in this subthreshold mania risk group. These relatively low prevalence rates may help allay concerns about the medicalization of normative emotions in large proportions of the population. Another important consideration is that risk research for subthreshold participants is largely confined to help-seeking individuals, where again their choices and autonomous decisions regarding their care improves the balance of harms to benefits.

Even in carefully identified subthreshold groups with a relatively low false positive rate, there are potential risks of stigma and labeling of HR youth. Few studies have examined perceptions of stigma or internalized stigma in young people who are either at risk or experiencing early-stage BD.[86] However, in a recently published study that provided a description of a young person with an "at-risk mental state" (ARMS) for psychosis to other young people, 41% of the participants labeled the hypothetical young person with words associated with psychosis,[87] indicating the potential for peer stigmatization. The stigma of BD is reported to be comparable to that of other severe mental illnesses such as schizophrenia and the psychoses,[88] and it is possible that at-risk states of BD may be viewed with stigmatized attitudes in the general population, and thus among peers of those identified to be at risk.

The answer to these concerns about stigma may be in the specific provision and culture of EI programs.[89] Youth-friendly, stigma-free models of care are being developed across the world that seek to provide EI programs with a holistic and optimistic stance.[5] In Australia, a tiered approach is being implemented nationwide as part of a new wave of mental health reform. Communities of Youth Services or headspace programs work in partnership with local communities and general practitioner networks and aim to provide stigma-free, evidence-based, preventive care for higher prevalence disorders and at-risk groups (likely in Stage 0 or 1). These programs are also colocated with other youth-focused services, such as those for vocational support or educational assistance, which then decreases the stigma of accepting help for mental illnesses. One of the earliest intervention services for the ARMS associated with the Early Psychosis Prevention and Intervention Centre in Melbourne, Australia, was deliberately generically termed the "Personal Assessment and Crisis Evaluation" (PACE) clinic to at least publicly avoid the labels associated with psychosis. In one of its early iterations this clinic was based at a popular shopping mall in an attempt to improve the accessibility and acceptance of help seeking for psychosis.[90] This became the template for the later universal primary care approach of headspace. Similarly, the Headstrong program in Ireland and the Youthspace program in Birmingham, UK, are examples of youth access initiatives that are community-linked, streamed separately from traditional mental health care by location, and holistic and optimistic in culture. They have all proven successful in engaging and providing care to young people with early-stage and high prevalence mental health difficulties.[5]

Principles of Justice: Who Deserves More Help and When?

The notion of justice can often be complicated for clinicians and doctors, where the patient in front of them may assume the most significance. It is noted that in many countries, physicians are oriented toward the beneficence of the individual patient, rather than that of the ethics of resource distribution in a population.[91] A better understanding of principles of justice can help appreciate the significance of research and clinical endeavors in EI and place this in the context of the needs of the community and its mental health.

The term *distributive justice* refers to fair, equitable, and appropriate distribution in society, determined by justified norms of distribution, and based on the terms of social cooperation.[59] This includes both the benefits, such as clinical care and funds for research, as well as the burdens, such as the cost of health care or insurance. The distribution of benefits and burdens may then depend on various social norms across societies. Cost-effectiveness research has the potential to identify the relative benefits of health care costs (burdens) to achieve better health outcomes for the population (benefits). A strong argument for EI in mood and psychotic disorders would be cost-effectiveness research that could demonstrate a reduction in the burden of care (direct costs) or an improvement in the productivity of the population at risk (indirect costs). In the field of EI in psychosis, a number of studies have now shown that EI is cost effective,[90,91] although this has been disputed by certain critics.[92] Despite some methodological issues, the overall picture from the cost-effectiveness literature in EI is strongly supportive of this, representing a cost-effective and value-for-money approach.[90,91] Given that EI in BD is yet to advance to a stage where cost-effectiveness may need to be considered, it may be argued that distributive justice would suggest that the resources are better spent elsewhere. However, the substantial economic burden of BD, which was ranked to be among the leading causes of loss of life years to disability[92] among the economically productive 15- to 44-year-old age group, may offer a strong argument for investment in research and clinical endeavors that might help limit the magnitude of this disability.

Another issue that may need to be considered in the "justice" of health care provision is the prevalence of subthreshold hypomanic symptoms in the general population. In a prevalence study of a stratified sample of college-level Korean students, the prevalence of bipolar spectrum disorder (BSD) was identified to be approximately 18.6% using the Korean version of the Mood Disorder Questionnaire,[93] although that instrument has been shown to be of questionable reliability, especially in population studies.[94] If preventive interventions needed to be provided to nearly a fifth of the population, as indicated by this study, finite resources available for health care provision would suggest that other groups requiring care might not receive that care. However, the study by Bae et al.[94] is unusual in that it included participants with minimal impairment due to their symptoms and hence may have identified the inflated prevalence of BSD. Other previously cited studies have consistently identified the prevalence of BSD to be approximately 2.4% in general population samples. In addition, the identified BSD participants in the study were not help seeking. The process of help seeking may be an exercise of individual autonomy, and in addition, creates the demand for care, which in turn creates an ethical necessity to provide care. For policymakers in health, this process of help seeking (and arguing for resources) may set apart the population that receives care from those who do not. One such group may be those at high risk for serious mental illnesses and who are unable to seek help, or face barriers to accessing health care. Proactive policies driven by strong advocacy may help preventative efforts for such vulnerable groups. Another driver of such policy changes could be arguments based on economic measures of population health outcomes.

Policymakers use measures of the unit cost of improving quality of life, measured as cost per quality-adjusted life year (QALY) saved by interventions across broad areas of health interventions. For example, the cost per QALY of a left ventricular assist device was 258,922 UK pounds in 2012,[95] while the same measure for a social recovery-based CBT intervention for psychosis was 18,844 UK pounds in 2009.[96] This would suggest that the CBT-based intervention could be a better investment over the assist device when decision makers consider priorities in health investment. However, such simple comparisons of costs may be deceptive, as a number of variables, including the measures of costs, the analysis methods, and the setting in which the studies are done, could make significant differences in the derived cost figures. To date, there have been no published cost utility studies on EI in BD. This may partly be due to the paucity of intervention research in general. However, research on cost utility in mental health has lagged behind other areas of medicine. An analysis of studies published up until 2001[97] suggested that though depression and BD contributed to the greatest DALYs (12.2% of total) in the United States, the number of cost utility analyses (CUAs) registered amounted only to 1.7% of the total. Osteoarthritis, on the other hand, despite contributing to only 2.2% of total DALYs, had a similar proportion of CUAs (1.5%). The study also identified that the CUAs focused more on pharmaceutical products and surgical procedures as opposed to psychological and behavioral interventions. This points to the need for greater economic evaluation of interventions in mental health in general, and EI in particular, to help direct resource allocation.

Respect for Autonomy and Choice

Though discussed last in this chapter, the principle of autonomy is often considered the most central of the four ethical principles. As detailed in the earlier sections, when conflicts between beneficence, nonmaleficence, and justice exist in the need to provide care in a variety of different settings, the concept of individual autonomy may help decide in favor of one or more of the other principles. In providing clinical interventions for at-risk youth, respect for autonomy is paramount, and informed consent and choice should at all points be the prime considerations. This section will attempt to address the issues of informed consent in young people, and in particular, the consent process for intervention research in BD.

As discussed previously, the highest risk age range for the development of BD and schizophrenia appears to be in the 15- to 25-year age group. Unfortunately, the age of consent, which varies between 16 and 21 years in many jurisdictions across the world, falls in the middle of this range and creates unique difficulties in research and clinical care for these at-risk young people. Even more problematic is the notion of Gillick competence,[98] where children under the age of 16 can be considered competent to make decisions regarding their medical treatment if they can be demonstrated to be able to do so. One of the specific issues involving consent from underage, at-risk young people relates to the need to involve guardians, often parents, in the consent process. Though for most part, this should improve the rigor of consent, there is a possibility that there may be competing interests that may compel young people to become involved in intervention or research studies. One of these may be the sense of guilt and responsibility that parents of at-risk children sometimes carry for the genes or psychosocial risks that may have conferred the vulnerability to their children, as demonstrated in recent interviews of mothers of children with serious mental illnesses, as opposed to medical problems.[99] The other may be that these parents themselves may be receiving care in affiliated clinical institutions that then places additional conflicts in their decision to include their children. In such a setting, it may well be possible that the nuances of the risk for BD, including the very high false-positive rate and the difficulties in separating symptoms from normal development, could be problematic for parents of enrolled children. In addition, if the parents are themselves unwell, subthreshold symptoms, cognitive difficulties associated with the illness, and the fear of the illness may also contribute to parents' choices for their children. In these situations, particular care must be taken in the informed consent process, and this should attempt to take additional steps that could help improve the autonomy and foster the best interests of the children included. These may include consenting over multiple sessions, detailed discussions of the risks and benefits of participation in studies, assessing various factors that may impede the consent process and thorough documentation of the capacity to consent. In addition, assent has been sought from participating children in intervention studies in BD,[55] which improves the autonomy of children in such studies. This is consistent with the guidance of the Royal College of Paediatrics and Child Health, UK, which suggests that children with sufficient capacity to understand what is proposed to them can consent to participate in research.[100]

Ensuring that the consent process is valid may be even more complicated in situations where young people may be enrolled in the military. In countries such as Singapore or Israel, mandatory conscription can mean that a substantial proportion of at-risk or control participants may be in military training or service. This is exemplified by the ethical problems associated with the LYRIKs project[101] in Singapore, which aimed to follow at-risk (for psychosis) participants over a period of time. In that study, the authors report that there was lack of clarity on whether conscripted youth under the age of 21 were under the guardianship of their parents or that of the military. However, informed consent was sought from parents in this study.

The ethical difficulties inherent in such research should not detract from these efforts, and research on vulnerable populations is justifiable if there is a reasonable likelihood that they stand to benefit from the results of the research, and if the research is responsive to the health needs and priorities of these populations, consistent with the Declaration of Helsinki (DoH).[102] This conclusion by the DoH exemplifies situations where the possibility of significant benefit may override the risks of infringement of autonomy, if the possible harm is relatively low. Such interplay of these major ethical principles, though formalized by IRBs for research, often needs careful reflection by clinicians in formulating difficult decisions in the everyday clinical care of at-risk youth.

Conclusions and Future Directions

BD is a chronic condition that is one of world's leading causes of disability in the young adult population. The efforts to diminish the clinical, emotional, and economic impact of this condition have prompted a shift to earlier intervention, in line with the approach for the serious psychotic illnesses. There have been efforts to identify familial and symptomatic at-risk groups for BD so that preventive interventions can be trialed in these groups. Early studies in at-risk familial and symptomatic youth have indicated the potential benefits but also the risks of interventions in these groups. Apart from the clinical improvements noted in these studies, the findings of normal cognitive function in earlier stages of BD and deterioration later are strong arguments for the benefits of intervention in at-risk groups. However, the risks of such interventions may primarily be that of labeling and stigma, as well as the toxicity of antipsychotics or mood stabilizers. These are issues that nevertheless have existing solutions as described earlier. Research in these subgroups also faces difficulties in achieving impartial consent from relevant guardians in the face of competing concerns, as well as the difficulties of identifying manic symptoms in childhood. Efforts to minimize harm by the use of stigma-free, youth-friendly models of care and lower risk interventions may represent the avenues ahead for navigating these potential ethical concerns among at-risk youth. Among older adolescents, the validity of subthreshold manic symptoms as at-risk states for BD is unclear, especially in the absence of depressive symptoms. In addition, the risk of medicalizing normal and potentially useful emotions in large proportions of the population is a particular concern in the subthreshold mania group. However, research that suggests that a smaller proportion of the population can be identified to have subthreshold or BSD disorder allays some of this concern.

A consideration of the balance of the *probability* as well as the *magnitude* of beneficence and nonmaleficence to the participants and the population may help determine the right course of action in many of these ethically challenging situations. Fostering autonomy and choice may also help moderate the balance of beneficence and nonmaleficence in some of these situations. This may be best done by providing help when it is sought and by providing adequate and comprehensive information of the risks and benefits, thereby helping young people and their guardians make the most reasonable decisions for themselves. The cost-effectiveness of interventions, measured in studies that consider both direct and indirect costs and benefits, will help determine the place of at-risk interventions for BD in decreasing the impact of this illness. It is likely that if safe and simple interventions can be introduced early, and followed up with stepwise or sequential adaptive interventions for nonresponders, then the burden of this illness can be diminished, particularly in the challenging and productive early years of emerging adulthood.

Author Disclosures

Professor McGorry currently receives research support from a National Health and Medical Research Council of Australia in the form of a Program Grant (no 566529), and the Colonial Foundation. He has also received grant funding from NARSAD and unrestricted research funding from Astra Zeneca, Eli Lilly, Janssen-Cilag, Pfizer, and Novartis, as well as honoraria for educational activities with Astra Zeneca, Eli Lilly, Janssen-Cilag, Pfizer, Bristol Myer Squibb, Roche, and the Lundbeck Institute.

Dr. Berk has received grant/research support from the National Institutes of Health, Cooperative Research Centre, Simons Autism Foundation, Cancer Council of Victoria, Stanley Medical Research Foundation, MBF, NHMRC, Beyond Blue, Rotary Health, Geelong Medical Research Foundation, Bristol Myers Squibb, Eli Lilly, Glaxo SmithKline, Meat and Livestock Board, Organon, Novartis, Mayne Pharma, Servier, and Woolworths; has been a speaker for Astra Zeneca, Bristol Myers Squibb, Eli Lilly, Glaxo SmithKline, Janssen Cilag, Lundbeck, Merck, Pfizer, Sanofi Synthelabo, Servier, Solvay and Wyeth; and served as a consultant to Astra Zeneca, Bioadvantex, Bristol Myers Squibb, Eli Lilly, Glaxo SmithKline, Janssen Cilag, Lundbeck Merck, and Servier. He is supported by NHMRC Senior Principal Research Fellowship 1059660. He is a coinventor of two provisional patents regarding the use of NAC and related compounds for psychiatric indications, which, while assigned to the Mental Health Research Institute, could lead to personal remuneration upon a commercialization event.

Dr. Ratheesh has no conflicts to declare.

References

1. Sanchez-Moreno J, Martinez-Aran A, Tabares-Seisdedos R, Torrent C, Vieta E, Ayuso-Mateos JL. Functioning and disability in bipolar disorder: an extensive review. *Psychother Psychosom.* 2009;78:285–97.
2. Yung AR, Killackey E, Hetrick SE, et al. The prevention of schizophrenia. *Int Rev Psychiatry.* 2007;19:633–46.
3. Bloom D, Cafiero E, Jane- Llopis E. *The Global Economic Burden of Non-Communicable Disease.* Geneva, Switzerland: World Economic Forum; 2011.
4. McGorry P. Early clinical phenotypes and risk for serious mental disorders in young people: need for care precedes traditional diagnoses in mood and psychotic disorders. *Can J Psychiatry.* 2013;58:19–21.
5. McGorry P, Bates T, Birchwood M. Designing youth mental health services for the 21st century: examples from Australia, Ireland and the UK. *Br J Psychiatry.* 2013;202:s30–5.
6. Fusar-Poli P, Bonoldi I, Yung A, et al. Predicting psychosis: a meta-analysis of evidence. *Arch Gen Psychiatry.* 2012;in press.
7. Jacka FN, Reavley NJ, Jorm AF, Toumbourou JW, Lewis AJ, Berk M. Prevention of common mental disorders: what can we learn from those who have gone before and where do we go next? *Aust NZ J Psychiatry.* 2013;47:920–9.
8. Cuijpers P. Examining the effects of prevention programs on the incidence of new cases of mental disorders: the lack of statistical power. *Am J Psychiatry.* 2003;160:1385–91.
9. Cornblatt BA, Lencz T, Kane JM. Treatment of the schizophrenia prodrome: is it presently ethical? *Schizophr Res.* 2001;51:31–8.
10. McGorry PD, Yung A, Phillips L. Ethics and early intervention in psychosis: keeping up the pace and staying in step. *Schizophr Res.* 2001;51:17–29.

11. Yung AR, McGorry PD. The prodromal phase of first-episode psychosis: past and current conceptualizations. *Schizophr Bull*. 1996;22:353–70.

12. Yung AR, McGorry PD, McFarlane CA, Jackson HJ, Patton GC, Rakkar A. Monitoring and care of young people at incipient risk of psychosis. *Schizophr Bull*. 1996;22:283–303.

13. McGorry PD, Yung AR, Phillips LJ, et al. Randomized controlled trial of interventions designed to reduce the risk of progression to first-episode psychosis in a clinical sample with subthreshold symptoms. *Arch Gen Psychiatry*. 2002;59:921–8.

14. McGlashan TH, Zipursky RB, Perkins D, et al. Randomized, double-blind trial of olanzapine versus placebo in patients prodromally symptomatic for psychosis. *Am J Psychiatry*. 2006;163:790–9.

15. van der Gaag M, Smit F, Bechdolf A, et al. Preventing a first episode of psychosis: meta-analysis of randomized controlled prevention trials of 12 month and longer-term follow-ups. *Schizophr Res*. 2013;149:56–62.

16. Lin A, Wood SJ, Nelson B, et al. Neurocognitive predictors of functional outcome two to 13 years after identification as ultra-high risk for psychosis. *Schizophr Res*. 2011;132:1–7.

17. Nelson B, Yuen HP, Wood SJ, et al. Long-term follow-up of a group at ultra high risk ("prodromal") for psychosis: the PACE 400 study. *JAMA Psychiatry*. 2013;70:793–802.

18. Berk M, Kapczinski F, Andreazza AC, et al. Pathways underlying neuroprogression in bipolar disorder: focus on inflammation, oxidative stress and neurotrophic factors. *Neurosci Biobehav Rev*. 2011;35:804–17.

19. Dodd S, Maes M, Anderson G, Dean OM, Moylan S, Berk M. Putative neuroprotective agents in neuropsychiatric disorders. *Prog Neuropsychopharmacol Biol Psychiatry*. 2013;42:135–45.

20. Anand S, Pennington-Smith PA. Compulsory treatment: rights, reforms and the role of realism. *Aust NZ J Psychiatry*. 2013;47:895–8.

21. Duffy A, Alda M, Hajek T, Grof P. Early course of bipolar disorder in high-risk offspring: prospective study. *Br J Psychiatry*. 2009;195:457–8.

22. Conus P, Ward J, Lucas N, et al. Characterisation of the prodrome to a first episode of psychotic mania: results of a retrospective study. *J Affect Disord*. 2010;124:341–5.

23. Bechdolf A, Ratheesh A, Cotton SM, Nelson B, Chanen AM, Betts J, et al. The predictive validity of bipolar at-risk (prodromal) criteria in help-seeking adolescents and young adults: a prospective study. *Bipolar Disord*. 2014. doi:10.1111/bdi.12205

24. Berk M, Conus P, Lucas N, et al. Setting the stage: from prodrome to treatment resistance in bipolar disorder. *Bipolar Disord*. 2007;9:671–8.

25. Scott J, Leboyer M, Hickie I, et al. Clinical staging in psychiatry: a cross-cutting model of diagnosis with heuristic and practical value. *Br J Psychiatry*. 2013;202:243–5.

26. Post RM, Leverich GS, Kupka RW, et al. Early-onset bipolar disorder and treatment delay are risk factors for poor outcome in adulthood. *J Clin Psychiatry*. 2010;71:864–72.

27. Berk M, Brnabic A, Dodd S, et al. Does stage of illness impact treatment response in bipolar disorder? Empirical treatment data and their implication for the staging model and early intervention. *Bipolar Disord*. 2011;13:87–98.

28. Colom F, Reinares M, Pacchiarotti I, et al. Has number of previous episodes any effect on response to group psychoeducation in bipolar patients? A 5-year follow-up post hoc analysis. *Acta Neuropsychiatrica*. 2010;22:50–3.

29. Smoller JW, Finn CT. Family, twin, and adoption studies of bipolar disorder. *Am J Med Genet C Semin Med Genet*. 2003;123C:48–58.

30. Gottesman, II, Laursen TM, Bertelsen A, Mortensen PB. Severe mental disorders in offspring with 2 psychiatrically ill parents. *Arch Gen Psychiatry*. 2010;67:252–7.

31. Duffy A. The early natural history of bipolar disorder: what we have learned from longitudinal high-risk research. *Can J Psychiatry*. 2010;55:477–85.

32. Duffy A, Alda M, Hajek T, Sherry SB, Grof P. Early stages in the development of bipolar disorder. *J Affect Disord*. 2010;121:127–35.

33. Akiskal HS, Downs J, Jordan P, Watson S, Daugherty D, Pruitt DB. Affective disorders in referred children and younger siblings of manic-depressives. Mode of onset and prospective course. *Arch Gen Psychiatry*. 1985;42:996–1003.

34. Hillegers MH, Reichart CG, Wals M, Verhulst FC, Ormel J, Nolen WA. Five-year prospective outcome of psychopathology in the adolescent offspring of bipolar parents. *Bipolar Disord*. 2005;7:344–50.
35. Duffy A, Alda M, Crawford L, Milin R, Grof P. The early manifestations of bipolar disorder: a longitudinal prospective study of the offspring of bipolar parents. *Bipolar Disord*. 2007;9:828–38.
36. Shaw JA, Egeland JA, Endicott J, Allen CR, Hostetter AM. A 10-year prospective study of prodromal patterns for bipolar disorder among Amish youth. *J Am Acad Child Adolesc Psychiatry*. 2005;44:1104–11.
37. Egeland JA, Endicott J, Hostetter AM, Allen CR, Pauls DL, Shaw JA. A 16-year prospective study of prodromal features prior to BPI onset in well Amish children. *J Affect Disord*. 2012;142:186–92.
38. Alda M. Bipolar disorder: from families to genes. *Can J Psychiatry*. 1997;42:378–87.
39. McNamara RK, Nandagopal JJ, Strakowski SM, DelBello MP. Preventative strategies for early-onset bipolar disorder: towards a clinical staging model. *CNS Drugs*. 2010;24:983–96.
40. Correll CU, Penzner JB, Frederickson AM, et al. Differentiation in the preonset phases of schizophrenia and mood disorders: evidence in support of a bipolar mania prodrome. *Schizophr Bull*. 2007;33:703–14.
41. Lewinsohn PM, Klein DN, Seeley JR. Bipolar disorder during adolescence and young adulthood in a community sample. *Bipolar Disord*. 2000;2:281–93.
42. Cannon M, Caspi A, Moffitt TE, et al. Evidence for early-childhood, pan-developmental impairment specific to schizophreniform disorder: results from a longitudinal birth cohort. *Arch Gen Psychiatry*. 2002;59:449–56.
43. Shankman SA, Lewinsohn PM, Klein DN, Small JW, Seeley JR, Altman SE. Subthreshold conditions as precursors for full syndrome disorders: a 15-year longitudinal study of multiple diagnostic classes. *J Child Psychol Psychiatry*. 2009;50:1485–94.
44. Tijssen MJ, van Os J, Wittchen HU, et al. Prediction of transition from common adolescent bipolar experiences to bipolar disorder: 10-year study. *Br J Psychiatry*. 2010;196:102–8.
45. Duffy A. The nature of the association between childhood ADHD and the development of bipolar disorder: a review of prospective high-risk studies. *Am J Psychiatry*. 2012;169:1247–55.
46. Skirrow C, Hosang GM, Farmer AE, Asherson P. An update on the debated association between ADHD and bipolar disorder across the lifespan. *J Affect Disord*. 2012;141:143–59.
47. Bechdolf A, Nelson B, Cotton SM, et al. A preliminary evaluation of the validity of at-risk criteria for bipolar disorders in help-seeking adolescents and young adults. *J Affect Disord*. 2010;127:316–20.
48. Brietzke E, Mansur RB, Soczynska JK, Kapczinski F, Bressan RA, McIntyre RS. Towards a multifactorial approach for prediction of bipolar disorder in at risk populations. *J Affect Disord*. 2012;140:82–91.
49. Frey BN, Andreazza AC, Houenou J, et al. Biomarkers in bipolar disorder: a positional paper from the International Society for Bipolar Disorders Biomarkers Task Force. Aust NZ J Psychiatry. 2013;47:321–32.
50. Berk M, Kapczinski F, Andreazza AC, et al. Pathways underlying neuroprogression in bipolar disorder: focus on inflammation, oxidative stress and neurotrophic factors. *Neurosci Biobehav Rev*. 2009;35:804–17.
51. Ratheesh A, Lin A, Nelson B, et al. Neurocognitive functioning in the prodrome of mania—an exploratory study. *J Affect Disord*. 2013;147:441–5.
52. Geller B, Cooper TB, Sun K, et al. Double-blind and placebo-controlled study of lithium for adolescent bipolar disorders with secondary substance dependency. *J Am Acad Child Adolesc Psychiatry*. 1998;37:171–8.
53. Findling RL, Frazier TW, Youngstrom EA, et al. Double-blind, placebo-controlled trial of divalproex monotherapy in the treatment of symptomatic youth at high risk for developing bipolar disorder. *J Clin Psychiatry*. 2007;68:781–8.
54. DelBello MP, Adler CM, Whitsel RM, Stanford KE, Strakowski SM. A 12-week single-blind trial of quetiapine for the treatment of mood symptoms in adolescents at high risk for developing bipolar I disorder. *J Clin Psychiatry*. 2007;68:789–95.
55. Miklowitz DJ, Schneck CD, Singh MK, et al. Early intervention for symptomatic youth at risk for bipolar disorder: a randomized trial of family-focused therapy. *J Am Acad Child Adolesc Psychiatry*. 2013;52:121–31.
56. Nemets H, Nemets B, Apter A, Bracha Z, Belmaker RH. Omega-3 treatment of childhood depression: a controlled, double-blind pilot study. *Am J Psychiatry*. 2006;163:1098–100.

57. Clayton EH, Hanstock TL, Hirneth SJ, Kable CJ, Garg ML, Hazell PL. Reduced mania and depression in juvenile bipolar disorder associated with long-chain omega-3 polyunsaturated fatty acid supplementation. *Eur J Clin Nutr.* 2009;63:1037–40.

58. Beauchamp TL, Childress JF. *Principles of Biomedical Ethics.* 5th ed. New York, NY: Oxford University Press; 2001.

59. Beauchamp TL. The philosphical basis of psychiatric ethics. In: Bloch S, Green S, eds. *Psychiatric Ethics.* New York, NY: Oxford University Press; 2009:25–48.

60. Hirschfeld RM, Vornik LA. Recognition and diagnosis of bipolar disorder. *J Clin Psychiatry.* 2004;65(Suppl. 15):5–9.

61. Berk M, Dodd S, Callaly P, et al. History of illness prior to a diagnosis of bipolar disorder or schizoaffective disorder. *J Affect Disord.* 2007;103:181–6.

62. Baldessarini RJ, Tondo L, Baethge CJ, Lepri B, Bratti IM. Effects of treatment latency on response to maintenance treatment in manic-depressive disorders. *Bipolar Disord.* 2007;9:386–93.

63. Grande I, Magalhaes PV, Kunz M, Vieta E, Kapczinski F. Mediators of allostasis and systemic toxicity in bipolar disorder. *Physiol Behav.* 2012;106:46–50.

64. Post RM, Fleming J, Kapczinski F. Neurobiological correlates of illness progression in the recurrent affective disorders. *J Psychiatr Res.* 2012;46:561–73.

65. Schneider MR, DelBello MP, McNamara RK, Strakowski SM, Adler CM. Neuroprogression in bipolar disorder. *Bipolar Disord.* 2012;14:356–74.

66. Lewandowski KE, Cohen BM, Ongur D. Evolution of neuropsychological dysfunction during the course of schizophrenia and bipolar disorder. *Psychol Med.* 2011;41:225–41.

67. Berk M, Conus P, Kapczinski F, et al. From neuroprogression to neuroprotection: implications for clinical care. *Med J Aust.* 2010;193:S36–40.

68. Magalhaes PV, Dodd S, Nierenberg AA, Berk M. Cumulative morbidity and prognostic staging of illness in the Systematic Treatment Enhancement Program for Bipolar Disorder (STEP-BD). *Aust NZ J Psychiatry.* 2012;46:1058–67.

69. Franchini L, Zanardi R, Smeraldi E, Gasperini M. Early onset of lithium prophylaxis as a predictor of good long-term outcome. *Eur Arch Psychiatry Clin Neurosci.* 1999;249:227–30.

70. Swann AC, Bowden CL, Calabrese JR, Dilsaver SC, Morris DD. Differential effect of number of previous episodes of affective disorder on response to lithium or divalproex in acute mania. *Am J Psychiatry.* 1999;156:1264–6.

71. Scott J, Paykel E, Morriss R, et al. Cognitive-behavioural therapy for severe and recurrent bipolar disorders: randomised controlled trial. *Br J Psychiatry.* 2006;188:313–20.

72. Meiser B, Mitchell PB, McGirr H, Van Herten M, Schofield PR. Implications of genetic risk information in families with a high density of bipolar disorder: an exploratory study. *Soc Sci Med.* 2005;60:109–18.

73. Nwulia EA, Hipolito MM, Aamir S, Lawson WB, Nurnberger JI Jr. Ethnic disparities in the perception of ethical risks from psychiatric genetic studies. *Am J Med Genet B Neuropsychiatr Genet.* 2011;156B:569–80.

74. LaRoche RB, Morgan RE. Adolescent fluoxetine exposure produces enduring, sex-specific alterations of visual discrimination and attention in rats. *Neurotoxicol Teratol.* 2007;29:96–107.

75. Youngs RM, Chu MS, Meloni EG, Naydenov A, Carlezon WA Jr., Konradi C. Lithium administration to preadolescent rats causes long-lasting increases in anxiety-like behavior and has molecular consequences. *J Neurosci.* 2006;26:6031–9.

76. Stringaris A, Stahl D, Santosh P, Goodman R. Dimensions and latent classes of episodic mania-like symptoms in youth: an empirical enquiry. *J Abnorm Child Psychol.* 2011;39:925–37.

77. Arnold LE, Demeter C, Mount K, et al. Pediatric bipolar spectrum disorder and ADHD: comparison and comorbidity in the LAMS clinical sample. *Bipolar Disord.* 2012;13:509–21.

78. Duffy A, Carlson GA. How does a developmental perspective inform us about the early natural history of bipolar disorder? *J Can Acad Child Adolesc Psychiatry.* 2013;22:6–12.

79. Carlson GA, Meyer SE. Phenomenology and diagnosis of bipolar disorder in children, adolescents, and adults: complexities and developmental issues. *Dev Psychopathol.* 2006;18:939–69.

80. Gamma A, Angst J, Ajdacic-Gross V, Rossler W. Are hypomanics the happier normals? *J Affect Disord.* 2008;111:235–43.

81. Angst J, Cui L, Swendsen J, et al. Major depressive disorder with subthreshold bipolarity in the National Comorbidity Survey Replication. *Am J Psychiatry*. 2010;167:1194–201.

82. Dubovsky SL, Leonard K, Griswold K, et al. Bipolar disorder is common in depressed primary care patients. *Postgrad Med*. 2011;123:129–33.

83. Bechdolf A, Ratheesh A, Wood SJ, et al. Rationale and first results of developing at-risk (prodromal) criteria for bipolar disorder. *Curr Pharm Des*. 2012;18:358–75.

84. Merikangas KR, Akiskal HS, Angst J, et al. Lifetime and 12-month prevalence of bipolar spectrum disorder in the National Comorbidity Survey replication. *Arch Gen Psychiatry*. 2007;64:543–52.

85. Merikangas KR, Jin R, He JP, et al. Prevalence and correlates of bipolar spectrum disorder in the world mental health survey initiative. *Arch Gen Psychiatry*. 2011;68:241–51.

86. Latalova K, Ociskova M, Prasko J, Kamaradova D, Jelenova D, Sedlackova Z. Self-stigmatization in patients with bipolar disorder. *Neuro Endocrinol Lett*. 2013;34:265–72.

87. Anglin DM, Greenspoon MI, Lighty Q, Corcoran CM, Yang LH. Spontaneous labelling and stigma associated with clinical characteristics of peers "at-risk" for psychosis. *Early Interv Psychiatry*. 2013. Epub ahead of print; doi: 10.1111/eip.12047

88. Hawke LD, Parikh SV, Michalak EE. Stigma and bipolar disorder: a review of the literature. *J Affect Disord*. 2013;150:181–91.

89. Macneil CA, Hasty M, Cotton S, et al. Can a targeted psychological intervention be effective for young people following a first manic episode? Results from an 18-month pilot study. *Early Interv Psychiatry*. 2012;6:380–8.

90. Phillips LJ, Leicester SB, O'Dwyer LE, et al. The PACE Clinic: identification and management of young people at "ultra" high risk of psychosis. *J Psychiatr Pract*. 2002;8:255–69.

91. Everett A, Huffine C. Ethics in contemporary community psychiatry. *Psychiatr Clin North Am*. 2009;32:329–41.

92. Whiteford HA, Degenhardt L, Rehm J, et al. Global burden of disease attributable to mental and substance use disorders: findings from the Global Burden of Disease Study 2010. *Lancet*. 2013;382(9904):1574–86.

93. Bae SO, Kim MD, Lee JG, et al. Prevalence of bipolar spectrum disorder in Korean college students according to the K-MDQ. *Neuropsychiatr Dis Treat*. 2013;9:869–74.

94. Dodd S, Williams LJ, Jacka FN, Pasco JA, Bjerkeset O, Berk M. Reliability of the Mood Disorder Questionnaire: comparison with the Structured Clinical Interview for the DSM-IV-TR in a population sample. *Aust NZ J Psychiatry*. 2009;43:526–30.

95. Moreno SG, Novielli N, Cooper NJ. Cost-effectiveness of the implantable HeartMate II left ventricular assist device for patients awaiting heart transplantation. *J Heart Lung Transplant*. 2012;31:450–8.

96. Barton GR, Hodgekins J, Mugford M, Jones PB, Croudace T, Fowler D. Cognitive behaviour therapy for improving social recovery in psychosis: cost-effectiveness analysis. *Schizophr Res*. 2009;112:158–63.

97. Neumann PJ, Rosen AB, Greenberg D, et al. Can we better prioritize resources for cost-utility research? *Med Decis Making*. 2005;25:429–36.

98. Larcher V, Hutchinson A. How should paediatricians assess Gillick competence? *Arch Dis Child*. 2010;95:307–11.

99. Lautenbach DM, Hiraki S, Campion MW, Austin JC. Mothers' perspectives on their child's mental illness as compared to other complex disorders in their family: insights to inform genetic counseling practice. *J Genet Couns*. 2012;21:564–72.

100. McIntosh N, Bates P, Brykczynska G, et al. Guidelines for the ethical conduct of medical research involving children. Royal College of Paediatrics, Child Health: Ethics Advisory Committee. *Arch Dis Child*. 2000;82:177–82.

101. Lysaght T, Capps B, Subramaniam M, Chong SA. Translational and clinical research in Singapore: ethical issues in a longitudinal study of the prodromal phase of schizophrenia. *Early Interv Psychiatry*. 2012;6:3–10.

102. World Medical Association: World Medical Association Declaration of Helsinki: ethical principles for medical research involving human subjects. *JAMA*. 2013;310(20):2191–4.

Medical Treatment Strategies for Young People With Bipolar Disorder

Sarah M. Lytle, Sonal K. Moratschek,
and Robert L. Findling

Overview of Treatment Considerations

Treatments for bipolar disorder have been primarily studied in adults. Given the developmental differences across the life cycle, the treatments that are most effective for adults may not be the best interventions for children. A number of medications are approved by the United States Food and Drug Administration (FDA) for the treatment of pediatric bipolar disorder, including lithium, risperidone, olanzapine, aripiprazole, and quetiapine (Table 8.1). Empirical evidence for their use, dosing guidelines, potential side effects, and suggestions for monitoring are addressed. Additionally, there are medications that do not have FDA approval but have been studied in children and adolescents with bipolar disorder. Available information with regard to these medications is provided as well.

Recommendations vary depending on the stage of bipolar disorder for which patients are being treated. Therefore, agents studied in acute manic and mixed states, bipolar depression, and maintenance treatment are discussed. Combination therapy may be warranted under certain conditions, and the available evidence is examined. Special consideration must be taken in treating pregnant adolescents, and recommendations for working with pregnant youth are given. Finally, pediatric bipolar is often comorbid with other psychiatric conditions. Available research to guide the practitioner working with youth with comorbid disorders is also provided.

Psychopharmacological management of pediatric bipolar disorder requires an understanding of unique concerns when treating children and adolescents. First, the

TABLE 8.1 Medications Approved by the FDA for the Treatment of Manic or Mixed Episodes of Pediatric Bipolar Disorder

Medication	Age (years)	Dosing Range (mg/day)	Adverse Effects
Lithium	12–17	300–2,400 (divided)	Abdominal pain, gastrointestinal distress, insomnia, dizziness, polyuria
Risperidone	10–17	0.25–2.5	Weight gain; EPS; increased LDL, cholesterol, and prolactin
Olanzapine	13–17	2.5–20	Weight gain; increased cholesterol, triglycerides and hepatic enzymes, and prolactin
Aripiprazole	10–17	2–30	Sedation, somnolence, gastrointestinal distress, and akathisia
Quetiapine	10–17	50–600 (divided)	Weight gain, increased fasting glucose, cholesterol, and thyrotropin

parent or guardian is ultimately responsible for giving consent to start the medication. Involving the child, especially if they are older, in the decision-making process may help increase patient understanding and adherence to treatment plans. Risks, benefits, and side effects of medications should be discussed with both guardian and child using developmentally appropriate language. Furthermore, addressing the ability of the child to swallow pills and coordination with school officials who may be dispensing these medications may be necessary to increase medication adherence.

While a comprehensive discussion of the pharmacodynamic and pharmacokinetic differences between youth and adults is beyond the scope of this chapter, practitioners are encouraged to gain an understanding of this area before prescribing medications to children and adolescents.

Monotherapy in Acute Mania/Mixed States

Lithium

Lithium was the first medication approved by the FDA for treatment of bipolar I disorder in children ages 12–17 years. Since few methodologically rigorous studies had been conducted in youth with this condition, approval was based on evidence of lithium from the adult literature. However, dosing guidelines, efficacy, safety, and monitoring guidelines had not been definitively established in children and adolescents at the time that approval was given. Thus, more recent focus has been on developing evidence-based dosing strategies and supplementing existing preliminary evidence that suggests that lithium may be effective in treating bipolar I disorder in this population. Studies comparing lithium to other medications used in the treatment of bipolar disorder, as well as lithium in bipolar disorder comorbid with other psychiatric disorders, have also been conducted and are discussed in other sections.

Empirical Support

A number of studies have examined lithium for the treatment of bipolar disorder, acute manic and mixed states in children and adolescents. An open-label trial of divalproex, carbamazepine, and lithium reported that lithium was effective in the treatment of youth with bipolar I and II disorder.[1] Acute stabilization of manic symptoms in youth with bipolar I disorder was also reported in a short-term open-label study.[2] Effectiveness of lithium in the treatment of bipolar I disorder in children and adolescents was also described in an 8-week open-label study of lithium, although remission was not achieved in a majority of patients.[3]

A randomized, double-blind, placebo-controlled trial of lithium and divalproex suggested that lithium might be efficacious in the treatment of acute mania in pediatric bipolar disorder, although a statistically significant difference from placebo was not observed.[4] This study may have had inadequate statistical power to detect an effect size similar to what has been observed in adults. The results of a more definitive study sponsored by the National Institute of Child Health and Human Development on the acute efficacy of lithium versus placebo are not yet published but are expected to be available soon.[5] When considered in its entirety, the extant evidence provides preliminary support for the use of lithium in the treatment of acute manic and mixed states in bipolar disorder in children and adolescents.

Dosing Guidelines

Initially, lithium dosing in children and adolescents was based on extrapolations from dosing used in adults. As a part of a larger initiative to examine the use of lithium in youth more definitively, a number of evidence-based dosing studies have been recently conducted to help guide treatment in this population.

An open-label trial examining the pharmacokinetic profile of lithium in pediatric bipolar I disorder provided support for starting lithium at 300 mg twice or three times daily for youth weighing greater than 30 kg and a dose of 300 mg once daily for youth weighing less than 30 kg.[6] Increases of 300 mg of lithium per week (with an additional 300 mg increase during the first week of treatment) were found to be safe and efficacious.[7]

Side Effects

While efficacy of lithium has not yet been definitively established, the side effect profile, as well as potential for toxicity, requires that the prescribing physician be well informed and follow guidelines for dosing and monitoring. In addition, patients and their parents must be informed of potential side effects.

In children and adolescents, commonly reported side effects include abdominal pain, nausea, vomiting, headache, insomnia, dizziness, polyuria, and enuresis.[6,8] Taking lithium with food, dividing doses during the day, and administration of the liquid formulation of lithium may reduce gastrointestinal side effects. However, potential toxicity must be considered, as gastrointestinal symptoms may be a sign that lithium levels are excessive.[9]

Elevated thyrotropin levels are a potential side effect and were reported to be significantly elevated compared to baseline when pediatric patients were treated with a combination of lithium and divalproex for up to 20 weeks.[10] Other potential side effects reported in adult studies include hyperparathyroidism,[11] nephrogenic diabetes insipidus, nephrotic syndrome/proteinuria,[12] and cardiac conduction problems (AV blocks and irregular sinus rhythm).[13] Leukocytosis may occur but is generally benign.[14] Adverse effects, including neurological side effects, may be more common in preschool age children treated with lithium[15] warranting even closer monitoring in this population.

Lithium undergoes renal excretion; therefore, dehydration or other circumstances in which sodium is depleted, and drug interactions that affect renal function, may alter serum lithium concentrations and must be closely monitored. In youth who develop polyuria and/or enuresis, it is important to avoid fluid restriction as this could lead to dehydration and toxicity. Potential interactions may occur with a number of medications, including nonsteroidal anti-inflammatory medications, which can increase the risk of lithium toxicity.[16]

Monitoring

Lithium has a narrow therapeutic index and appropriate dosing parameters are critical. An open-label trial of children and adolescents with bipolar I disorder showed that variability in serum levels of lithium after a single dose of 600 or 900 mg of lithium was significant, suggesting the need for monitoring of serum lithium levels throughout the course of treatment.[6] Obtaining serum trough levels is recommended to maintain an effective dose and maintain serum levels below 1.4 mEqL.[7] Toxicity can occur when serum lithium levels are too high. Early signs of lithium toxicity may include listlessness, dysarthria, and tremor that can advance to increased tremors, decreased motor coordination and ataxia, confusion, and delirium possibly resulting in coma and/or death.

Other laboratory assessment, including complete blood counts, thyroid function tests, urinalysis, blood urea nitrogen, creatinine, and serum calcium levels, should be obtained prior to initiating lithium therapy (Table 8.2). Monitoring of serum electrolytes, renal and thyroid function studies, and a urinalysis is recommended every 3 months while the patient remains on lithium.[17] A pregnancy test in adolescent females is advised prior to initiation of lithium therapy due to an increased risk of Ebstein's anomaly in women taking lithium during their first trimester. In addition, discussions regarding pregnancy and birth-control options prior to the initiation of lithium therapy are warranted. Due to potential cardiac effects, electrocardiograms (EKGs) are recommended prior to lithium initiation, after 2–3 months and then yearly. Additionally, since weight gain is a potential side effect, weight monitoring prior to initiation of and periodically during lithium therapy is advised. Referrals to and consultations with appropriate specialists such as nephrologists, cardiologists, or endocrinologists is recommended as necessary if laboratory studies are found to be abnormal.

In summary, a number of open-label and one double-blind study have suggested that lithium might have efficacy in the treatment of bipolar disorder in children and

TABLE 8.2 Monitoring Suggestions During Lithium Treatment

	Baseline	6–8 Weeks Postinitiation	Every 3 Months	As Indicated by Signs/Symptoms
Lithium level*	X	X	X	X
Complete blood count	X	X		X
Thyrotropin	X		X	X
Urinalysis	X		X	X
Blood urea nitrogen/creatinine	X	X	X	X
Serum calcium levels	X			X
Pregnancy test	X			X
Electrocardiogram	X		X	X
Weight/height	X		X	X

*More frequent monitoring of lithium levels during initiation of treatment and when medication dosage adjustments are made is recommended.

adolescents. Results of a more definitive study should be available in the near future. As described later in this chapter, studies of other agents have been more definitive in terms of their efficacy and for that reason they should probably be considered prior to using lithium. Close monitoring due to lithium's side effect profile and potential for toxicity is required and may limit its use.

Anticonvulsants

With the success of anticonvulsants in treating bipolarity in adult populations, the use of these medications has received attention as possible treatments in children and adolescents. The following is a discussion of the current research in the acute treatment of manic, hypomanic, or mixed symptoms in pediatric bipolar disorder with anticonvulsants.

Divalproex Sodium

Divalproex sodium, first marketed as an antiepileptic medication, is FDA approved for the treatment of the manic and/or mixed states of adult bipolar. While not approved for the treatment of bipolar disorder in children and adolescents, it is used by clinicians for this indication.

Empirical Support

Based on the efficacy of divalproex for the treatment of bipolar mania in adults, researchers have performed studies in children and adolescents to examine its efficacy and safety in this population. A short-term, random assignment, open-label prospective study of divalproex, lithium, and carbamazepine reported that divalproex might be effective in the acute treatment of manic and/or mixed states of bipolar I and II disorder in children and adolescents, with a response rate of 53%.[1] A subsequent chart review of the long-term use of divalproex found a 53% response rate as measured by the Clinical Global Impression- Improvement Scale (CGI-I), but 40% of participants discontinued the medication, with the most commonly cited reason being weight gain (27%).[18] Additional open-label trials have supported the putative effectiveness and safety of divalproex in pediatric bipolar disorder.[19,20]

An acute double-blind placebo-controlled trial of divalproex extended-release of 150 patients (age 10–17 years) was conducted with a subsequent open-label extension phase. The acute study failed to show separation from placebo[21] (Table 8.3). However, another double-blind comparison study of lithium, divalproex, and placebo demonstrated effectiveness of divalproex over placebo for acute manic symptoms.[4] The explanation for these discrepant results is not entirely clear. However, the study by Wagner et al.[21] was an industry-sponsored multisite study, whereas the other study by Kowatch et al.[4] was conducted at fewer sites, thereby potentially minimizing the between-site variability that could potentially obscure positive results. In addition, the multisite, industry-sponsored trial used the extended-release formulation, in comparison to the work of Kowatch and colleagues that did not. This difference in formulation may also have contributed to the observed differences in results. Overall, these studies suggest that monotherapy may be beneficial for the symptomatic treatment of pediatric bipolar disorder.

Studies comparing divalproex to quetiapine and risperidone suggests that these second-generation antipsychotics (SGAs) may be more efficacious than divalproex and are reviewed in the section on SGAs.

Dosing Guidelines

Currently, divalproex is available in capsules, syrup, intravenous, and sprinkle forms. It is also available in an extended-release formulation. General dosing approach is patterned after pediatric epilepsy with recommended starting doses of 10–15 mg/kg per day, divided into twice or thrice a day dosing, and may be increased by 250 mg to 500 mg per day as tolerated. Titration of divalproex is based on symptom response. Therapeutic serum levels are between 80 to 125 µg/ml, and dosage should not exceed 60 mg/kg per day.[9]

Side Effects

Divalproex is absorbed through the gut and metabolized in the liver, allowing for potential significant drug interactions. These interactions are discussed in more detail later.

Common side effects noted in studies with divalproex include weight gain, gastrointestinal upset, sedation, increased appetite, and tremor.[22] Significant weight gain has also been observed.[23] Polycystic ovary syndrome (PCOS) may be a consequence of treatment with divalproex. Symptoms of PCOS include weight gain, menstrual changes, hirsutism, and acne. Uncommon, but serious side effects of divalproex may include pancreatitis, liver toxicity, and thrombocytopenia.

TABLE 8.3 Select Acute Placebo-Controlled Trials for Monotherapy in Manic and/or Mixed States of Pediatric Bipolar Disorder

Study (Drug)	No. of Participants	Ages (years)	Study Design	Results	Side Effects
Haas 2009[1] Risperidone	n = 169	10–17	Randomized, double-blind, placebo-controlled	Mean change in YMRS significantly greater for risperidone 3–6 mg (−16.5) and risperidone 0.5–2.5 mg (−18.5) versus placebo (−9.1)	Somnolence; headache; fatigue
Tohen 2007[1] Olanzapine	n =161	13–17	Randomized, double-blind, placebo-controlled	Mean change in YMRS significantly greater for olanzapine (−17.65) versus placebo (−9.99)	Increased appetite; weight increase; somnolence; sedation; increased blood pressure, fasting glucose and total cholesterol; increased prolactin
Pathak 2013[1] Quetiapine	n = 277	10–17	Randomized, double-blind, placebo-controlled, parallel-group	Mean change in YMRS for quetiapine 400 mg/d (−14.25) and quetiapine 600 mg/d (−15.60) significantly greater than placebo (−9.04)	Somnolence; sedation; dizziness; headache
Findling 2013 Ziprasidone	n = 237	10–17	Randomized, double-blind, placebo-controlled	Mean change in YMRS significantly greater for ziprasidone (−13.83) versus placebo (−8.61)	Sedation; somnolence; headache; fatigue; nausea
Findling 2009[1] Aripiprazole	n = 296	10–17	Randomized, double-blind, placebo-controlled	Mean change in YMRS significantly greater for aripiprazole 10 mg and 30 mg (−14.2 and −16.5, respectively) versus placebo (−8.2 and −8.2, respectively)	Somnolence and EPS greater in aripiprazole 30 mg compared to 10 mg group; fatigue; headache; akathisia
Wagner 2009 Divalproex Extended Release	n = 150	10–17	Randomized, double-blind, placebo-controlled	No statistically significant difference on YMRS between placebo (mean change = −7.9) and divalproex (mean change = −8.8)	Weight gain, headache
DelBello 2005 Topiramate	n = 56	6–17	Double-blind, placebo- controlled	Premature termination of study. Inconclusive secondary to small sample size	Decreased appetite; nausea; diarrhea; paresthesias
Wagner 2006 Oxcarbazepine	n = 116	7–18	Randomized, placebo-controlled	No statistically significant difference between placebo (mean change = −9.79) versus oxcarbazepine (mean change = −10.90) on YMRS	Dizziness; nausea; somnolence; rash; diplopia

[1]Used for FDA approval.

Monitoring

When starting divalproex in the pediatric population, baseline height, weight, liver enzymes, and complete blood counts are recommended. Subsequent follow-up of weight and height are recommended secondary to potential for weight gain, and they should be followed every 2 to 3 months. Follow-up monitoring of liver enzymes and complete blood counts are suggested every 3 to 6 months or when clinically indicated. Educating patients on signs of liver failure, pancreatitis, and thrombocytopenia, including abdominal pain, jaundice, and bruising or prolonged bleeding, respectively, is advised.

Divalproex is potentially toxic at high doses and care must be taken to monitor serum levels to prevent toxicity. Divalproex levels should be maintained within the range of 50–125 µl/ml. Divalproex toxicity is rare and may occur at any blood level, but it more commonly occurs at levels over 125 µg/ml. Signs of toxicity range from nausea and vomiting to confusion, ataxia, and tremor with more severe symptoms including acute liver failure and coma.

It is recommended that a serum trough level be drawn 4 to 5 days after initiating divalproex, as well as relatively frequently until a therapeutic dose and blood concentration are achieved. Subsequently, the level can be monitored every 6 months thereafter, or more frequently, if necessary.[9] Additional monitoring is recommended when the divalproex dose is changed or if there are concerns for toxicity.

As mentioned earlier, divalproex has the potential for multiple drug interactions. Divalproex increases serum levels of a number of medications, including carbamazepine, lamotrigine, topiramate, phenytoin, phenobarbital, amitriptyline, and warfarin. Increased serum drug levels of carbamazepine and lamotrigine increase the risk of toxic side effects from these medications, including Stevens-Johnson syndrome, a serious systemic reaction.

Furthermore, carbamazepine, phenytoin, and combined oral contraceptives can decrease divalproex serum levels whereas risperidone, fluoxetine, and aspirin are known to increase serum divalproex levels. These changes can potentially affect symptom stabilization in patients who are taking the medications concomitantly.

Specific considerations must be taken with adolescent females using divalproex. A pregnancy test in adolescent females is recommended prior to the initiation of divalproex therapy due to the potential for teratogenic effects on the developing fetus, specifically neural tube defects. Due to this risk, prior to initiation of divalproex, discussions with adolescents of childbearing age regarding pregnancy and birth control options are recommended. It is recommended that clinicians monitor for symptoms of PCOS, including menstrual irregularities, hirsutism, acne, and changes in weight.[22] Appropriate referrals to gynecology and endocrinology may be considered as necessary.

Carbamazepine

Initially used in pediatric epilepsy, carbamazepine is an anticonvulsant with mood-stabilizing properties. It is currently approved by the FDA for manic or mixed episodes in adult bipolar disorder, but it is not currently approved by the FDA for use in pediatric bipolar disorder.

Empirical Support

In a chart review of 300 pediatric patients using carbamazepine extended release as either monotherapy or adjunctive therapy (mean dose 541 + /1,328.1 mg/day), 76% reported improvement of symptoms as measured by the CGI-I. However, 119 patients eventually discontinued the drug, most commonly secondary to poor response.[24]

To date, there are a limited number of prospective open-label trials of carbamazepine in pediatric mania. The previously discussed 8-week open-label study (n = 42) of divalproex, lithium, and carbamazepine showed a modest response rate with carbamazepine (38%).[1] A second 8-week open-label trial of carbamazepine extended-release monotherapy (n = 27) reported a modestly significant improvement, but not a remission of symptoms, with a mean serum level of 6.6 +/- 3.5 μl/ml.[25] In this study, 41% of participants dropped out, with the most common reason cited as lack of response.[25] An additional open-label trial of the effectiveness, safety, and tolerability of carbamazepine extended-release in 161 children and adolescents supported effectiveness and safety in this population.[26]

While the available research suggests possible effectiveness and safety of carbamazepine in pediatric bipolar disorder, there are currently no randomized, placebo-controlled studies in this population. Furthermore, the dosing schedule, multiple drug interactions, and need for close monitoring may make the practical implications of its use in pediatric bipolar disorder challenging.

Dosing Guidelines

Dosing of carbamazepine is patterned largely after pediatric epilepsy studies, with initial dosing of 15 mg/kg, divided up to four times a day, with a maximum dose of 1,200 mg per day. In adolescents, doses may be increased by 200 mg weekly, but slower titration in younger children is recommended.[9] Target serum drug levels are between 4 and 12 μg/ml.

Side Effects

Overall, carbamazepine is generally well tolerated in the pediatric population. Common side effects include nausea, somnolence, dizziness, and rash.[22,24] In adult populations, carbamazepine has been associated with Stevens-Johnson syndrome and aplastic anemia.[22] As a result, caution is advised when initiating and titrating this medication.

Monitoring

A baseline history and physical is recommended with specific attention to cardiac, hematologic, and hepatic illness. Serum blood levels and monitoring of complete blood counts and liver enzymes are recommended at baseline, every 2 weeks for the first 2 months, and then every 3 months.[9] Furthermore, monitoring is recommended during any dose adjustments and with addition or removal of medications.[22]

Carbamazepine is extensively metabolized by the cytochrome P450 enzyme in the liver and has numerous drug interactions. It induces its own metabolism, thereby decreasing its own serum levels.[22] Considering its potential for multiple drug interactions, and potential serious dermatological and hematologic side effects, care is advised when using carbamazepine in the pediatric population.

Lamotrigine

Lamotrigine is FDA approved for maintenance treatment in adult bipolar disorder, but it does not have approval for use in pediatric bipolar disorder.

Empirical Support

A 12-week open-label study of 39 youth, ages 12–17 years, was performed to assess effectiveness and safety of lamotrigine monotherapy for acute manic and mixed episodes of pediatric bipolar disorder. Results showed a statistically significant reduction in manic, depressed, attention deficit, and psychotic symptoms. While 13 of the subjects developed skin rashes, there were no cases of Stevens-Johnson syndrome.[27] A 14-week open-label trial of lamotrigine in 46 youth (ages 8–12 years) with acute manic or mixed episode of bipolar I disorder or hypomanic episode of bipolar II was conducted. During the initial 8 weeks of this study, lamotrigine was initiated and slowly uptitrated. As a result of this slow titration during the initial 8-week period, patients were started on and treated with an atypical antipsychotic (risperidone, aripiprazole, quetiapine, or ziprasidone) for acute symptom stabilization. The atypical antipsychotic was slowly withdrawn between 4 and 8 weeks, with every patient on lamotrigine monotherapy at the end of the 8-week period. At the end of 8 weeks, there was a significant improvement of manic/hypomanic symptoms (as measured by the Young Mania Rating Scale [YMRS]). Lamotrigine monotherapy was then continued for another 6 weeks. At the end of the 14 weeks, the response rate of manic symptoms was 71% (as measured by YMRS), the response rate of depressive symptoms was 82% (as measured by the Child Depression Rating Scale-Revised [CDRS-R]), and the remission rate was 56%. Of those patients who had obtained remission at 8 weeks, 23% relapsed by week 14. Benign rash was noted in 6.4% of patients.[28]

An open-label study of lamotrigine in bipolar depression is reviewed in the section on bipolar depression. There are currently no published randomized, placebo-controlled trials studying the efficacy or safety of lamotrigine in the acute treatment of pediatric bipolar disorder. The available research suggests that lamotrigine may be effective in manic and mixed episodes of pediatric bipolar disorder; however, further trials are needed.

Dosing Guidelines

Caution is advised when dosing lamotrigine in children and adolescents due to the concern for Stevens-Johnson syndrome. It is recommended to generally start at 25 mg/day, slowly titrating by 25 mg every 2 weeks targeting symptom reduction, usually to a total dose of 200 mg/day.[29]

Side Effects

Common side effects of lamotrigine include gastrointestinal upset, headache, sedation, and rash. Biederman et al.[27] measured metabolic parameters and noted a small but significant increase in platelets, sodium, and creatinine levels, and a decrease in QTC interval, associated with use of lamotrigine.

Monitoring

Prior to starting lamotrigine, a baseline history and physical examination are recommended. While there are no specific recommendations regarding baseline laboratory studies, a complete blood count and liver enzymes are suggested.

Lamotrigine is metabolized via glucuronidation and susceptible to medications that either induce or inhibit this action in the liver. Concomitant use with divalproex requires slower titration and lower doses secondary to inhibition of lamotrogine's metabolism by divalproex, whereas coadministration with carbamazepine can decrease concentrations of lamictal. Higher serum lamotrigine levels increase the risk of serious dermatological reactions. Monitoring for rash is necessary. Traditionally, if within 2 months of starting or changing the dose of lamotrigine, a rash appears without alternate explanation, the medication should be discontinued.[29]

Topiramate

Case studies of adjunctive topiramate for acute manic symptoms in pediatric bipolar disorder have described overall improvement in the patients.[30,31] A double-blind, placebo-controlled trial of topiramate monotherapy in youth was stopped prior to the end of the trial, after ongoing trials in adults failed to show separation from placebo (Table 8.3).[32] When the data obtained prior to termination of the study were analyzed, it provided preliminary, albeit inconclusive evidence for possible effectiveness. Commonly reported side effects of topiramate in these studies include decreased appetite, weight loss, sedation, paresthesias, and gastrointestinal upset. Further studies are needed to assess more definitively the effectiveness and safety of topiramate in pediatric bipolar disorder.

Oxcarbazepine

Oxcarbazepine, a derivative of carbamazepine, was first used in children with epilepsy.[33] There are few studies examining its use in pediatric bipolar disorder. Initial preliminary case reports described improvement in the manic, hypomanic, and mixed phases of bipolar illness.[33] However, a subsequent randomized, placebo-controlled ($n = 116$) trial demonstrated that oxcarbazepine monotherapy did not separate from placebo for the acute treatment of manic and/or mixed states of bipolar disorder in children and adolescents (Table 8.3).[34] Common side effects included dizziness, gastrointestinal upset, fatigue, diplopia, and rash.[34] Based on available data, oxcarbazepine is not recommended for the treatment of bipolar disorder in children and adolescents.

Gabapentin

Gabapentin is approved by the FDA for adjunctive therapy in pediatric seizure disorders, but it does not have an indication for bipolar disorder in adult or pediatric populations. There are two case reports[35,36] describing an improvement in mood swings and irritability in two children with bipolar disorder. However, there are no other published studies of gabapentin in pediatric bipolar disorder.

With minimal hepatic metabolism, gabapentin has few interactions with other medications. Side effects are generally thought to be mild, with sedation being the most common. Other side effects include dizziness, tremor, and weight gain.[22] However, due to the absence of rigorous studies in children, gabapentin is not recommended for use in pediatric bipolar disorder.

Second-Generation Antipsychotics

Studies of SGAs in the treatment of acute manic or mixed states of pediatric bipolar disorder include clozapine, risperidone, olanzapine, quetiapine, ziprasidone, aripiprazole, and paliperidone. Research on the SGAs asenapine, iloperidone, and lurasidone has not been published in the child and adolescent population. Many of the SGAs have evidence supporting their use in the treatment of bipolar disorder, and an overview of these data is provided in this section.

Clozapine

There are no placebo-controlled reports of clozapine in pediatric bipolar disorder. A case series in which a small number of youth with treatment-resistant bipolar disorder received clozapine, suggested that it might have antipsychotic and antimanic effects in this population.[37] One retrospective chart review of clozapine treatment in 10 adolescents with bipolar disorder, acute manic or mixed episode, suggested that a significant improvement in symptoms may occur. The most common side effects noted were increased appetite and weight gain, sedation, enuresis, and sialorrhea.[38]

Clozapine is not used as a first-line agent for treatment of pediatric bipolar disorder due to lack of rigorous methodological studies and its potential for serious adverse side effects, including agranulocytosis and seizures.

Risperidone

Risperidone is an SGA approved by the FDA for the short-term treatment of manic or mixed episodes of bipolar I disorder in children and adolescents ages 10–17 years.

Empirical Support

A number of reports have provided evidence that risperidone may be a safe and effective option for the treatment of acute manic and mixed states of pediatric bipolar disorder. A short-term, open-label study of risperidone or olanzapine monotherapy showed that both had effectiveness in treating bipolar disorder in children aged 4–6 years.[39] Another open-label study of risperidone in children and adolescents ages 6–17 years described a significant improvement in manic symptoms at doses of both 0.5–2.5 mg/day and 3–6 mg/day.[40]

Randomized controlled trials have also demonstrated efficacy. A 3-week, randomized, placebo-controlled, double-blind trial of 169 youth (ages 10–17 years) demonstrated that risperidone in doses of 0.5 to 2.5 mg/d or 3–6 mg/d were significantly more effective than placebo in reducing symptoms in subjects with bipolar I disorder, manic or mixed episode (Table 8.3).[41] A short-term, double-blind, randomized trial of risperidone versus divalproex in pediatric bipolar disorder showed that the group receiving risperidone improved more quickly than those receiving divalproex. Remission and response rates were significantly greater in the risperidone group as compared to the divalproex group. In addition, the dropout rate in the risperidone group was 24% versus a dropout rate of 48% in the divalproex group, suggesting that risperidone was better tolerated.[42]

Most recently, the Treatment of Early Age Mania (TEAM) study was a randomized, controlled 8-week, parallel comparison study of risperidone, lithium carbonate, and divalproex in manic or mixed states of pediatric bipolar disorder. Subjects treated with risperidone showed a significantly higher response rate (as measured by the clinical global impressions for bipolar illness improvement—mania scale) than those treated with lithium or divalproex. The response rates were 68.5%, 35.6%, and 24%, respectively. The difference between response rates in lithium and divalproex was not statistically significant. These results suggest that risperidone may be superior to both lithium and divalproex sodium in the treatment of acute manic and mixed states of bipolar disorder in children and adolescents.[43]

These data provide support for the use of risperidone in acute manic and mixed episodes of bipolar disorder in children and adolescents.

Dosing Guidelines

FDA labeling for the short-term treatment of manic or mixed episodes of bipolar I disorder in youth ages 10–17 years recommends initiating risperidone at doses of 0.5 mg/day. Doses may be increased by 0.5 mg/day to a total of 2.5 mg/day, as tolerated. Doses of risperidone equal to or less than 2.5 mg have been shown to carry a better safety profile than higher doses.[41] Adverse side effects, including sedation and extrapyramidal side effects (EPS), may limit rapid titration. Clinical experience suggests that young children may benefit from an initial dose of 0.25 mg/d with a slower titration schedule and lower overall daily doses to minimize adverse side effects. In addition, doses may be divided to increase tolerability.[9]

Side Effects

Common side effects include somnolence, headache, and fatigue.[41] The potential for weight gain and increase in body mass index (BMI) can be significant and may be greater than that seen with other medications, such as divalproex and lithium.[40,43] In addition, EPS has been observed in youth who are taking risperidone at rates that may be higher than that in adults, especially at doses greater than 3 mg/d.

Effects on cholesterol have been observed as well. In the TEAM study described earlier, low-density cholesterol was increased in the risperidone group as compared to the divalproex group and high-density cholesterol was decreased as compared to the divalproex group.[43] Prolactin elevation has also been noted in children and adolescents treated with risperidone.[39,40,42,43] Signs of hyperprolactinemia can include galactorrhea, gynecomastia, and amenorrhea. The rates of hyperprolactinemia appear to be higher than that of other SGAs.

Olanzapine

Olanzapine is an SGA that is FDA approved for the treatment of acute manic or mixed episodes of bipolar I disorder in adolescents ages 13–17 years.

Empirical Support

Two 8-week, open-label trials of olanzapine in youth (ages 5–14 and 6–17 years, respectively) reported significant improvement in symptoms of mania.[44,45] As mentioned earlier, a short-term, open-label study of risperidone or olanzapine monotherapy described that both agents were effective in treating bipolar disorder in children aged 4–6 years.[39]

A randomized, double-blind, placebo-controlled trial of 161 adolescents with bipolar disorder randomized to either olanzapine or placebo reported that improvements in manic symptoms were significantly greater in patients who received olanzapine as compared to placebo (Table 8.3).[46] Together, these studies suggest that olanzapine may be effective for the treatment of acute manic and mixed episodes of pediatric bipolar disorder.

Dosing Guidelines

FDA labeling for the treatment of acute manic or mixed episodes in adolescents aged 13–17 years with bipolar disorder recommends initial doses of 2.5 mg/d or 5 mg/d. Titration by 2.5 mg/d or 5 mg/d as tolerated, up to a maximum daily dose of 20 mg/d, is advised.

Side Effects

The most commonly reported adverse effects with olanzapine are increased appetite, weight gain, somnolence, and sedation. In addition, increases in prolactin, total cholesterol, high-density lipoprotein cholesterol, triglycerides, and hepatic enzymes have been reported to be significantly greater than placebo in patients treated with olanzapine.

Extrapyramidal symptoms were not found to be higher in patients treated with olanzapine as compared to placebo.[46] Treatment is most commonly limited by the potential for weight gain and related changes in lipids and glucose metabolism.

While studies have indicated that olanzapine may be effective for acute or mixed episodes of pediatric bipolar disorder, its safety profile suggests caution. FDA guidelines indicate that olanzapine should not be used as a first-line treatment due to potential increases in weight and hyperlipidemia. Therefore, clinicians are advised to consider alternative agents for first-line treatment of pediatric bipolar disorder.

Aripiprazole

Aripiprazole is an SGA that has been approved by the FDA for treatment of acute manic or mixed episodes of bipolar I disorder in children aged 10–17 years.

Empirical Support

A chart review of 41 youth (mean age 11.4 ± 3.5 years) with bipolar spectrum disorder treated with aripiprazole at an average mean daily dose of 16.0 ± 7.9 mg/d indicated that 71% showed improvement in manic symptoms.[47] An open-label, pilot study of aripiprazole in 19 children and adolescents (ages 6–17 years) reported a significant reduction in symptoms of mania.[48] An open-label, dose-escalation study reported that aripiprazole at doses of 20, 25, and 30 mg/d was safe and effective in youth (ages 10–17 years) with primary psychiatric disorders that preferentially included bipolar or schizophrenia spectrum disorder diagnoses.[49] Symptomatic youth ages 4–9 years with bipolar spectrum disorders were treated in an open-label trial for up to 16 weeks with aripiprazole. In all, 62.5% of patients were considered responders and the authors suggest that aripiprazole may be effective in the acute treatment of bipolar disorder in children.[50]

A short-term, randomized, double-blind, placebo-controlled trial of aripiprazole for the treatment of manic or mixed episodes of pediatric bipolar disorder in youth ages 10–17 years reported superiority of aripiprazole as compared to placebo at doses of 10 mg and 30 mg. This data suggested that doses of aripiprazole up to 30 mg/d for the treatment of pediatric bipolar disorder may be effective and safe (Table 8.3).[51]

These studies provide support for the use of aripiprazole in the treatment of acute manic and mixed episodes of pediatric bipolar disorder.

Dosing Guidelines

Current FDA labeling for manic or mixed episodes of bipolar I disorder in children aged 10 to 17 years of age suggest starting aripiprazole at a daily dose of 2 or 5 mg/d. Gradual titration to a maximum of 30 mg/d is recommended. One study demonstrated that although aripiprazole doses of both 10 mg and 30 mg were effective, rates of adverse side effects, including weight gain, somnolence, and extrapyramidal symptoms, were higher at the 30 mg dose.[51] Thus, as with other medications, the minimum effective dose should be used.

Side Effects

Common adverse effects of aripiprazole include sedation/somnolence, gastrointestinal symptoms, cold symptoms, headache, dizziness, and extrapyramidal symptoms.[48, 51] Decreases in serum prolactin have been observed in youth treated with aripiprazole. The implications for this finding are not known. Aripiprazole may be less likely to affect metabolic parameters such as weight gain and lipid profiles, as compared to other SGAs.[51]

Quetiapine

Quetiapine is approved for the treatment of acute mania in children and adolescents ages 10–17 years with bipolar disorder.

Empirical Support

A retrospective chart review of patients (mean age 10.8 ± 3.9 years) receiving monotherapy for bipolar disorder type I and II, cyclothymia and bipolar disorder NOS reported a response rate of 78.6% for those receiving quetiapine monotherapy.[52] Two prospective open-label trials of quetiapine monotherapy in 30 preschool and 19 school-age children were conducted that reported a significant improvement in manic symptoms in both age groups.[53]

A double-blind, randomized, pilot study comparing quetiapine and divalproex in adolescents (ages 12–18 years) described comparable efficacy in the treatment of manic symptoms. However, a reduction in manic symptoms was observed to occur more quickly in patients treated with quetiapine as compared to divalproex.[54] A double-blind, randomized, placebo-controlled, parallel-group study of 277 youth (ages 10–17 years) with bipolar disorder, currently manic, was conducted. Patients treated with quetiapine at doses of 400 mg/d and 600 mg/d were reported to show a significantly greater improvement (as measured by the YMRS) than patients treated with placebo (Table 8.3).[55]

These studies suggest that quetiapine may be effective in the treatment of acute mania in pediatric bipolar disorder.

Dosing Guidelines

FDA labeling suggests a starting dose of 25 mg divided twice daily titrated to 200 mg divided twice daily by day five, with increases of no more than 100 mg/d. The maximum recommended dose is 600 mg/d, divided twice or three times daily for tolerability.

Side Effects

Small, but significant increases in posttreatment pulse and blood pressure have been noted in youth ages 4–15 years treated with quetiapine. In addition, patients treated with quetiapine were noted to experience significant weight gain.[53] The most commonly reported side effects were cold symptoms, sedation, gastrointestinal disturbance, and headache in this report.[53] Pathak et al.[55] reported that the most common side effects in patients treated with quetiapine were somnolence, sedation, dizziness, and headache. Increases in weight, fasting glucose, total cholesterol, triglycerides, low-density lipoprotein, and thyrotropin were noted in patients treated with quetiapine as compared to those treated with placebo.[55]

Ziprasidone

While ziprasidone does have FDA approval for the treatment of acute mania in adult bipolar disorder, it does not have FDA approval for the treatment of bipolar disorder in children and adolescents.

Empirical Support

Four case reports of youth with bipolar disorder were described in which the authors observed that ziprasidone up to 60 mg/d in divided doses was safe and effective.[56] An 8-week, prospective, open-label trial of ziprasidone in pediatric bipolar disorder (youth ages 6–17 years) reported significant improvement in symptoms and the medication was well tolerated.[57] A short-term, open-label study of 63 children and adolescents (aged 10–17 years), 73% of whom had bipolar disorder, followed by a 24-week, open-label extension suggested that ziprasidone may be useful in the treatment of bipolar disorder in children and adolescents.[58]

A randomized, double-blind, placebo-controlled, 4-week trial of ziprasidone was conducted. Youth ages 10–17 years ($n = 237$) with acute manic or mixed episodes of bipolar disorder were randomized in a 2:1 fashion (ziprasidone:placebo). A significant improvement in manic symptoms (as measured by the YMRS) was reported in the ziprasidone group as compared to the placebo group. This short-term trial was followed by an open-label, extension trial, which is described in the section on maintenance treatments (Table 8.3).[59]

These data suggest that ziprasidone may be efficacious in the treatment of acute manic and mixed episodes of pediatric bipolar disorder.

Dosing Guidelines

Results of the study conducted by Findling et al.[59] suggest that doses of 40–160 mg/day are effective and generally well tolerated for children and adolescents ages 10–17 years with bipolar disorder. A starting dose of 20 mg/day, with 20 mg/day increases every second day, was used in this study.

Side Effects

Common side effects of ziprasidone include sedation, somnolence, headache, fatigue, and nausea and occur at similar rates across the dosing range.[59] They have also been noted to occur at a higher frequency than that seen in adults.[58] A statistically significant increase in weight was not observed in one study[57]; however, in another study 33.3% of patients had a greater than 7% increase in weight.[58] Metabolic parameters including serum lipid and fasting glucose levels were not significantly changed, EPS was infrequent, and EKG changes were minimal.[58,59]

Ziprasidone has, however, been associated with prolongation of the heart rate-corrected QT interval (QTc) on EKGs in youth treated with ziprasidone.[60,61]

Others (Paliperidone, Iloperidone, Asenapine, Lurasidone)

There is one study in the child and adolescent population available for paliperidone. This 8-week, prospective, open-label trial of paliperidone in pediatric bipolar disorder reported a statistically significant improvement in manic symptoms in 73% of patients (aged 16–17 years).[62] The most common reported side effects of paliperidone were decreased energy, cold/infection/allergy symptoms, increased appetite, and headache. In addition, a significant increase in weight was observed.[62] There are no published studies of iloperidone, lurasidone, or asenapine in pediatric bipolar disorder. Due to a paucity of data for these antipsychotics, as well as the evidence to support the administration of other compounds, the use of these four agents is not recommended for children and adolescents with bipolar disorder.

Monitoring of Children and Adolescents Treated With Second-Generation Antipsychotics

Regular monitoring of patients prescribed SGAs is important, and suggested monitoring intervals to guide clinical practice are noted (Table 8.4). At baseline, a personal and family history, as well as a physical exam, is recommended. Monthly monitoring

TABLE 8.4 Suggested Monitoring Guidelines for Second-Generation Antipsychotics Used in the Treatment of Acute Manic and Mixed Episodes of Pediatric Bipolar Disorder

	Baseline	Monthly	Every 3 Months	As Indicated by Signs/Symptoms
Weight/height/waist circumference	X	X**	X	X
Blood pressure	X		X	X
Fasting glucose and lipid profile/HgA1C	X		X	X
AIMS	X	X		X
Prolactin level*	X			X
Electrocardiogram	X			X

*Prolactin level monitoring is suggested for risperidone and olanzapine, but it is not indicated for other antipsychotic medications unless there are signs or symptoms of hyperprolactinemia.

**Monitoring of weight, height, and metabolic parameters may need to be more frequent in patients treated with olanzapine.

of weight, body mass index, height, and waist circumference for the first 3 months and then every 3 months thereafter is recommended. Blood pressure, fasting plasma glucose, HgA1C, and a fasting lipid profile at baseline, at 12 weeks after initiation of treatment, and less frequently thereafter if weight gain is not substantive are advised. Other recommended baseline screening includes an Abnormal Involuntary Movements Scale (AIMS)[63] to monitor for tardive dyskinesia and other involuntary movements. The AIMS examination may be repeated monthly and as needed if there are concerns regarding new involuntary movements. These guidelines apply to the SGAs discussed in this section. Also, additional recommendations apply to specific medications as noted next.

Due to the potential for hyperprolactinemia with risperidone, obtaining a baseline serum prolactin level is advised. The baseline prolactin level can be used as a comparison if prolactin levels need to be drawn in the future secondary to symptoms of hyperprolactinemia.[9] Since the potential for weight gain for patients treated with olanzapine is greater than for other antipsychotics, practitioners may consider more frequent monitoring of weight and other metabolic parameters. Finally, due to potential EKG changes in youth treated with ziprasidone, it is recommended that an EKG be done at baseline and as necessary during treatment to assess for QTc prolongation, particularly if it is combined with other medications that may prolong the QTc.

Monotherapy in Other Stages
Bipolar Depression

The previously mentioned studies focus on the treatment of acute manic, hypomanic, or mixed states of bipolar disorder. Children with bipolar disorder also experience depressive episodes as part of their illness. However, the depressed phase appears to be less often recognized in youth than adults, with it being more common in adolescents than younger children.[64] Currently, the olanzapine/fluoxetine combination is approved by the FDA for treatment of bipolar I disorder, acute depressive episode in youth ages 10 to 17 years old. The following section focuses on the available research in this area.

Antidepressants

As in adults, there is concern that antidepressants may trigger or exacerbate symptoms of mania. Biederman et al.[65] conducted a prospective chart review of 59 youth, which demonstrated a significant improvement in depressive symptoms in children using selective serotonin reuptake inhibitors (SSRIs). However, this study also found a significantly increased risk of manic symptoms after starting an SSRI. Currently, there are no published prospective studies of antidepressants in patients with pediatric bipolar disorder. Therefore, the use of antidepressants is not recommended in pediatric bipolar disorder without prior mood stabilization and use of concurrent mood stabilizer.[64, 66]

Lithium

Currently, the treatment guidelines for children and adolescents with bipolar disorder recommend the use of lithium during the depressed phase based largely on the adult literature.[66] An open-label trial of lithium in 27 adolescents with bipolar depression demonstrated an improvement in mean depressive scores from baseline to endpoint, with an effect size of 1.7. Response and remission rates were 48% and 30%, respectively.[67] These results suggest that lithium may be effective in treating the depressed phase of pediatric bipolar disorder, but more definitive studies are needed.

Anticonvulsants

Data on anticonvulsants in the depressed phase of pediatric bipolar disorder are also limited. Due to its promise in adults, lamotrigine has been studied in the pediatric population. A case report of five adolescents with bipolar depression described improvement in depressive symptoms with the use of adjunctive lamotrigine.[68] Chang and colleagues[29] conducted a prospective, open-label trial of lamotrigine monotherapy and lamotrigine as adjunctive therapy in adolescent bipolar depression. Of the 19 patients, 63% saw an improvement in the depressive symptoms, and there were no significant differences in response between monotherapy and adjunctive therapy. None of the participants developed a rash or manic symptoms during this 8-week trial.[29] These studies suggest that lamotrigine may be effective in bipolar depression, but further clinical trials are needed to support its use.

Second-Generation Antipsychotics

An improvement in depressive symptoms in adults has been observed with quetiapine.[69,70] To examine this in youth, DelBello et al.[71] performed a double-blind, placebo-controlled study of quetiapine in 32 adolescents with bipolar depression. The study failed to demonstrate significant differences in improvement of depressive symptoms between quetiapine and placebo. The authors concluded that quetiapine was no more effective than placebo for depressed adolescents with bipolar disorder. However, a high placebo response was evident and may have made it difficult to find a statistically significant difference.[71] Subsequently, a large, multisite randomized placebo controlled trial further examined the efficacy of extended-release quetiapine. In a study in which 193 patients with bipolar depression between the ages of 10–17 years were randomized, active treatment was not found to be superior to placebo.[72]

However, it should be noted that in an 8-week, randomized, double-blind, placebo-controlled study ($n = 291$) comparing olanzapine/fluoxetine combination (OFC) in youth ages 10–17 years who met criteria for bipolar I disorder, current episode depressed was conducted. As measured by the CDRS-R, significantly more patients (59%) in the OFC group achieved remission as compared to patients (43.4%) in the placebo group. Adverse events that were more likely in the OFC group included weight gain; increased appetite; somnolence; QTc prolongation; and elevations in lipids, hepatic enzymes, and prolactin.

The authors concluded that OFC is efficacious for the acute treatment of depressive epi-sodes in patients 10 to 17 years of age with bipolar I disorder.[73] Olanzapine/fluoxetine combination was approved by the FDA in 2013 for treatment of bipolar I disorder, acute depressive episode, in youth ages 10- to 17-years-old.

Overall, open-label studies of antidepressants, lithium, and lamotrigine show promise. However, since patients in these trials may be responding to factors other than pharmacological treatment, it is important that placebo-controlled trials are per-formed in order to confirm or refute the putative efficacy of agents and better guide the treating clinician.

Maintenance Therapy

As pediatric bipolar disorder is a chronic illness, the use of medication to maintain symp-tom remission is an important consideration. However, the available research for the long-term treatment of pediatric bipolar disorder is limited. The following is a discussion of the relevant studies of monotherapy for the maintenance treatment of pediatric bipolar disorder.

Open-Label Studies

Open-label, extension-phase trials in pediatric bipolar disorder have been published in regards to lithium, divalproex, and several antipsychotics. In general, these studies sug-gest a sustained effectiveness following the acute phase, and tolerability of these medica-tions in pediatric bipolar disorder.

Specifically, a 16-week, open-label trial of lithium in 41 patients with pediatric bipo-lar disorder found the response achieved in the acute 8-week phase was maintained dur-ing the 16-week follow-up. The authors found lithium was generally well tolerated.[3]

While most tolerability data in divalproex come from studies of pediatric epilepsy, a 6-month, open-label trial of divalproex extended release ($n = 226$) reported weight gain (16%) as the most common side effect, with other side effects including increased appe-tite and nausea. There were no serious side effects.[74]

As previously mentioned, a recent double-blind, randomized placebo-controlled trial for the acute treatment (4 weeks) of bipolar disorder in youth (ages 10–17 years) with ziprasidone was conducted. It was followed by a 26-week, open-label, extension phase to evaluate for the long-term efficacy and safety of ziprasidone. The study found that the response achieved in the acute phase was maintained. The most commonly reported side effects included somnolence, sedation, headache, and insomnia with no significant changes in metabolic parameters, including weight gain, fasting lipids, and glucose, over the course of this study.[59] In addition, tolerability of ziprasidone in a 27-week, open-label study ($n = 63$) for treatment of pediatric bipolar mania, schizophrenia, or schizoaffective disorder was performed. The authors concluded the side effect profile was similar to that found in adults, and overall the drug was well tolerated with most common side effects being sedation, somnolence, nausea, and headache.[58]

Blinded Studies

A limited number of blinded studies have been performed to assess the efficacy of these agents for maintenance therapy in pediatric bipolar disorder. Following is a discussion of these studies.

A randomized, placebo-controlled, lithium discontinuation study in 108 children (ages 12–18 years) diagnosed with bipolar disorder, currently manic, was performed. In this study, if the patient was severely aggressive or psychotic, he or she received an anti-psychotic for acute stabilization over a 4-week period, and then received lithium mono-therapy for an additional 4 weeks. Those patients who were classified as responders after 8 weeks of pharmacotherapy were randomly assigned to either continue lithium or pla-cebo for an additional 2 weeks. Of the 40 participants who continued into discontinua-tion phase, 57.5% experienced a significant worsening of symptoms (52.6% and 61.9% for lithium and placebo, respectively). The difference between lithium and placebo was not statistically significant, suggesting that lithium may not be adequate for maintaining remission of mood symptoms in pediatric bipolar disorder.[75]

A long-term double-blind study comparing the use of lithium and divalproex in pediatric bipolar disorder (ages 5–17 years) was performed. After stabilization with a combination of lithium and divalproex, the participants ($n = 139$) were randomized to either lithium or divalproex monotherapy. There were no significant differences between the two agents, as measured by days until relapse or discontinuation over 18 months. The authors concluded that divalproex monotherapy was no more efficacious than lithium monotherapy for maintenance treatment of pediatric bipolar disorder. Time to symp-toms of mood relapse and time to study discontinuation did not differ between the two groups. This study also suggested that both agents were relatively well tolerated during long-term use.[8]

Two blinded studies for the use of aripiprazole in maintenance treatment of pedi-atric bipolar disorder have been conducted. Findling et al.[74] performed a double-blind, randomly assigned trial of aripiprazole (placebo versus 10 mg/day or 30 mg/day) in chil-dren (age 10–17 years) for the acute treatment of bipolar I disorder ($n = 296$). Those who completed the acute phase were eligible to be enrolled in a 26-week extension phase ($n = 211$) and were continued in the same treatment arm. A statistically significant improve-ment in symptoms as compared to placebo, as measured by YMRS, was observed at the endpoint for both doses of aripiprazole. Aripiprazole was generally well tolerated, and side effects appeared to be dose related.[76]

A second randomized, double-blind, placebo-controlled trial studying the efficacy of aripiprazole for maintenance therapy of bipolar disorder for children ages 4 to 9 years was conducted. After an acute phase of symptom stabilization, 30 patients were random-ized to continue aripiprazole and 30 children were randomized to placebo. During the 72-week maintenance phase, patients on aripiprazole had a significantly longer time to discontinuation secondary to a mood state and time to discontinuation for any reason. However, there was a significant dropout rate for both aripiprazole (50%) and placebo

(90%). The authors cited concerns for a nocebo effect in this study, meaning that if parents felt their child was switched from active medication to placebo, they may have had concern about a poor response, leading to high discontinuation rates. Despite the high dropout rate, these findings suggest possible efficacy of aripiprazole in maintenance treatment of pediatric bipolar.[77]

Overall, the limited available research for maintenance treatment in pediatric bipolar disorder suggests that symptom response is maintained from the acute phase trials and treatment is generally well tolerated. However, the limited number of blinded studies warrants further research in this area.

Combination Therapy

Treatment of acute manic and mixed states of pediatric bipolar disorder with a single agent often does not lead to remission of mood symptoms. Monotherapy with a mood stabilizer has been shown to be effective in only about 50% of youth with bipolar disorder.[1,51,78,79] While, the American Psychiatric Association guidelines recommend that a 6–8 week trial of a mood stabilizer at therapeutic dosage be used before adding or changing to another mood stabilizer,[17] combination therapy may sometimes be needed for bipolar disorder in children and adolescents. Several studies have examined combination therapy in the treatment of pediatric bipolar disorder and are described next.

A 6-week, randomized, parallel-group, double-blind, placebo-controlled study of divalproex combined with quetiapine versus divalproex combined with placebo in adolescents with manic or mixed episodes of bipolar disorder was conducted. A significantly greater reduction in manic symptoms in the divalproex plus quetiapine group as compared to the divalproex plus placebo group was noted. In addition, a significantly greater response rate (as measured by the YMRS) in the divalproex plus quetiapine group compared to the divalproex plus placebo group was noted (87% versus 53%, respectively). Safety measures were noted to be similar between the two groups with the most common side effects in both groups being sedation, nausea, headache, and gastrointestinal distress. Sedation was significantly more common in the divalproex plus quetiapine group. The authors concluded that quetiapine in combination with divalproex is more effective than divalproex alone for the treatment of pediatric bipolar disorder.[80]

An open-label study in which 90 youth with bipolar disorder (who had experienced a manic or hypomanic episode within the 3 months prior to the study) were treated with a combination of lithium and divalproex for up to 20 weeks was conducted. The remission rate (as measured by the YMRS) was reported as 46.7%. The combination treatment was well tolerated with the most common side effects being emesis, enuresis, stomach pain, and tremor. The authors concluded that a combination of divalproex and lithium may be useful in the treatment of pediatric bipolar disorder, but they were careful to not imply that combination therapy was superior to monotherapy, as this was not explored in their study.[81]

Patients in the aforementioned study who achieved symptom remission for 4 consecutive weeks were enrolled in a double-blind, randomized, maintenance phase in which they received monotherapy with either lithium or divalproex for up to 76 weeks.[8] Patients who relapsed during the maintenance phase of the trial ($n = 38$) were eligible to enroll in an 8-week, open-label trial in which they again received a combination of lithium and divalproex. Results from the open-label trial suggested that patients could be safely and effectively (89.5% response rate as measured by the YMRS) restabilized with reinitiation of a combination of lithium and DVPX.[82]

A 6-month, prospective, open-label trial of youth with pediatric bipolar disorder, manic or mixed episode, was conducted in which patients were treated with either combination lithium and risperidone or a combination divalproex and risperidone. Both groups showed a significant improvement in manic symptoms (as measured by the YMRS), but there was no difference between groups, suggesting that either combination may be useful in treating pediatric bipolar disorder. Patients in both groups were noted to have gained weight beyond what would be expected for normal growth.[83]

Other research has focused on augmenting one medication with a second medication. A 12-month, prospective, open-label trial of children and adolescents with preschool age onset of bipolar disorder was conducted in which patients were treated with lithium and subsequently augmented with risperidone if they had not responded sufficiently to lithium (55.3% were considered nonresponders). The response rate in the augmented group was 85.7% at the end of the 12-month study with 53% achieving remission (as measured by the YMRS).[84]

A recent comparison trial of adjunctive topiramate with olanzapine versus olanzapine monotherapy in 40 youth with bipolar disorder, manic, hypomanic, or mixed phases was conducted. Patients in both groups were reported to have a significant reduction in manic symptoms (as measured by the YMRS), with no significant difference noted between the two groups. Patients in both groups had significant increases in weight, but weight gain was significantly less in the combination group.[85]

Based on research, at this time it is impossible to predict at treatment initiation which patients will or will not respond to monotherapy for acute manic and mixed episodes of pediatric bipolar disorder. In addition, the available evidence does not provide guidelines with regard to if and when combination treatment should be considered. The available evidence does suggest that combining two medications may be useful in the treatment of pediatric bipolar disorder, particularly in patients who do not obtain symptom remission or who become less responsive to medication over time. We recommend considering combination therapy at the initiation of treatment in patients who are severely symptomatic and for patients requiring inpatient hospitalization for safety.

Special Considerations for Pregnant Adolescents

In adolescence, females with bipolar disorder who would benefit from pharmacotherapy may also be postmenarche and at an increased risk for pregnancy.[86] Due to their childbearing potential, specific consideration should be given to this particular population. Discussion of sexual activity, the use of birth control, and the teratogenic potential of specific medications is recommended prior to initiation of any medication in the adolescent female. Risky behaviors that can accompany elevated mood and/or mixed states, including hypersexual behaviors and substance use, can put these patients at risk of unintended pregnancy.[87] Therefore, clinicians may need to consider medication management of bipolar disorder during pregnancy.

When prescribing medications in pregnancy, there are several basic principles to consider. First, an examination of the risks of a specific agent versus the risks of the untreated mental illness is recommended. This includes a discussion with both the patient and the guardian of these risks and benefits, a judgment of severity of illness, trimester of fetal development, past psychiatric history, and response to different medications.[88,89] If possible, pregnancy is not the ideal time for therapeutic trials of new medications.[89] As pregnancies during adolescence may be unplanned, a fetus may be exposed to medication during the first trimester, before discovery of the pregnancy. Abruptly stopping the medication may precipitate relapse and may not provide any further protection to the fetus.[88]

When choosing a treatment, monotherapy is ideal if possible.[89,90] Furthermore, the lowest effective dose and doses divided into multiple daily doses to decrease peak serum levels is suggested.[90] Close coordination with obstetricians, pediatricians, family, and case managers for monitoring of mood and side effects is indicated. Specific medications and their use for bipolar disorder during pregnancy are beyond the scope of this chapter and are discussed elsewhere.[88,90]

Comorbidities

Psychiatric conditions, including attention-deficit/hyperactivity disorder (ADHD), disruptive behavior disorders, anxiety disorders, autism spectrum disorder (ASD), and substance use disorders, are often comorbid with pediatric bipolar disorder.[84] It is strongly recommended that patients who present with symptoms of pediatric bipolar disorder be evaluated for the possibility of other psychiatric disorders. Treatment of comorbid conditions may also be necessary to allow the best outcome for the patient. The evidence with regards to treatment of comorbid psychiatric disorders in patients with pediatric bipolar disorder is presented next.

Attention-Deficit/Hyperactivity Disorder

Children and adolescents with ADHD have been reported to be at an increased risk of developing bipolar disorder.[91] Some evidence suggests that response to medications used in the treatment of bipolar disorder may be less robust in patients with comorbid ADHD as compared to those with pediatric bipolar disorder alone. Strober et al.[92] compared lithium responsiveness in 30 inpatients with pediatric bipolar disorder and a diagnosis of early childhood ADHD to lithium responsiveness in 30 inpatients with pediatric bipolar disorder alone. The latter group was noted to have a significantly greater reduction in manic symptoms (as measured by the Bech-Rafaelsen Mania Scale) as compared to the former group. The authors suggested that early childhood ADHD could represent a risk factor for treatment nonresponsiveness in pediatric bipolar disorder.[92]

In a retrospective chart review of 42 adolescents hospitalized with a discharge diagnosis of bipolar disorder (index episode of mania), 34.1% had a diagnosis of ADHD. These patients were treated with either lithium or divalproex. Those with a diagnosis of comorbid ADHD had a significantly decreased response rate to either medication than those with bipolar disorder alone (57.1% and 92.6%, respectively).[93]

Researchers have attempted to determine whether medications used in the treatment of pediatric bipolar disorder may also treat comorbid disorders such as ADHD, and conversely if medications for ADHD can be used safely in patients with pediatric bipolar disorder. An 8-week, open-label trial of divalproex was followed by a 4-week, double-blind, placebo-controlled, crossover trial of mixed amphetamine salts versus placebo in 40 children and adolescents in manic, mixed, or hypomanic episodes of bipolar disorder. The initial phase was designed to examine whether divalproex had an effect on ADHD symptoms. There was a significant reduction in manic symptoms, but ADHD symptoms were not significantly improved. The subsequent stage was to examine whether mixed amphetamine salts were safe and effective in pediatric bipolar disorder patients ($n = 30$) who had been previously stabilized on divalproex. Mixed amphetamine salts were significantly more effective than placebo in reducing ADHD symptoms and were well tolerated. The authors suggested that pediatric bipolar patients could be safely and effectively treated with mixed amphetamine salts after stabilization of manic symptoms, but that divalproex was not sufficient to treat ADHD.[94]

A 4-week, double blind, placebo-controlled study of 16 youth with a diagnosis of bipolar disorder and comorbid ADHD was conducted. In this study, patients were required to receive at least 5 days of a mood stabilizer, and then given either methylphenidate or placebo. Results suggested that concomitant treatment with methylphenidate in patients with pediatric bipolar disorder was well tolerated and beneficial.[95]

A 6-week randomized, double-blind trial of aripiprazole or placebo in children ages 8–17 years with bipolar I or II disorder and comorbid ADHD demonstrated a response rate of 88.9% (as measured by the YMRS) in the aripiprazole group and 52% in the placebo group. Remission rates were 72% and 32% in the aripiprazole group and placebo groups, respectively. There was no significant difference in change from baseline to endpoint in ADHD symptoms (as measured by the SNAP-IV) between the two groups. The authors concluded that aripiprazole was effective in reducing manic symptoms in juvenile bipolar disorder, but that adjunctive medications might be needed for treatment of ADHD after mood stabilization.[96]

These studies suggest that medications used for the treatment of pediatric bipolar disorder may not be effective or sufficient to treat comorbid ADHD. The presence of comorbid ADHD may increase the likelihood for treatment nonresponsiveness in patients treated with lithium or divalproex. The research suggests that following stabilization of manic symptoms, the use of stimulant medications when prescribed concomitantly with mood stabilizers in pediatric patients with bipolar disorder may be safe and effective for treating comorbid ADHD.

Substance Use Disorders

Comorbid substance use disorders may be present in adolescents with bipolar disorder. A limited number of studies have looked at treatment considerations when they occur concurrently. A short-term, double-blind study of youth with bipolar I disorder or II or major depressive disorder (with risk factors for developing bipolar disorder, including delusions, switching to bipolar disorder during tricyclic antidepressant treatment, marked psychomotor retardation, or bipolar disorder in a first-degree relative) and comorbid substance dependence demonstrated a significant reduction in positive urine toxicology screens and a significant improvement in global assessment of functioning when they were treated with lithium as compared to placebo.[97] Future studies are needed to assess the best treatment options for youth with comorbid pediatric bipolar disorder and substance use disorders.

Autism Spectrum Disorders

Bipolar disorder and autism spectrum disorders (ASDs) may also co-occur. A secondary analysis of identically designed short-term, open-label trials of atypical antipsychotic monotherapy (including risperidone, olanzapine, quetiapine, ziprasidone, or aripiprazole) was conducted. Of the 151 patients with manic, hypomanic, or mixed episodes of pediatric bipolar disorder, 15% had comorbid ASD. The study reported that there was no difference in response rate or tolerability in patients with comorbid ASD (as measured by YMRS) compared to patients without comorbid ASD.[98] Further studies are needed to better define safe and effective treatment options for patients with comorbid acute manic and mixed states of bipolar disorder and ASD.

Conclusion

This chapter reviewed the available research on the psychopharmacologic management of pediatric bipolar disorder. Based on the current efficacy data, clinicians may initially consider a trial of an atypical antipsychotic or lithium monotherapy. Anticonvulsants are recommended as second-line or adjunctive therapies. As previously discussed, monotherapy may not be sufficient for remission of mood symptoms, and combination therapy may be necessary in severe or treatment refractory cases. Furthermore, certain populations of patients, including those with bipolar depression, psychosis, comorbid psychopathology, and pregnant adolescents, may require specific considerations for treatment. Stabilization of acute manic and psychotic symptoms is recommended prior to treatment of comorbid conditions such as ADHD. In addition, consistent monitoring of metabolic and other parameters is recommended.

While the available research for the treatment of pediatric bipolar disorder has expanded over the last decade, ongoing research is imperative to further inform treating clinicians. Expanding our understanding of psychopharmacologic treatments, both as monotherapy and as combination treatments, for children and adolescents with bipolar disorder is necessary to continue to provide the safest and most effective treatments to this vulnerable group of youths.

Author Disclosures

Dr. Lytle and Dr. Moratschek have no conflicts to disclose. Dr. Findling receives or has received research support, acted as a consultant, and/or served on a speaker's bureau for Alexza Pharmaceuticals, American Academy of Child & Adolescent Psychiatry, American Physician Institute, American Psychiatric Press, AstraZeneca, Bracket, Bristol-Myers Squibb, Clinsys, Cognition Group, Coronado Biosciences, Dana Foundation, Forest, GlaxoSmithKline, Guilford Press, Johns Hopkins University Press, Johnson & Johnson, KemPharm, Lilly, Lundbeck, Merck, NIH, Novartis, Noven, Otsuka, Oxford University Press, Pfizer, Physicians Postgraduate Press, Rhodes Pharmaceuticals, Roche, Sage, Seaside Pharmaceuticals, Shire, Stanley Medical Research Institute, Sunovion, Supernus Pharmaceuticals, Transcept Pharmaceuticals, Validus, and WebMD.

References

1. Kowatch RA, Suppes T, Carmody TJ, et al. Effect size of lithium, divalproex sodium, and carbamazepine in children and adolescents with bipolar disorder. *J Am Acad Child Adolesc Psychiatry.* 2000;39:713–20.
2. Kafantaris V, Coletti D, Dicker R, Padula G, Kane JM. Lithium treatment of acute mania in adolescents: a large open trial. *J Am Acad Child Adolesc Psychiatry.* 2003;42:1038–45.
3. Findling RL, Kafantaris V, Pavuluri M, et al. Post-acute effectiveness of lithium in pediatric bipolar I disorder. *J Child Adolesc Psychopharmacol.* 2013;23:80–90.
4. Kowatch RA, Findling RL, Scheffer RE, et al. Pediatric bipolar collaborative mood stabilizer trial. Poster presented at: Annual Meeting of the American Academy of Child and Adolescent Psychiatry; October 23–28, 2007; Boston, MA.
5. Findling RL, Frazier JA, Kafantaris V, et al. The collaborative lithium trials (CoLT): specific aims, methods, and implementation. *Child Adolesc Psychiatry Ment Health.* 2008;2:21.
6. Findling RL, Landersdorfer CB, Kafantaris V, et al. First-dose pharmacokinetics of lithium carbonate in children and adolescents. *J Clin Psychopharmacol.* 2010;30:404–10.
7. Findling RL, Kafantaris V, Pavuluri M, et al. Dosing strategies for lithium monotherapy in children and adolescents with bipolar I disorder. *J Child Adolesc Psychopharmacol.* 2011;21:195–205.
8. Findling RL, McNamara NK, Youngstrom EA, et al. Double-blind 18-month trial of lithium versus divalproex maintenance treatment in pediatric bipolar disorder. *J Am Acad Child Adolesc Psychiatry.* 2005;44:409–17.
9. Thomas T, Kuich KW, Findling RL. Bipolar disorders. In: McVoy M, Findling RL, eds. *Clinical Manual of Child and Adolescent Psychopharmacology.* Washington, DC: American Psychiatric Publishing; 2013:227–67.

10. Gracious BL, Findling RL, Seman C, Youngstrom EA, Demeter CA, Calabrese JR. Elevated thyrotropin in bipolar youths prescribed both lithium and divalproex sodium. *J Am Acad Child Adolesc Psychiatry*. 2004;43:215–20.

11. Mallette LE, Khouri K, Zengotita H, Hollis BW, Malini S. Lithium treatment increases intact and midregion parathyroid hormone and parathyroid volume. *J Clin Endocrinol Metab*. 1989;68:654–60.

12. Markowitz GS, Radhakrishnan J, Kambham N, Valeri AM, Hines WH, D'Agati VD. Lithium nephrotoxicity: a progressive combined glomerular and tubulointerstitial nephropathy. *J Am Soc Nephrol*. 2000;11:1439–48.

13. Madaan V, Chang KD. Pharmacotherapeutic strategies for pediatric bipolar disorder. *Expert Opin Pharmacother*. 2007;8:1801–19.

14. Oyewumi LK, McKnight M, Cernovsky ZZ. Lithium dosage and leukocyte counts in psychiatric patients. *J Psychiatry Neurosci*. 1999;24:215–21.

15. Hagino OR, Weller EB, Weller RA, Washing D, Fristad MA, Kontras SB. Untoward effects of lithium treatment in children aged four through six years. *J Am Acad Child Adolesc Psychiatry*. 1995;34:1584–90.

16. Finley PR, Warner MD, Peabody CA. Clinical relevance of drug interactions with lithium. *Clin Pharmacokinet*. 1995;29:172–191.

17. McClellan J, Kowatch R, Findling RL, Work Group on Quality Issues. Practice parameter for the assessment and treatment of children and adolescents with bipolar disorder. *J Am Acad Child Adolesc Psychiatry*. 2007;46:107–25.

18. Henry CA, Zamvil LS, Lam C, Rosenquist KJ, Ghaemi SN. Long-term outcome with divalproex in children and adolescents with bipolar disorder. *J Child Adolesc Psychopharmacol*. 2003;13:523–9.

19. Wagner KD, Weller EB, Carlson GA, et al. An open-label trial of divalproex in children and adolescents with bipolar disorder. *J Am Acad Child Adolesc Psychiatry*. 2002;41:1224–30.

20. Papatheodorou G, Kutcher SP, Katic M, Szalai JP. The efficacy and safety of divalproex sodium in the treatment of acute mania in adolescents and young adults: an open clinical trial. *J Clin Psychopharmacol*. 1995;15:110–6.

21. Wagner KD, Redden L, Kowatch RA, et al. A double-blind, randomized, placebo-controlled trial of divalproex extended-release in the treatment of bipolar disorder in children and adolescents. *J Am Acad Child Adolesc Psychiatry*. 2009;48:519–32.

22. Kowatch RA, DelBello MP. Pharmacotherapy of children and adolescents with bipolar disorder. *Psychiatr Clin North Am*. 2005;28:385–97.

23. Pavuluri MN, Henry DB, Carbray JA, Naylor MW, Janicak PG. Divalproex sodium for pediatric mixed mania: a 6-month prospective trial. *Bipolar Disord*. 2005;7:266–73.

24. Ginsberg LD. Carbamazepine extended-release capsules: a retrospective review of its use in children and adolescents. *Ann Clin Psychiatry*. 2006;18(Suppl. 1):3–7.

25. Joshi G, Wozniak J, Mick E, et al. A prospective open-label trial of extended-release carbamazepine monotherapy in children with bipolar disorder. *J Child Adolesc Psychopharmacol*. 2010;20:7–14.

26. Findling RL, Gingsberg L. A phase IV, multi-center, open label study of extended-release carbamazepine in the treatment of manic or mixed states in youths aged 10–17 years. Poster presented at: Annual Meeting of the American Academy of Child and Adolescent Psychiatry; May 6, 2012, Philadelphia, PA.

27. Biederman J, Joshi G, Mick E, et al. A prospective open-label trial of lamotrigine monotherapy in children and adolescents with bipolar disorder. *CNS Neurosci Ther*. 2010;16:91–102.

28. Pavuluri MN, Henry DB, Moss M, Mohammed T, Carbray JA, Sweeney JA. Effectiveness of lamotrigine in maintaining symptom control in pediatric bipolar disorder. *J Child Adolesc Psychopharmacol*. 2009;19:75–82.

29. Chang K, Saxena K, Howe M. An open-label study of lamotrigine adjunct or monotherapy for the treatment of adolescents with bipolar depression. *J Am Acad Child Adolesc Psychiatry*. 2006;45:298–304.

30. DelBello MP, Kowatch RA, Warner J, et al. Adjunctive topiramate treatment for pediatric bipolar disorder: a retrospective chart review. *J Child Adolesc Psychopharmacol*. 2002;12:323–30.

31. Barzman DH, DelBello MP, Kowatch RA, et al. Adjunctive topiramate in hospitalized children and adolescents with bipolar disorders. *J Child Adolesc Psychopharmacol*. 2005;15:931–7.

32. Delbello MP, Findling RL, Kushner S, et al. A pilot controlled trial of topiramate for mania in children and adolescents with bipolar disorder. *J Am Acad Child Adolesc Psychiatry*. 2005;44:539–47.

33. Davanzo P, Nikore V, Yehya N, Stevenson L. Oxcarbazepine treatment of juvenile-onset bipolar disorder. *J Child Adolesc Psychopharmacol.* 2004;14:344–5.

34. Wagner KD, Kowatch RA, Emslie GJ, et al. A double-blind, randomized, placebo-controlled trial of oxcarbazepine in the treatment of bipolar disorder in children and adolescents. *Am J Psychiatry.* 2006;163:1179–86.

35. Soutullo CA, Casuto LS, Keck PE Jr. Gabapentin in the treatment of adolescent mania: a case report. *J Child Adolesc Psychopharmacol.* 1998;8:81–5.

36. Hamrin V, Bailey K. Gabapentin and methylphenidate treatment of a preadolescent with attention deficit hyperactivity disorder and bipolar disorder. *J Child Adolesc Psychopharmacol.* 2001;11:301–9.

37. Kowatch RA, Suppes T, Gilfillan SK, Fuentes RM, Grannemann BD, Emslie GJ. Clozapine treatment of children and adolescents with bipolar disorder and schizophrenia: a clinical case series. *J Child Adolesc Psychopharmacol.* 1995;5:241.

38. Masi G, Mucci M, Millepiedi S. Clozapine in adolescent inpatients with acute mania. *J Child Adolesc Psychopharmacol.* 2002;12:93–9.

39. Biederman J, Mick E, Hammerness P, et al. Open-label, 8-week trial of olanzapine and risperidone for the treatment of bipolar disorder in preschool-age children. *Biol Psychiatry.* 2005;58:589–94.

40. Biederman J, Mick E, Wozniak J, Aleardi M, Spencer T, Faraone SV. An open-label trial of risperidone in children and adolescents with bipolar disorder. *J Child Adolesc Psychopharmacol.* 2005;15:311–7.

41. Haas M, Delbello MP, Pandina G, et al. Risperidone for the treatment of acute mania in children and adolescents with bipolar disorder: a randomized, double-blind, placebo-controlled study. *Bipolar Disord.* 2009;11:687–700.

42. Pavuluri MN, Henry DB, Findling RL, et al. Double-blind randomized trial of risperidone versus divalproex in pediatric bipolar disorder. *Bipolar Disord.* 2010;12:593–605.

43. Geller B, Luby JL, Joshi P, et al. A randomized controlled trial of risperidone, lithium, or divalproex sodium for initial treatment of bipolar I disorder, manic or mixed phase, in children and adolescents. *Arch Gen Psychiatry.* 2012;69:515–28.

44. Frazier JA, Biederman J, Tohen M, et al. A prospective open-label treatment trial of olanzapine monotherapy in children and adolescents with bipolar disorder. *J Child Adolesc Psychopharmacol.* 2001;11:239–50.

45. Wozniak J, Mick E, Waxmonsky J, Kotarski M, Hantsoo L, Biederman J. Comparison of open-label, 8-week trials of olanzapine monotherapy and topiramate augmentation of olanzapine for the treatment of pediatric bipolar disorder. *J Child Adolesc Psychopharmacol.* 2009;19:539–45.

46. Tohen M, Kryzhanovskaya L, Carlson G, et al. Olanzapine versus placebo in the treatment of adolescents with bipolar mania. *Am J Psychiatry.* 2007;164:1547–56.

47. Biederman J, McDonnell MA, Wozniak J, et al. Aripiprazole in the treatment of pediatric bipolar disorder: a systematic chart review. *CNS Spectr.* 2005;10:141–8.

48. Biederman J, Mick E, Spencer T, et al. An open-label trial of aripiprazole monotherapy in children and adolescents with bipolar disorder. *CNS Spectr.* 2007;12:683–9.

49. Findling RL, Kauffman RE, Sallee FR, et al. Tolerability and pharmacokinetics of aripiprazole in children and adolescents with psychiatric disorders: an open-label, dose-escalation study. *J Clin Psychopharmacol.* 2008;28:441–6.

50. Findling RL, McNamara NK, Youngstrom EA, et al. An open-label study of aripiprazole in children with a bipolar disorder. *J Child Adolesc Psychopharmacol.* 2011;21:345–51.

51. Findling RL, Nyilas M, Forbes RA, et al. Acute treatment of pediatric bipolar I disorder, manic or mixed episode, with aripiprazole: a randomized, double-blind, placebo-controlled study. *J Clin Psychiatry.* 2009;70:1441–51.

52. Marchand WR, Wirth L, Simon C. Quetiapine adjunctive and monotherapy for pediatric bipolar disorder: a retrospective chart review. *J Child Adolesc Psychopharmacol.* 2004;14:405–11.

53. Joshi G, Petty C, Wozniak J, et al. A prospective open-label trial of quetiapine monotherapy in preschool and school age children with bipolar spectrum disorder. *J Affect Disord.* 2012;136:1143–53.

54. DelBello MP, Kowatch RA, Adler CM, et al. A double-blind randomized pilot study comparing quetiapine and divalproex for adolescent mania. *J Am Acad Child Adolesc Psychiatry.* 2006;45:305–13.

55. Pathak S, Findling RL, Earley WR, Acevedo LD, Stankowski J, Delbello MP. Efficacy and safety of quetiapine in children and adolescents with mania associated with bipolar I disorder: a 3-week, double-blind, placebo-controlled trial. *J Clin Psychiatry.* 2013;74:e100–9.

56. Barnett MS. Ziprasidone monotherapy in pediatric bipolar disorder. *J Child Adolesc Psychopharmacol.* 2004;14:471–7.

57. Biederman J, Mick E, Spencer T, Dougherty M, Aleardi M, Wozniak J. A prospective open-label treatment trial of ziprasidone monotherapy in children and adolescents with bipolar disorder. *Bipolar Disord.* 2007;9:888–94.

58. DelBello MP, Versavel M, Ice K, Keller D, Miceli J. Tolerability of oral ziprasidone in children and adolescents with bipolar mania, schizophrenia, or schizoaffective disorder. *J Child Adolesc Psychopharmacol.* 2008;18:491–9.

59. Findling RL, Cavus I, Pappadopulos E, et al. Efficacy, long-term safety, and tolerability of ziprasidone in children and adolescents with bipolar disorder. *J Child Adolesc Psychopharmacology.* 2013;23(8):545–57.

60. Blair J, Scahill L, State M, Martin A. Electrocardiographic changes in children and adolescents treated with ziprasidone: a prospective study. *J Am Acad Child Adolesc Psychiatry.* 2005;44:73–9.

61. Correll CU, Lops JD, Figen V, Malhotra AK, Kane JM, Manu P. QT interval duration and dispersion in children and adolescents treated with ziprasidone. *J Clin Psychiatry.* 2011;72:854–60.

62. Joshi G, Petty C, Wozniak J, et al. A prospective open-label trial of paliperidone monotherapy for the treatment of bipolar spectrum disorders in children and adolescents. *Psychopharmacology (Berl).* 2013;227:449–58.

63. Guy WA. Abnormal involuntary movement scale (AIMS). ECDEU assessment manual for psychopharmacology. 1976:534–7.

64. Chang K. Challenges in the diagnosis and treatment of pediatric bipolar depression. *Dialogues Clin Neurosci.* 2009;11:73–80.

65. Biederman J, Mick E, Spencer TJ, Wilens TE, Faraone SV. Therapeutic dilemmas in the pharmacotherapy of bipolar depression in the young. *J Child Adolesc Psychopharmacol.* 2000;10:185–92.

66. Kowatch RA, Fristad M, Birmaher B, et al. Treatment guidelines for children and adolescents with bipolar disorder. *J Am Acad Child Adolesc Psychiatry.* 2005;44:213–35.

67. Patel NC, DelBello MP, Bryan HS, et al. Open-label lithium for the treatment of adolescents with bipolar depression. *J Am Acad Child Adolesc Psychiatry.* 2006;45:289–97.

68. Soutullo CA, Diez-Suarez A, Figueroa-Quintana A. Adjunctive lamotrigine treatment for adolescents with bipolar disorder: retrospective report of five cases. *J Child Adolesc Psychopharmacol.* 2006;16:357–64.

69. Thase ME, Macfadden W, Weisler RH, et al. Efficacy of quetiapine monotherapy in bipolar I and II depression: a double-blind, placebo-controlled study (the BOLDER II study). *J Clin Psychopharmacol.* 2006;26:600–9.

70. Young AH, McElroy SL, Bauer M, et al. A double-blind, placebo-controlled study of quetiapine and lithium monotherapy in adults in the acute phase of bipolar depression (EMBOLDEN I). *J Clin Psychiatry.* 2010;71:150–62.

71. DelBello MP, Chang K, Welge JA, et al. A double-blind, placebo-controlled pilot study of quetiapine for depressed adolescents with bipolar disorder. *Bipolar Disord.* 2009;11:483–93.

72. Findling RL, Pathak S, Earley WR, Liu S, DelBello MP. Efficacy and safety of extended-release quetiapine fumarate in youth with bipolar depression: an 8-week, double-blind, placebo-controlled trial. *J Child Adolesc Psychopharmacol.* in press.

73. Detke HC, Delbello M, Landry J, Usher R, Dingankar M. Safety and efficacy of olanzapine/fluoxetine combination vs. placebo in patients ages 10 to 17 in the acute treatment of major depressive episodes associated with bipolar I disorder. Poster presented at: Annual meeting of the American College of Neuropsychopharmacology; December 2–6, 2012; Hollywood, FL.

74. Redden L, DelBello M, Wagner KD, et al. Long-term safety of divalproex sodium extended-release in children and adolescents with bipolar I disorder. *J Child Adolesc Psychopharmacol.* 2009;19:83–9.

75. Kafantaris V, Coletti DJ, Dicker R, Padula G, Pleak RR, Alvir JM. Lithium treatment of acute mania in adolescents: a placebo-controlled discontinuation study. *J Am Acad Child Adolesc Psychiatry*. 2004;43:984–93.

76. Findling RL, Correll CU, Nyilas M, et al. Aripiprazole for the treatment of pediatric bipolar I disorder: a 30-week, randomized, placebo-controlled study. *Bipolar Disord*. 2013;15:138–49.

77. Findling RL, Youngstrom EA, McNamara NK, et al. Double-blind, randomized, placebo-controlled long-term maintenance study of aripiprazole in children with bipolar disorder. *J Clin Psychiatry*. 2012;73:57–63.

78. Kafantaris V, Dicker R, Coletti DJ, Kane JM. Adjunctive antipsychotic treatment is necessary for adolescents with psychotic mania. *J Child Adolesc Psychopharmacol*. 2001;11:409–13.

79. Geller B, Luby JL, Joshi P, et al. A randomized controlled trial of risperidone, lithium, or divalproex sodium for initial treatment of bipolar I disorder, manic or mixed phase, in children and adolescents. *Arch Gen Psychiatry*. 2012;69:515–28.

80. Delbello MP, Schwiers ML, Rosenberg HL, Strakowski SM. A double-blind, randomized, placebo-controlled study of quetiapine as adjunctive treatment for adolescent mania. *J Am Acad Child Adolesc Psychiatry*. 2002;41:1216–23.

81. Findling RL, McNamara NK, Gracious BL, et al. Combination lithium and divalproex sodium in pediatric bipolarity. *J Am Acad Child Adolesc Psychiatry*. 2003;42:895–901.

82. Findling RL, McNamara NK, Stansbrey R, et al. Combination lithium and divalproex sodium in pediatric bipolar symptom re-stabilization. *J Am Acad Child Adolesc Psychiatry*. 2006;45:142–8.

83. Pavuluri MN, Henry DB, Carbray JA, Sampson G, Naylor MW, Janicak PG. Open-label prospective trial of risperidone in combination with lithium or divalproex sodium in pediatric mania. *J Affect Disord*. 2004;82(Suppl. 1):S103–11.

84. Pavuluri MN, Henry DB, Carbray JA, Sampson GA, Naylor MW, Janicak PG. A one-year open-label trial of risperidone augmentation in lithium nonresponder youth with preschool-onset bipolar disorder. *J Child Adolesc Psychopharmacol*. 2006;16:336–50.

85. Wozniak J, Mick E, Waxmonsky J, Kotarski M, Hantsoo L, Biederman J. Comparison of open-label, 8-week trials of olanzapine monotherapy and topiramate augmentation of olanzapine for the treatment of pediatric bipolar disorder. *J Child Adolesc Psychopharmacol*. 2009;19:539–45.

86. Heffner JL, Delbello MP, Fleck DE, Adler CM, Strakowski SM. Unplanned pregnancies in adolescents with bipolar disorder. *Am J Psychiatry*. 2012;169(12):1319.

87. Joshi G, Wilens T. Comorbidity in pediatric bipolar disorder. *Child Adolesc Psychiatr Clin N Am*. 2009;18:291–319, vii–viii.

88. Viguera AC, Whitfield T, Baldessarini RJ, et al. Risk of recurrence in women with bipolar disorder during pregnancy: prospective study of mood stabilizer discontinuation. *Am J Psychiatry*. 2007;164:1817–24; quiz 1923.

89. Cohen LS. Treatment of bipolar disorder during pregnancy. *J Clin Psychiatry*. 2007;68(Suppl. 9):4–9.

90. Yonkers KA, Wisner KL, Stowe Z, et al. Management of bipolar disorder during pregnancy and the postpartum period. *Am J Psychiatry*. 2004;161:608–20.

91. Biederman J, Faraone S, Mick E, et al. Attention-deficit hyperactivity disorder and juvenile mania: an overlooked comorbidity? *J Am Acad Child Adolesc Psychiatry*. 1996;35:997–1008.

92. Strober M, DeAntonio M, Schmidt-Lackner S, Freeman R, Lampert C, Diamond J. Early childhood attention deficit hyperactivity disorder predicts poorer response to acute lithium therapy in adolescent mania. *J Affect Disord*. 1998;51:145–51.

93. State RC, Frye MA, Altshuler LL, et al. Chart review of the impact of attention-deficit/hyperactivity disorder comorbidity on response to lithium or divalproex sodium in adolescent mania. *J Clin Psychiatry*. 2004;65:1057–63.

94. Scheffer RE, Kowatch RA, Carmody T, Rush AJ. Randomized, placebo-controlled trial of mixed amphetamine salts for symptoms of comorbid ADHD in pediatric bipolar disorder after mood stabilization with divalproex sodium. *Am J Psychiatry*. 2005;162:58–64.

95. Findling RL, Short EJ, McNamara NK, et al. Methylphenidate in the treatment of children and adolescents with bipolar disorder and attention-deficit/hyperactivity disorder. *J Am Acad Child Adolesc Psychiatry*. 2007;46:1445–53.

96. Tramontina S, Zeni CP, Ketzer CR, Pheula GF, Narvaez J, Rohde LA. Aripiprazole in children and adolescents with bipolar disorder comorbid with attention-deficit/hyperactivity disorder: a pilot randomized clinical trial. *J Clin Psychiatry*. 2009;70:756–64.

97. Geller B, Cooper TB, Sun K, et al. Double-blind and placebo-controlled study of lithium for adolescent bipolar disorders with secondary substance dependency. *J Am Acad Child Adolesc Psychiatry*. 1998;37:171–8.

98. Joshi G, Biederman J, Wozniak J, et al. Response to second generation antipsychotics in youth with comorbid bipolar disorder and autism spectrum disorder. *CNS Neurosci Ther*. 2012;18:28–33.

Psychotherapeutic Strategies for Treating Youth With or At Risk for Bipolar Disorder

David J. Miklowitz

Why Psychotherapy?

Pharmacotherapy is the first-line treatment for patients with bipolar disorder, young or old. However, drug treatment by itself has been shown to be less effective in hastening recovery from episodes than the combination of drug treatment and disorder-specific forms of psychotherapy.[1] Psychotherapeutic interventions may provide an effective supplement to medication management without adding to the overall burden of side effects.

Considerable evidence is accumulating for the effectiveness of specific psychotherapeutic interventions in bipolar disorder. Most of the randomized controlled trials (RCTs) of adjunctive psychotherapy, however, have been conducted in adult populations. The extension of many of these methods to children or adolescents is new. This chapter will review the existing findings from RCTs in adult populations and, when possible, their extension to children with or at risk for bipolar disorder.

The chapter begins with a review of stress factors that play a role in the onset or recurrences of bipolar disorder in adults and children. Stress variables may define targets for psychotherapy, in the same way that new drugs are developed to alter specific biological targets.[2] Next, the chapter reviews the major models of psychotherapy for bipolar disorder in adults and (when available) adolescents or children. The major schools of therapy include family-based treatments, including family-focused therapy (FFT) and multifamily psychoeducation groups; individual cognitive-behavioral therapy (CBT); interpersonal and social rhythm therapy (IPSRT); various forms of group psychoeducation; and systematized (collaborative) care management.

The Role of Stress in Bipolar Disorder
Life Events Research

Negative life events (i.e., loss experiences) have been examined most extensively in studies of bipolar depression among adults. The most methodologically sound studies use interview-based measurements rather than questionnaire measures. Prospective studies with interview measures indicate that stressful life events are correlated with slow recovery from bipolar depression among adults[3] and increases in depression over several months.[4]

Research on life stress and mania highlights two sets of predictors: goal attainment events and sleep/schedule disruption. The goal dysregulation model suggests that people with bipolar illness show more extreme responses to rewarding stimuli.[5] Indeed, people with bipolar disorder place a stably high emphasis on goal pursuit, even when they are not in an episode.[6] This reward sensitivity would be expected to influence reactions to life events that involve major successes. In fact, life events involving goal attainment (such as new relationships) predict increases in manic symptoms, but not depressive symptoms.[4,7]

Wehr[8] proposed that sleep disruption mediates the pathway between life events and episodes of bipolar disorder, noting that illness episodes are often preceded by events that interfere with sleep or changed sleep/wake cycles (e.g., transmeridian flights, physical illnesses, childbearing). Ehlers and colleagues postulated that social disruptions lead to circadian rhythm disruptions (for example, the body's natural light/dark cycles), leading to the onset or worsening of mood symptoms.[9-10] In parallel, removing a previously stabilizing influence, such as when a parent begins traveling more frequently for a job, may disrupt a child's or teen's mood.

There is now considerable evidence from laboratory studies[11] and naturalistic/longitudinal studies[12] that sleep deprivation is an important precursor of manic symptoms. In two studies, Malkoff-Schwartz et al.[13-14] found that bipolar individuals reported more life events that affect sleep or wake times, patterns of social stimulation, or daily routines in the 8 weeks before manic episodes compared to the 8 weeks before depressive episodes. Furthermore, Jones et al.[15] found using actigraph assessments that people with bipolar disorder had more variability in their daily schedules than healthy participants.

The role of life events in childhood samples has received less attention. In one study of adolescents with bipolar I, II, or not otherwise specified (NOS) disorder, discrete life events were not associated with symptom change. However, adolescents with more chronic, ongoing stress in family and romantic relationships had more sustained depressive symptoms over time.[16] Among the offspring of parents with bipolar illness, negative life events were associated with the onset of depressive disorders.[17]

Thus, life events (negative, goal attainment, or schedule/sleep disrupting events) play a role in the onset of depressive and manic episodes. Although stressful events cannot be prevented, the ways in which individuals respond to events are targets for change, in the hopes of enhancing resilience. For example, IPSRT teaches people with bipolar disorder the strategy of stabilizing sleep/wake and social rhythms, especially when there are events that provoke changes.[18] CBT examines individuals' distorted attitudes about goal attainment events, such as risk underestimation and benefit overestimation.[19,20]

Stress Sensitization

Responses to stress may change at different points of development in the progression of bipolar disorder. Thus, one must consider the point in the illness in which stress will have its largest effects on recurrence. The "stress sensitization" model postulates that, as the illness becomes more and more recurrent, less stress is needed to provoke episodes.[21] Two studies have supported this idea[22,23] and one has not.[24] One study found that childhood adversity (i.e., parental neglect, emotional, abuse, or physical abuse) and life stress interacted in predicting mood recurrences in bipolar I disorder, such that those with a history of adversity reported lower levels of stress prior to recurrences than those without a history of adversity. Thus, childhood adversity may create a vulnerability to life events such that less severe events can provoke mood episodes.[23]

Family Environment

Another body of research—and one that is particularly relevant to pediatric populations—concerns the role of family relationships in the onset and course of bipolar illness. In a study of young adult patients living with parents, Miklowitz et al.[25] found that young adult manic patients who returned after a hospitalization to families rated high on expressed emotion (EE) (high levels of criticism or hostility or emotional involvement toward the patient) or who showed high levels of caregiver-to-patient affective negativity (criticism, hostility, or guilt induction) during family interactions were highly likely to relapse within 9 months (94%), whereas those whose families rated low on both EE and affective negativity were unlikely to relapse within this time frame (17%). The association between EE and the course of bipolar disorder was replicated in a small sample of bipolar adolescents.[26]

EE is only one means of measuring the family environment. For example, in an 8-year follow-up of children with a bipolar I, manic or mixed episode, children's and parents' ratings of maternal warmth were associated with time to recurrence.[27] More generally, mother–child relationships in pediatric bipolar disorder are associated with higher tension, conflict, and hostility compared to families with a healthy child or a child with attention-deficit/hyperactivity disorder (ADHD).[28,29] Other studies have reported low levels of cohesion and adaptability in families with a bipolar offspring.[30,31] In one large-scale cross-sectional study ($n = 272$) of families with parents with mood disorders, the association between parental and child bipolar disorder was mediated by the level of family conflict reported by parents.[32]

What factors explain why some parents of bipolar offspring are high in EE (or high in conflict or low in warmth), whereas others are not? One study of adults with bipolar disorder found that high-EE families (usually spousal or parent/adult offspring pairs) were characterized by high levels of reciprocal affective negativity, such that criticisms were often returned by the bipolar person, leading to long "volleys" of caregiver/bipolar individual conflict.[33] Another study found that high levels of criticism and conflict are related to behavioral outbursts among children with bipolar disorder that are not easily attributed to an illness state.[29] In these cases, parents or other caregivers may attribute aversive behavior to oppositionality rather than a true biologically based disorder.[34] Finally, parental conflict with bipolar adolescents is more strongly related to hostility expressed by the adolescent than to the concurrent severity of depressive or manic symptoms, suggesting that parents are often reciprocating the child's affective state.[35]

The cause–effect relationship between parental attitudes/behaviors and aversive child behavior is not known, but it is likely to be bidirectional. Overall, research on family processes suggests multiple targets for family interventions, including dyadic communication patterns, parental attributions about the causes of the proband's behavior, and factors that lead to low maternal warmth.

Research on Psychosocial Treatments

The research on life events and family processes suggests the importance of developing individual or family therapies aimed to change these processes. However, psychotherapies for bipolar disorder have not been developed in direct response to findings about psychosocial predictors. In fact, most of the psychotherapies currently in use for childhood bipolar disorder are derived from treatments already in use for depression or schizophrenia. A few investigators have arrived at post-hoc explanations for a treatment's mechanisms of change by referencing the stress literature. For example, CBT is based on the assumption that bipolar individuals have distorted cognitions that distinguish them from patients with other disorders or healthy subjects, and predispose them to depressive or manic states. This assumption has not been examined in bipolar individuals followed longitudinally.

All of the empirically tested forms of psychotherapy for bipolar disorder share common assumptions. They are (1) conceived as adjuncts to ongoing medication maintenance; (2) present focused and skill oriented, and (3) psychoeducational (i.e., oriented toward learning about and coping with the disorder). Most have included some form of monitoring of prodromal symptoms, sleep/wake cycle stabilization, and addressing medication adherence They also have distinctive elements, such as format (i.e., group, family, individual, or, more broadly, whether or not caregivers are involved), length and frequency, and whether people begin treatment during or shortly after an episode or during remission.[36] In the next sections, the different forms of psychotherapy are described, with an emphasis on those that have been tested in at least one RCT.

Family-Focused Treatment

Family-oriented treatments were among the first forms of therapy to be described in bipolar disorder. The earliest treatments were psychoanalytically informed,[37] with small-scale randomized trials of couple-based treatments appearing in the early to mid-1990s.[38–40] The move toward developing and manualizing family psychoeducational treatments for schizophrenia, based in part on the emerging expressed emotion findings, spawned a similar movement in bipolar disorder. The model that has received the most empirical attention in bipolar disorder—family-focused treatment (FFT)—is based on Falloon et al.'s[41] behavioral family management for schizophrenia patients and Anderson, Reiss, and Hogarty's psychoeducational family therapy for schizophrenia.[42]

FFT proceeds in up to 21 sessions for up to 9 months. In the first treatment module, *psychoeducation*, bipolar individuals and their caregivers (usually parents or, when possible, spouses, older siblings, or grandparents) are encouraged to describe their experiences with the person's manic or depressive symptoms. The person with bipolar disorder is often given the role of "expert" in this discussion. The objective is to encourage the family to develop a common perception of what bipolar disorder is and to generate a list of prodromal symptoms of episodes. The latter will be essential to a contract for preventing mania, consisting of a list of common triggers for prior episodes (e.g., sleep-disrupting events), early warning signs (e.g., irritability, anxiety), and preventative maneuvers (e.g., calling the physician for a medication reevaluation; changing family routines to encourage more regular bedtimes).

As FFT proceeds, the family engages in communication enhancement training to improve daily exchanges (see Box 9.1). Using role-playing and between-session rehearsal,

---

BOX 9.1

Carl, a 14-year-old boy who had been diagnosed with bipolar I disorder, was becoming increasingly agitated at night, working on a series of computer programs that, he claimed, would coalesce into an extension of Google Earth to allow the viewer to see into people's houses. His parents noticed that he began to "tool around the house," looking for loose camera equipment in the middle of the night. Although Carl fell short of agreeing that he was manic or hypomanic, he did describe a feeling of increased energy and mental acuity. He had been manic once before. In an FFT session, Carl and his parents developed a list of his current prodromal signs, the likely precipitants (in his case, the beginning of high school; a computer science class), and treatment or preventative strategies. These included an appointment with his psychiatrist (who added risperidone to his valproate regimen), agreements about when computers were to be shut off at night (and a reward from his parents when he followed the plan consistently), and use of relaxation and meditation exercises (his suggestion) before he went to bed.

clinicians guide family members and individuals with bipolar disorder in how to listen actively (i.e., keep eye contact, ask questions, paraphrase the speaker), balance positive and negative feedback, and diplomatically ask for changes in each others' behaviors. These exercises often reduce the tension level in the household and create an atmosphere of collaboration. Finally, sessions of problem-solving skills training—in which families and affected individuals identify a list of specific problems, generate possible solutions, review the advantages and disadvantages of each solution, and choose an implementation plan—round out the treatment. Each session is accompanied by homework assignments that encourage family members and patients to practice communication and problem-solving skills.

FFT has been tested in a number of randomized trials in adults (for review, see ref. 2). These trials have compared FFT and pharmacotherapy to individual therapy and pharmacotherapy or case management and pharmacotherapy. The trials consistently indicate a benefit for adult individuals with bipolar disorder who begin treatment shortly after an acute episode, in terms of time to recovery, time to recurrence, and symptom severity over time. One study—the multisite Systematic Treatment Enhancement Program for Bipolar Disorder (STEP-BD)—found that pharmacotherapy plus weekly and biweekly sessions of FFT over 9 months were more effective than pharmacotherapy plus brief therapy (three sessions of psychoeducation) in terms of time to recovery from depression, amount of time spent well, and psychosocial functioning over 1 year.[43] This study also found benefits for interpersonal and social rhythm therapy (IPSRT) and cognitive-behavioral therapy (CBT) compared to brief treatment; none of the intensive therapies differed in terms of primary outcomes over 1 year.[1]

Randomized trials of FFT for youth with bipolar disorder are few. In a randomized trial of 58 bipolar adolescents treated in two sites, FFT-Adolescent version (FFT-A) and pharmacotherapy were more effective than enhanced care (three sessions of family education) and pharmacotherapy in hastening time to remission from depressive episodes and maintaining stability over 2 years. The effects of FFT-A were moderated by the EE level of the family at randomization: those adolescents who had high-EE families showed greater reductions in depressive and manic symptoms over 2 years if they received FFT-A than if they received EC. Thus, adolescents in high-conflict, high-criticism families (and possibly, those in families with high levels of enmeshment) may show greater clinical benefits from intensive family treatment than adolescents in low-conflict/low-involvement families.

A second trial found that FFT, in abbreviated form (12 sessions), was effective in stabilizing youth (mean age: 12 years) at high risk for bipolar disorder.[44] These youth had clinical presentations that have been found to predict the onset of bipolar I or II disorder when a positive family history of mania is also present.[45–46] Youth with bipolar disorder not otherwise specified (NOS) and major depressive disorder showed more rapid recovery from depression, more improvement in hypomania symptoms, and more weeks well over a 1-year follow-up than those who received 1–2 sessions of family psychoeducation. The psychosocial results could not be explained by concurrent medications taken by children.

In summary, FFT, given in 12–21 sessions over 4–9 months (depending on the population) is an effective adjunct to pharmacotherapy for youth in the earliest stages of bipolar disorder, and in adults who have more established illnesses. It has not been shown that FFT is more (or less) effective than disorder-specific individual therapies of equal intensity, such as IPSRT. One trial of adults[47] found that FFT was more effective in delaying recurrences and rehospitalizations than an individual psychoeducational therapy of the same intensity (21 sessions in 9 months). Involving family members in the identification of prodromal symptoms may hasten the process by which patients receive emergency treatment to prevent recurrences; enhancing the family relational context may contribute to long-term mood stability.

Family-Focused Treatment for Adolescents With Substance Abuse

A version of FFT has been developed to reduce the frequency and amount of substance use among bipolar adolescents.[48] Although the same structure (psychoeducation, communication training, and problem solving) is used, the focus of sessions is on preventing and/or minimizing negative outcomes related to substance use, including medication nonadherence, legal problems, accidents, suicide attempts, and risky sexual behavior. In part, this is done through promoting "substance-free homes" in which parents are coached to avoid using alcohol or substances themselves or making access to substances easy for adolescents.

In a pilot study,[48] 10 adolescents with bipolar disorder who had a substance use disorder and a recent exacerbation of mood symptoms were given up to 21 FFT sessions. Over 12 months, those who completed all or most of the treatment showed significant reductions in manic and depressive symptoms and improved global functioning, along with nonsignificant reductions in cannabis use. Interestingly, 3 of 3 subjects who dropped out of treatment early had parents with an active substance use disorder. The results suggest the viability of a family approach to dual diagnosis in adolescents, as well as the importance of considering the parents' sobriety as a key mediator of adolescents' treatment engagement.

Multifamily Group Approaches

Several investigators have examined psychoeducational interventions in multifamily group contexts in which parents of bipolar children have the opportunity to interact with one another. Fristad and colleagues[49,50] conducted an 18-month waitlist control study of multifamily group psychoeducation with 165 school-aged bipolar (70%) and depressed (30%) children. The groups included didactic information about mood management, communication skills, and coping strategies to avert mood escalation. Over 1 year, children whose families participated in the groups had greater improvement in mood symptoms than children whose families were assigned to the waitlist. The clinical benefits of the groups were mediated by improvements in parents' ability to advocate for the child's mental health care needs.[50]

Another model, the "RAINBOW" program (which also goes by a less enticing title, "child and family-focused cognitive behavioral therapy") consists of 12 sessions of family psychoeducation and individual CBT (i.e., cognitive restructuring and pleasurable events scheduling). In a sample of 34 bipolar children (ages 5–17 years), West and associates[51] reported that gains in mania, aggression, psychosis, depression, and global functioning during a 12-week open trial were maintained over a 3-year follow-up. A model using multifamily groups produced similar changes in 26 bipolar youth, although the effects did not appear to be as consistent.[52] The RAINBOW program is currently being evaluated in a randomized trial.[53]

Individual Cognitive-Behavioral Therapy

CBT assumes that bipolar depression is associated with negative attributional styles and mania with excessively optimistic styles; these attributions are a major target of treatment. A reanalysis of the STEP-BD dataset indicated that "extreme attributions" (excessively pessimistic or optimistic causal explanations for events) measured shortly after onset of a depressive episode predicted a longer interval prior to recovery and a shorter time to manic or mixed recurrences, independently of the severity of depressive or manic symptoms.[54–55]

The record for individual CBT in the treatment of BD is mixed. One randomized trial in the United Kingdom found that remitted individuals ($n = 103$) who received an average of 14 sessions of CBT in 6 months were less likely to have depressive episodes and had better social functioning over 30 months than those in routine care.[56] The STEP-BD trial found that individual CBT given after a bipolar depressive episode, like FFT and IPSRT, was associated with faster time to recovery than a three-session comparator.[1] However, results of a five-site effectiveness trial in the United Kingdom ($n = 252$) found no advantage for CBT versus usual care in time to recurrence over 18 months. A secondary analysis indicated that individuals with fewer than 12 prior episodes had longer survival times prior to recurrence in CBT than usual care, although the reverse pattern was observed in people with more than 12 prior episodes.[57]

The recently published CANMAT (Canadian Mood and Anxiety Treatment) multisite trial compared 20 sessions of individual CBT to 6 group psychoeducation sessions, both with standard pharmacotherapy, in 204 bipolar individuals who were in full or partial remission.[58] There were no differences in recurrence or symptom severity over an average of 72 weeks. Thus, the evidence for adjunctive CBT for recovery or relapse prevention in adult bipolar disorder is inconclusive.

Dialectical Behavior Therapy in Adolescent Patients

There have been no published randomized trials of CBT for childhood or adolescent bipolar subjects, although a small-scale ($n = 8$) open trial found that adolescents who received individual CBT showed greater mood improvement than eight matched controls who did not received CBT.[59]

A treatment development trial[60] demonstrated the feasibility and acceptability of a dialectical behavior therapy (DBT) adaptation of the Linehan model.[61] The approach consisted of an average of 33–36 sessions over 1 year of mindfulness, emotion regulation, distress tolerance, and interpersonal effectiveness skills, taught in alternating individual and family sessions. In a 10-case open trial, adolescents with BD showed significant improvement over 1 year in suicidality, nonsuicidal self-injurious behavior, emotional dysregulation, and depressive symptoms. Thus, DBT may be an important option for adolescents with suicidal or self-injurious behavior or thinking.

Interpersonal and Social Rhythm Therapy

Interpersonal and social rhythm therapy (IPSRT) is an adaptation of the interpersonal psychotherapy for depression, an exploratory, insight-oriented approach to solving interpersonal problems.[62] Unique to IPSRT is the focus on encouraging bipolar individuals to maintain daily routines and sleep/wake rhythms.[18] In an RCT involving 175 acutely ill bipolar I subjects, random assignment was conducted during an acute phase to IPSRT (given weekly) or equally intensive clinical management, both with pharmacotherapy. Following episode recovery, random assignment was conducted again (IPSRT vs. clinical management) and treatment continued monthly over 2 years. IPSRT was not associated with faster recovery from the acute episode than clinical management. However, significant differences emerged during the 2-year maintenance phase: Individuals who had received IPSRT in the acute phase had longer intervals prior to recurrence and better occupational functioning than those who had received clinical management during the acute phase.[63] Importantly, the effects of IPSRT in delaying recurrences were mediated by whether subjects had been able to stabilize their daily or nightly routines during acute IPSRT.[18] Thus, assisting bipolar individuals in stabilizing sleep/wake rhythms after an acute episode may help prevent future episodes. A strength of this study is the matching of the two treatments on amount of clinical contact in both study phases.

IPSRT has been re-manualized for adolescents with BD I or II, who have considerable difficulty with sleep/wake cycles. Although no randomized trials have been conducted, an open trial involving 12 adolescents treated for 16–18 sessions showed high rates of treatment acceptance, decreases in manic and depressive symptoms, and improvements in global functioning over 20 weeks.[64]

Given the level of disruption observed in adolescents' sleep patterns, future studies of IPSRT or other psychosocial interventions should clarify whether improvements in symptoms or functioning can be attributed to improvements in sleep consistency. In a randomized trial of FFT-A, sleep impairment was associated with the severity of manic and depressive symptoms and level of functional impairment among bipolar adolescents followed over 2 years, independently of psychosocial interventions.[65]

Group Psychoeducation

A potentially cost-effective alternative are group approaches for people with bipolar disorder who cannot afford individual therapy and/or do not have access to family caregivers. Most of the existing models of group treatment use predesigned curricula, with sessions devoted to illness awareness, early detection of recurrences, treatment adherence, sleep/wake regularity, and in some models, substance/alcohol abuse.[66–69]

A group at the University of Barcelona has developed a 6-month group psychoeducational treatment that emphasizes illness coping strategies. In a trial of 120 euthymic bipolar I and II individuals, subjects were assigned to pharmacotherapy and 20 sessions of structured group psychoeducation or 20 sessions of an unstructured support group. The results indicated that, at 2 and 5 years after randomization, those who received the structured groups had fewer relapses and less time ill than those in the unstructured groups.[66,69,70] Moreover, secondary analyses indicated that, at 5 years, the reduction in hospital days translated into a cost savings of €5,000 (about $6,800) per patient.[70]

A psychoeducation group based on CBT principles has been developed for bipolar adults who have substance abuse disorders.[67,71] The groups proceed with sessions on identifying risk factors for mood and substance abuse recurrence, learning to decline drugs when offered by others, and the importance of medication consistency. The position of the group leaders is that bipolar disorder and substance abuse are one disorder. This position is not supported by research—for example, the course of the two disorders is known to diverge in many cases.[72] Nonetheless, the CBT groups were found to reduce alcohol use in comorbid bipolar I individuals.[67] No studies of this group approach have been undertaken with adolescents.

Systematic Care Management

Two research groups have examined systematic or "collaborative care" programs that combine protocol-driven pharmacotherapy, group psychoeducation, and clinical monitoring by a nurse care manager. These models usually assume a level of illness chronicity that justifies careful oversight to minimize recurrences and noncompliance. In trials at a group health cooperative ($n = 441$)[73] and in 11 Veterans Administration (VA) sites ($n = 306$),[74] subjects were randomly assigned to systematic care or usual care. Those in systematic care had fewer weeks in manic episodes than those in usual care, and in the VA study, better social functioning and quality of life over 2 years. Neither study found that systematic care reduced rates of relapse. Cost-effectiveness analyses indicated that the care programs saved money despite the personnel costs of a nurse care manager.[73–74]

Future Directions

At this stage, we have considerable evidence that targeted forms of psychotherapy are effective adjuncts to medication management in bipolar disorder. The evidence for the utility of these approaches in children and adolescents is growing. Evidence suggests that family interventions—FFT and multifamily psychoeducational groups—are effective for bipolar youth; the effects of DBT, IPSRT, and the RAINBOW approach are still being tested.

Psychotherapy studies of bipolar disorder are not far enough along to justify offering youth psychotherapy alone, given the considerable evidence that mood stabilizers and second-generation antipsychotics are effective for mania in children.[75] It may make sense to begin treating youth at risk for bipolar disorder (for example, those with depression or BD-NOS and a familial history of mania) with psychotherapy alone at the earliest stages of symptom development, with introduction of pharmacotherapy if symptoms worsen. However, even high-risk conditions present with multiple comorbidities, and the use of psychostimulants (for ADHD) or mood stabilizers/antipsychotics with anxiolytic properties must be considered in any treatment plan.

Many promising treatments for adult mood disorders have not been tested in pediatric bipolar samples. One example is mindfulness-based cognitive therapy (MBCT), an eight-session group treatment in which participants learn mindfulness meditation (i.e., nonjudgmental observation of internal processes) and cognitive-behavioral skills such as identification of pessimistic thoughts. MBCT has a specific skill training agenda: to teach participants to incorporate an accepting stance toward their illness and its challenges. Results from six RCTs of remitted or subsyndromally ill patients with recurrent major depressive disorder (i.e., three or more episodes) indicate that, when compared to usual care, treatment with MBCT is highly effective in preventing depressive recurrences over 12–18 months.[76–80] In a 15-month maintenance trial, MBCT was as effective and cost-effective as maintenance antidepressants in preventing recurrence in multiepisode depressed patients, and more effective than antidepressants in reducing residual depressive symptoms and improving quality of life.[79] An 18-month trial found that MBCT offered protective effects against relapse or recurrence in major depressive disorder that were comparable to the effects offered by maintenance pharmacotherapy.[80]

There are five small-scale open trials suggesting the applicability of MBCT to remitted or subsyndromally ill adults with bipolar disorder,[81–85] including improvements in anxiety, cognition, and in one study, suicidal ideation. However, the only randomized study of MBCT in bipolar disorder found no effects on time to recurrence or on depression or mania scores compared to usual care.[86] Randomized trials of mindfulness treatment in children or adolescents with bipolar disorder, perhaps using adaptations of MBCT for childhood anxiety,[87] are an important direction for future research.

Many questions remain about the appropriate timing and format of psychosocial interventions for pediatric-onset patients, as well as what variables moderate clinical response. Studies of depression prevention among adolescents have found that the clinical status of the parent (i.e., whether he or she also suffers from depression) moderates the efficacy of CBT groups in preventing first episodes of major depression.[88] The factors that moderate whether youth benefit from family versus individual or group interventions warrants study—it is possible, for example, that group psychoeducational approaches are more beneficial for older teens than for younger children.

Several studies indicate that bipolar individuals in high-EE families benefit more from FFT than those in low-EE families.[44,89,90] It may be that youth in high-EE families are more emotionally reactive and have a more difficult time with self-regulation but show greater clinical benefits when attributes of the family context (e.g., the degree to which families engage in productive interchanges) improve. Research has not examined whether family contextual variables moderate the responses of pediatric bipolar individuals to other kinds of psychotherapy.

Related to the issue of treatment moderation is the role of comorbid disorders in explaining the variability in outcomes of psychotherapy. A reanalysis of the STEP-BD trial found that comorbid anxiety disorders predicted a better response among bipolar depressed patients to intensive individual or family therapy compared to brief treatment.[91] No comparable data are available for pediatric populations. The difficulties inherent in treating children with bipolar disorder who also have ADHD, oppositional defiant disorders, or autism spectrum disorders are well known to clinicians, although the reasons why these disorders raise additional challenges—or whether they simply mean that the child will be less cooperative—are unclear.

Finally, we must consider the complexity of implementing evidence-based treatments in community settings. Although community practitioners are becoming more familiar with manual-based treatments, there are significant differences between the populations seen in community mental health centers (CMHCs) versus academic centers. Lengthy protocols may be impossible to deliver in CMHCs where clinicians must carry a minimum caseload and in which the number of sessions is capped. Thus, researchers will need to work closely with community administrators and practitioners to engage CMHCs in a partnership regarding evidence-based practice, where communication is reciprocal and mutually informative.[92]

Author Disclosures

Dr. Miklowitz has received grant funding from the National Institute of Mental Health, the National Alliance for Research on Schizophrenia and Depression, the Attias Family Foundation, the Danny Alberts Foundation, the Carl and Roberta Deutsch Foundation, the Kayne Family Foundation, and the Knapp Foundation. He receives book royalties from Guilford Press and John Wiley and Sons.

References

1. Miklowitz DJ, Otto MW, Frank E, et al. Psychosocial treatments for bipolar depression: a 1-year randomized trial from the Systematic Treatment Enhancement Program. *Arch Gen Psychiatry*. 2007;64:419–27.
2. Geddes JR, Miklowitz DJ. Treatment of bipolar disorder. *Lancet*. 2013;381(9878):1672–82.
3. Johnson SL, Miller I. Negative life events and time to recovery from episodes of bipolar disorder. *J Abnorm Psychol*. 1997;106:449–57.

4. Johnson SL, Cuellar A, Ruggero C, et al. Life events as predictors of mania and depression in bipolar I disorder. *J Abnorm Psychol.* 2008;117:268–77.

5. Johnson SL, Edge MD, Holmes MK, Carver CS. The behavioral activation system and mania. *Annu Rev Clin Psychol.* 2012;8:143–67.

6. Johnson SL, Eisner L, Carver CS. Elevated expectancies among persons diagnosed with bipolar disorders. *Br J Clin Psychol.* 2009;48:217–22.

7. Johnson SL, Sandrow D, Meyer B, et al. Increases in manic symptoms following life events involving goal-attainment. *J Abnorm Psychol.* 2000;109:721–7.

8. Wehr TA, Sack DA, Rosenthal NE. Sleep reduction as a final common pathway in the genesis of mania. *Am J Psychiatry.* 1987;144:210–14.

9. Ehlers CL, Frank E, Kupfer DJ. Social zeitgebers and biological rhythms: a unified approach to understanding the etiology of depression. *Arch Gen Psychiatry.* 1988;45:948–52.

10. Ehlers CL, Kupfer DJ, Frank E, Monk TH. Biological rhythms and depression: the role of zeitgebers and zeitstorers. *Depression.* 1993;1:285–93.

11. Barbini B, Bertelli S, Colombo C, Smeraldi E. Sleep loss, a possible factor in augmenting manic episode. *Psychiatry Res.* 1996;65(2):121–5.

12. Leibenluft E, Albert PS, Rosenthal NE, Wehr TA. Relationship between sleep and mood in patients with rapid-cycling bipolar disorder. *Psychiatry Res.* 1996;63:161–8.

13. Malkoff-Schwartz S, Frank E, Anderson B, et al. Stressful life events and social rhythm disruption in the onset of manic and depressive bipolar episodes: a preliminary investigation. *Arch Gen Psychiatry.* 1998;55:702–7.

14. Malkoff-Schwartz S, Frank E, Anderson BP, et al. Social rhythm disruption and stressful life events in the onset of bipolar and unipolar episodes. *Psychol Med.* 2000;30:1005–16.

15. Jones SH, Hare DJ, Evershed K. Actigraphic assessment of circadian activity and sleep patterns in bipolar disorder. *Bipolar Disorder.* 2005;7(2):176–86.

16. Kim EY, Miklowitz DJ, Biuckians A, Mullen K. Life stress and the course of early-onset bipolar disorder. *J Affect Disord.* 2007;99(1):37–44.

17. Hillegers MH, Burger H, Wals M, et al. Impact of stressful life events, familial loading and their interaction on the onset of mood disorders. *Br J Psychiatry.* 2004;185:97–101.

18. Frank E, Kupfer DJ, Thase ME, et al. Two-year outcomes for interpersonal and social rhythm therapy in individuals with bipolar I disorder. *Arch Gen Psychiatry.* 2005;62(9):996–1004.

19. Newman C, Leahy RL, Beck AT, Reilly-Harrington N, Gyulai L. *Bipolar Disorder: A Cognitive Therapy Approach.* Washington, DC: American Psychological Association Press; 2001.

20. Johnson SL, Fulford D. Preventing mania: a preliminary examination of the GOALS Program. *Behav Ther.* 2009;40(2):103–13.

21. Post RM, Leverich GS. The role of psychosocial stress in the onset and progression of bipolar disorder and its comorbidities: the need for earlier and alternative modes of therapeutic intervention. *Dev Psychopathol.* 2006;18(4):1181–211.

22. Hammen C, Gitlin MJ. Stress reactivity in bipolar patients and its relation to prior history of the disorder. *Am J Psychiatry.* 1997;154:856–7.

23. Dienes KA, Hammen C, Henry RM, Cohen AN, Daley SE. The stress sensitization hypothesis: understanding the course of bipolar disorder. *J Affect Disord.* 2006;95(1–3):43–9.

24. Hlastala SA, Frank E, Kowalski J, et al. Stressful life events, bipolar disorder, and the "kindling model." *J Abnorm Psychol.* 2000;109:777–86.

25. Miklowitz DJ, Goldstein MJ, Nuechterlein KH, Snyder KS, Mintz J. Family factors and the course of bipolar affective disorder. *Arch Gen Psychiatry.* 1988;45:225–31.

26. Miklowitz DJ, Biuckians A, Richards JA. Early-onset bipolar disorder: a family treatment perspective. *Dev Psychopathol.* 2006;18(4):1247–65.

27. Geller B, Tillman R, Bolhofner K, Zimerman B. Child bipolar I disorder: prospective continuity with adult bipolar I disorder; characteristics of second and third episodes; predictors of 8-year outcome. *Arch Gen Psychiatry.* 2008;65(10):1125–133.

28. Geller B, Bolhofner K, Craney JL, Williams M, Delbello MP, Gunderson K. Psychosocial functioning in a prepubertal and early adolescent bipolar disorder phenotype. *J Am Acad Child Adolesc Psychiatry.* 2000;39:1543–8.

29. Schenkel LS, West AE, Harral EM, Patel NB, Pavuluri MN. Parent-child interactions in pediatric bipolar disorder. *J Clin Psychology*. 2008;64(4):422–37.

30. Sullivan AE, Miklowitz DJ. Family functioning among adolescents with bipolar disorder. *J Fam Psychol*. 2010;24(1):60–7.

31. Chang KD, Blaser C, Ketter TA, Steiner H. Family environment of children and adolescents with bipolar parents. *Bipolar Disorders*. 2001;3:73–8.

32. Du Rocher Schudlich TD, Youngstrom EA, Calabrese JR, Findling RL. The role of family functioning in bipolar disorder in families. *J Abnorm Child Psychology*. 2008;36(6):849–63.

33. Simoneau TL, Miklowitz DJ, Saleem R. Expressed emotion and interactional patterns in the families of bipolar patients. *J Abnorm Psychol*. 1998;107:497–507.

34. Wendel JS, Miklowitz DJ, Richards JA, George EL. Expressed emotion and attributions in the relatives of bipolar patients: an analysis of problem-solving interactions. *J Abnorm Psychol*. 2000;109:792–6.

35. Keenan-Miller D, Peris T, Axelson D, Kowatch RA, Miklowitz DJ. Family functioning, social impairment, and symptoms among adolescents with bipolar disorder. *J Am Acad Child Adolesc Psychiatry*. 2012;51(10):1085–094.

36. Miklowitz DJ, Goodwin GM, Bauer M, Geddes JR. Common and specific elements of psychosocial treatments for bipolar disorder: a survey of clinicians participating in randomized trials. *J Psychiatric Prac*. 2008;14(2):77–85.

37. Davenport YB, Ebert MH, Adland ML, Goodwin FK. Couples group therapy as adjunct to lithium maintenance of the manic patient. *Am J Orthopsychiatry*. 1977;47:495–502.

38. van Gent EM, Zwart FM. Psychoeducation of partners of bipolar-manic patients. *J Affect Disord*. 1991;21(1):15–8.

39. Clarkin JF, Carpenter D, Hull J, Wilner P, Glick I. Effects of psychoeducational intervention for married patients with bipolar disorder and their spouses. *Psychiatric Serv*. 1998;49:531–3.

40. Clarkin JF, Glick ID, Haas GL, et al. A randomized clinical trial of inpatient family intervention: V. Results for affective disorders. *J Affect Disord*. 1990;18:17–28.

41. Falloon IRH, Boyd JL, McGill CW, et al. Family management in the prevention of morbidity of schizophrenia. *Arch Gen Psychiatry*. 1985;42:887–96.

42. Anderson CM, Reiss DJ, Hogarty GE. *Schizophrenia and the Family*. New York, NY: Guilford Press; 1986.

43. Miklowitz DJ, Otto MW, Frank E, et al. Intensive psychosocial intervention enhances functioning in patients with bipolar depression: results from a 9-month randomized controlled trial. *Am J Psychiatry*. 2007;164(9):1–8.

44. Miklowitz DJ, Schneck CD, Singh MK, et al. Early intervention for symptomatic youth at risk for bipolar disorder: a randomized trial of family-focused therapy. *J Am Acad Child Adolesc Psychiatry*. 2013;52(2):121–31.

45. Birmaher B, Axelson D, Goldstein B, et al. Four-year longitudinal course of children and adolescents with bipolar spectrum disorders: the Course and Outcome of Bipolar Youth (COBY) study. *Am J Psychiatry*. 2009;166(7):795–804.

46. Luby JL, Navsaria N. Pediatric bipolar disorder: evidence for prodromal states and early markers. *J Child Psychol Psychiatry*. 2010;51(4):459–71.

47. Rea MM, Tompson M, Miklowitz DJ, Goldstein MJ, Hwang S, Mintz J. Family focused treatment vs. individual treatment for bipolar disorder: results of a randomized clinical trial. *J Consult Clin Psychol*. 2003;71:482–92.

48. Goldstein B, Goldstein TR, Collinger-Larson K, et al. Treatment development and feasibility study of family-focused treatment for adolescents with bipolar disorder and comorbid substance use disorders. *J Psychiatric Pract*. 2014; 20(3):237–48.

49. Fristad MA, Verducci JS, Walters K, Young ME. Impact of multifamily psychoeducational psychotherapy in treating children aged 8 to 12 years with mood disorders. *Arch Gen Psychiatry*. 2009;66(9):1013–21.

50. Mendenhall AN, Fristad MA, Early T. Factors influencing service utilization and mood symptom severity in children with mood disorders: effects of Multi-Family Psychoeducation Groups (MFPG). *J Consult Clin Psychol*. 2009;77(3):463–73.

51. West AE, Henry DB, Pavuluri MN. Maintenance model of integrated psychosocial treatment in pediatric bipolar disorder: a pilot feasibility study. *J Am Acad Child Adolesc Psychiatry.* 2007;46(2):205–12.

52. West AE, Jacobs RH, Westerholm R, et al. Child and family-focused cognitive-behavioral therapy for pediatric bipolar disorder: pilot study of group treatment format. *J Can Acad Child AdolescPsychiatry.* 2009;18(3):239–46.

53. West AE, Weinstein SM. A family-based psychosocial treatment model. *Israeli J Psychiatry Relat Sci.* 2012;49(2):86–93.

54. Stange JP, Sylvia LG, Vieira da Silva Magalhães P, et al. Extreme attributions predict the course of bipolar depression: results from the STEP-BD randomized controlled trial of psychosocial treatment. *J Clin Psychiatry.* 2013;74(3):249–55.

55. Stange JP, Sylvia LG, Magalhães PV, et al. Extreme attributions predict transition from depression to mania in bipolar disorder. *J Psychiatric Res.* 2013;47(10):1329–36.

56. Lam DH, Hayward P, Watkins ER, Wright K, Sham P. Relapse prevention in patients with bipolar disorder: cognitive therapy outcome after 2 years. *Am J Psychiatry.* 2005;162:324–9.

57. Scott J, Paykel E, Morriss R, et al. Cognitive behaviour therapy for severe and recurrent bipolar disorders: a randomised controlled trial. *Br J Psychiatry.* 2006;188:313–20.

58. Parikh SV, Zaretsky A, Beaulieu S, et al. A randomized controlled trial of psychoeducation or cognitive-behavioral therapy in bipolar disorder: a Canadian Network for Mood and Anxiety treatments (CANMAT) study. *J Clin Psychiatry.* 2012;73(6):803–10.

59. Feeny NC, Danielson CK, Schwartz L, Youngstrom EA, Findling RL. Cognitive-behavioral therapy for bipolar disorders in adolescents: a pilot study. *Bipolar Disord.* 2006;8(5 Pt. 1):508–15.

60. Goldstein TR, Axelson DA, Birmaher B, Brent DA. Dialectical behavior therapy for adolescents with bipolar disorder: a 1-year open trial. *J Am Acad Child Adolesc Psychiatry.* 2007;46(7):820–30.

61. Linehan M. *Cognitive-Behavioral Treatment of Borderline Personality Disorder.* New York, NY: Guilford Press; 1993.

62. Klerman GL, Weissman MM, Rounsaville BJ, Chevron RS. *Interpersonal Psychotherapy of Depression.* New York, NY: Basic Books; 1984.

63. Frank E, Soreca I, Swartz HA, et al. The role of interpersonal and social rhythm therapy in improving occupational functioning in patients with bipolar I disorder. *Am J Psychiatry.* 2008;165(12):1559–65.

64. Hlastala SA, Kotler JS, McClellan JM, McCauley EA. Interpersonal and social rhythm therapy for adolescents with bipolar disorder: treatment development and results from an open trial. *Depress Anxiety.* 2010;27(5):457–64.

65. Lunsford-Avery JA, Judd CM, Axelson DA, Miklowitz DJ. Sleep impairment, mood symptoms, and psychosocial functioning in adolescent bipolar disorder. *Psychiatry Res.* 2012;200(2–3):265–71.

66. Colom F, Vieta E, Martinez-Aran A, Reinares M, Goikolea JM, Martínez-Arán A. A randomized trial on the efficacy of group psychoeducation in the prophylaxis of bipolar disorder: a five year follow-up. *Br J Psychiatry.* 2009;194(3):260–65.

67. Weiss RD, Griffin ML, Kolodziej ME, et al. A randomized trial of integrated group therapy versus group drug counseling for patients with bipolar disorder and substance dependence. *Am J Psychiatry.* 2007;164(1):100–7.

68. Bauer MS, McBride L, Chase C, Sachs G, Shea N. Manual-based group psychotherapy for bipolar disorder: a feasibility study. *J Clin Psychiatry.* 1998;59:449–55.

69. Colom F, Vieta E, Martinez-Aran A, et al. A randomized trial on the efficacy of group psychoeducation in the prophylaxis of recurrences in bipolar patients whose disease is in remission. *Arch Gen Psychiatry.* 2003;60:402–7.

70. Scott J, Colom F, Popova E, et al. Long-term mental health resource utilization and cost of care following group psychoeducation or unstructured group support for bipolar disorders: a cost-benefit analysis. *J Clin Psychiatry.* 2009;70(3):378–86.

71. Weiss RD, Griffin ML, Jaffee WB, et al. A "community-friendly" version of integrated group therapy for patients with bipolar disorder and substance dependence: a randomized controlled trial. *Drug Alcohol Depend.* 2009;104(3):212–9.

72. Strakowski SM, DelBello MP, Fleck DE, Arndt S. The impact of substance abuse on the course of bipolar disorder. *Biol Psychiatry.* 2000;48:477–85.

73. Simon GE, Ludman EJ, Bauer MS, Unutzer J, Operskalski B. Long-term effectiveness and cost of a systematic care program for bipolar disorder. *Arch Gen Psychiatry*. 2006;63(5):500–8.

74. Bauer MS, McBride L, Williford WO, et al. Collaborative care for bipolar disorder: Part II. Impact on clinical outcome, function, and costs *Psychiatric Services*. 2006;57:937–45.

75. Pfeifer JC, Kowatch RA, DelBello MP. Pharmacotherapy of bipolar disorder in children and adolescents: recent progress. *CNS Drugs*. 2010;24(7):575–93.

76. Piet J, Hougaar E. The effect of mindfulness-based cognitive therapy for prevention of relapse in recurrent major depressive disorder: a systematic review and meta-analysis. *Clin Psychol Rev*. 2011;31:1032–40.

77. Teasdale JD, Segal ZV, Williams JM, Ridgeway VA, Soulsby JM, Lau MA. Prevention of relapse/recurrence in major depression by mindfulness-based cognitive therapy. *J Consult Clin Psychol*. 2000;68(4):615–23.

78. Ma SH, Teasdale J. Mindfulness-based cognitive therapy for depression: replication and exploration of differential relapse prevention effects. *J Consult Clin Psychol*. 2004;72(1):31–40.

79. Kuyken W, Byford S, Taylor RS, et al. Mindfulness-based cognitive therapy to prevent relapse in recurrent depression. *J Consult Clin Psychol*. 2008;76(6):966–78.

80. Segal ZV, Bieling P, Young T, et al. Antidepressant monotherapy v. sequyential pharmacotherapy and mindfulness-based cognitive therapy, or placebo, for relapse prophylaxis in recurrent depression. *Arch Gen Psychiatry*. 2010;67(12):1256–64.

81. Miklowitz DJ, Alatiq Y, Goodwin GM, et al. A pilot study of mindfulness-based cognitive therapy for bipolar disorder. *Int J Cog Ther*. 2009;2(4):373–82.

82. Williams JM, Alatiq Y, Crane C, et al. Mindfulness-based Cognitive Therapy (MBCT) in bipolar disorder: preliminary evaluation of immediate effects on between-episode functioning. *J Affect Disord*. 2008;107(1–3):275–79.

83. Weber B, Jermann F, Gex-Fabry M, Nallet A, Bondolfi G, Aubry JM. Mindfulness-based cognitive therapy for bipolar disorder: a feasibility trial. *Eur Psychiatry*. 2010;25(6):334–7.

84. Chadwick P, Kaur H, Swelam M, Ross S, Ellett L. Experience of mindfulness in people with bipolar disorder: a qualitative study. *Psychother Res*. 2011;21(3):277–85.

85. Deckersbach T, Hölzel BK, Eisner LR, et al. Mindfulness-based cognitive therapy for nonremitted patients with bipolar disorder. *CNS Neurosci Ther*. 2012;18(2):133–41.

86. Perich T, Manicavasagar V, Mitchell PB, Ball JR, Hadzi-Pavlovic D. A randomized controlled trial of mindfulness-based cognitive therapy for bipolar disorder. *Acta Psychiatr Scand*. 2013;127(5):333–43.

87. Semple R, Lee J, Williams M, Teasdale JD. *Mindfulness-Based Cognitive Therapy for Anxious Children: A Manual for Treating Childhood Anxiety*. New York, NY: New Harbinger; 2011.

88. Beardslee WR, Brent DA, Weersing VR, et al. Prevention of depression in at-risk adolescents: longer-term effects. *JAMA Psychiatry*. 2013;70(11):1161–70.

89. Kim EY, Miklowitz DJ. Expressed emotion as a predictor of outcome among bipolar patients undergoing family therapy. *J Affect Disord*. 2004;82:343–52.

90. Miklowitz DJ, Axelson DA, George EL, et al. Expressed emotion moderates the effects of family-focused treatment for bipolar adolescents. *J Am Acad Child Adolesc Psychiatry*. 2009;48:643–51.

91. Deckersbach T, Peters AT, Sylvia L, et al. Do comorbid anxiety disorders moderate the effects of psychotherapy for bipolar disorder? Results from STEP-BD. *Am J Psychiatry*. 2014;171(2):178–86.

92. Wells K, Jones L. "Research" in community-partnered, participatory research. *JAMA*. 2009;302(3):320–1.

Complementary and Alternative Medicine in Child and Adolescent Bipolar Disorder

Barbara L. Gracious, Sathyan Gurumurthy, Alexandra Cottle, and Taylor M. McCabe

Introduction: Definitions, Justification, Current Status and Challenges

The definitions of complementary and alternative medical treatments have been stated most clearly by Arnold.[1] A complementary treatment adds to the benefit of an established treatment by augmenting the primary response or working synergistically with an established primary treatment. Alternative treatment refers to use when substituted for an established treatment. Uses of the same treatment can be complementary or alternative.

Numerous challenges exist prior to justified dissemination of complementary and alternative medicine (CAM) for child and adolescent bipolar disorder (CABD), despite strong public interest. Safety, efficacy, and effectiveness research for CAM in CABD is in its infancy. This situation is despite a compelling rationale that includes concerns about serious metabolic and other adverse effects from conventional psychopharmacology, as well as broader issues of access to care, overall treatment costs, and differing health service delivery systems in an expanding global population with insufficient access to conventional child psychiatric diagnosis and treatment. As advances in understanding bipolar disorder continue through cell and animal studies, epidemiology, epigenetics, neuroimaging, and genomic approaches, these techniques will be increasingly applied to CAM studies for bipolar disorder, but funding sources for such research in mental health remain limited. CAM research overall is growing exponentially internationally, with mechanistic data and clinical trial results in other biologically based disorders informing potential central nervous system (CNS) uses. For example, testing CAM strategies that can alter oxidative stress and systemic inflammation processes documented in those with severe bipolar I disorder may be particularly informative. Another challenge for CAM is to integrate newer mechanistic findings into emerging data that support historical population-based public health strategies, known somewhat collectively and broadly as "healthy lifestyle." Study of lifestyle habit changes that mitigate symptom expression and encourage remission that may be defined as CAM includes the roles of diet, exercise, chronobiology, and meditative practices, among others. Combined, these approaches may offer more immediate hope for change to individuals and families facing an often devastating illness, toward reducing the suffering and violence commonly associated with CABD.

This chapter reports evidence published in the English literature for different CAM approaches that have potential applicability to CABD, grouped into dietary supplements, lifestyle, and healing practices modalities. Where possible, information from direct study in CABD cohorts is given; when not available, the closest information possible, for example, studies in adults with bipolar or unipolar illness or youth with unipolar depression, is provided. Known or potential mechanisms of action, as well as dose ranges and possible adverse effects, are briefly summarized (see Table 10.1), with implications for future research noted. Dose ranges are from both lay publication and research sources, typically from adult mental and physical health studies, and do not necessarily represent what should be used in an individual pediatric case. Expert consultation should be sought as needed for clinical practice. More focused reviews of CAM for CABD are provided in Sylvia et al. (dietary supplements and diet),[2] Sarris et al. (on adjunctive nutraceuticals),[3,4] and Nierenberg (mitochondrial modifiers).[5] These authors envision CAM treatments as adjunctive in alleviating residual symptoms and improving outcomes of standard therapies or, potentially, as primary therapy.

Dietary Supplements

Omega-3 Fatty Acids

Long-chain polyunsaturated fatty acids (LC-PUFAs) refer to fatty acids including subgroups known as omega n-3 and n-6 fatty acids, due to the position of the last double bond in their chemical structures. Omega-3 fatty acids are essential, meaning they are obtained only from naturally occurring dietary sources, as mammals are unable to synthesize them *de novo* and can only elongate and desaturate, changing plant-based alpha-linolenic acid (ALA) into eicosapentanoic acid (EPA) and EPA into docosahexaenoic acid (DHA). Western diets are deficient in omega-3 fats, due to relatively low seafood and higher processed food consumption coupled with food industry changes over the last century resulting in greater use of corn and soy oils high in the omega-6 fatty acid linoleic acid.[6] Insufficient dietary intake of LC-n-3 PUFAs has likely contributed to the rise of

TABLE 10.1

Supplement/Technique	Potential or Known Mechanisms	Dose[a]	Potential Side Effects[aa]
Dietary Supplements			
1. Omega-3 Fatty Acids	Improves neural cell fluidity; suppresses neuronal signaling, calcium channel and protein kinase C activity; lowers proinflammatory cytokines and oxidative stress; reduces kindling	1000 mg/day; see references for EPA/DHA amounts	nausea, diarrhea; possible bleeding in anticoagulated or those at risk for bleeding
2. Amino Acids & Their Derivatives			
a. Amino Acid Depletion Models	Lowers tyrosine which causes a decreased release of dopamine	varies; see references	unpalatable, vomiting
b. L-Tryptophan	Direct precursor in the synthesis of serotonin	150mg–8gm/day	mania, irritability, drowsiness
c. N-Acetyl Cysteine	Scavenges free radicals and protects neurons from oxidative stress; possibly modulates glutamatergic system, by increasing extracellular cysteine, which ultimately results in synaptic vesicular release of glutamate, decreasing the excitatory to inhibitory ratio.	up to 2700 mg/day	nausea, vomiting (uncommon)
d. S-Adenosyl Methionine	Augments CNS dopamine and norepinephrine levels, promotes serotonin release	600–1600 mg/day	GI complaints; dry mouth, headache, insomnia, sweating, dizziness, anxiety
e. acetyl-L-carnitine (ALCAR)	shuttles fatty acids into mitochondria for oxidation and energy generation; scavenges reactive oxygen species; acetylcholine precursor	1000–3000 mg/day	GI complaints; restlessness, 'fishy' odor
f. alpha-lipoic acid (ALA)	mitochondrial coenzyme; ↑ cellular glucose uptake for ATP synthesis; antioxidant effects; chelates heavy metals; anti-apoptotic, neuroprotective from glutamate-induced intracellular Ca++ increases	600–1800 mg/day	skin rash; potential for hypoglycemia
3. Other Mitochondrial Modifiers	Act along the electron transport chain		
a. Co-Enzyme Q10 (CoQ10)	neutralizes free radicals; reduces vitE to absorbable alpha-tocopherol; transfers electrons across mitochondrial electron transport chain complex I to III	50–1200 mg/day	GI upset; low blood pressure; rarely, skin rash
b. Creatine monohydrate (CM)	reduce markers of oxidative stress in neurodegenerative diseases	1–5 g/day	transient nausea, flatus, and constipation; mania or depression at higher doses
c. Melatonin	potent antioxidant; increases glutathione peroxidase and superoxide dismutase; stimulates GSH production; boosts mitochondrial functioning	0.25mg–10 mg/day	drowsiness, sleepwalking, and disorientation
4. Anti-Inflammatory Agents			
a. Minocycline	robust neuroprotective activities; promotes neurogenesis; antioxidant and antiglutamate exocitoxicity effects; may regulate pro-inflammatory cytokines	100–200 mg/day	tooth/skin discoloration; GI upset, diarrhea; thrush/fungal infection; hepatitis

(continued)

TABLE 10.2 Continued

Supplement/Technique	Potential or Known Mechanisms	Dose[a]	Potential Side Effects[**]
b. Aspirin	COX-1 prostaglandin inhibitor in CNS microglia	81 mg/day	stomach irritation, bleeding in at-risk individuals, dizziness
5. Vitamins and Minerals			
a. Magnesium	Blocks methylphenidate-induced hyperlocomotion	400 mg up to bid MgOx; in children, 15 mg/kg in 3 divided doses for up to 16 weeks.	GI complaints; can be toxic
b. Zinc	HGF modulates GABAergic activity and enhances NMDA action in the hippocampus	Zinc sulfate 55–150mg/day	GI complaints; can be toxic
c. Selenium	redox-active antioxidant mineral	RDA[2] (from diet): children 4-8 yrs, 30 mcg; 9–13 yrs, 40 mcg; > 13 yrs, 55 mcg	GI complaints; other; can be toxic
d. Chromium	facilitates making MAO neurotransmitters; hypothalamic sensitizer to insulin	800 ug/day	skin irritation; headaches; dizziness; nausea; mood, cognitive, coordination changes; avoid in renal/liver impairment
e. B Vitamins	synthesize neurotransmitters, including serotonin		
i. Folate/ Folic Acid	Coenzyme or cosubstrate in the single- carbon transfers in the synthesis of nucleic acids and metabolism of amino acids	800 mcg to 5 mg/day	in high doses: sleep disorders, irritability, confusion, GI complaints, behavior changes, skin reactions, seizures, other
ii. B12	one-carbon metabolism necessary for the production of monoamine transmitters	300–10,000 ug/day if deficient	diarrhea, blood clots, itching, serious allergic reactions, and other
iii. Inositol	Sensitizes serotonin receptors; precursor for intracellular second messenger system	10–25 g/day	headache, nausea, diarrhea, flatulence
iv. Choline and Lecithin (Phosphatidyl Choline)	Increases acetylcholine, membrane phospholipid synthesis	lecithin 15–30 mg/day; choline 50 mg/kg/day; Daily Upper Intake Levels are: 1 g/day in children 1–8 yrs, 2 grams in children 9–13 yrs, 3 g/day 14–18 yrs; 3.5 g/day in adults	GI complaints; sweating, 'fishy' odor

f. Vitamin D	neuroprotective, neurotrophic, regulate glucocorticoid signaling	variable; see references	GI complaints; if toxic, weakness, weight loss, anemia, confusion
g. Vitamin E	antioxidant	60–3,000 mg/day alpha-tocopherol	high dose: GI complaints; fatigue, weakness, headache, blurred vision, rash, bleeding/bruising
h. Multinutrient Vitamin Preparations	combined, as above	e.g. 8 EMPowerplus pills per day	nausea, vomiting, difficulty falling asleep

Lifestyle Modifications

1. Diet	reduces systemic inflammation, improves micro- and macronutrient status	see references	change in GI functioning
a. Ketogenic Diet	Lowers CNS glucose; reduces activity of N-methyl-D-aspartate receptors; elevates GABA and other neurotransmitter levels	see references	constipation, menstrual abnormalities, increased cholesterol and triglycerides, hemolytic anemia, elevated liver enzymes, renal and gallstones, alterations in cardiac conduction
b. Probiotic Diet	Influence behavior; effect on production of local GABA and other neurotransmitters as well as vagal nerve effects	varies; see references	GI bloating, gas, change in bowel habits
2. Light Therapy	suppresses melatonin	10,00 lux UV-blocked white light 1–2x a day as prescribed	headache, eyestrain, agitation, nausea; in more severely ill bipolar patients, worsening depression, ultrarapid cycling, mixed states, and suicidality
3. Exercise	improved blood flow, decreases oxidative stress, catecholamine release	daily or as directed	muscle soreness, dizziness
4. Trigger Identification	Provides personalized intervention and support toward early intervention	daily	emotional distress
5. Smoking Cessation	Reduces systemic inflammation; lessens depression, improves physical health	use gum, patches as appropriate	nicotine craving: irritability, stomach upset, headache, tremors

Healing Arts

1. Acupuncture	Upregulates neurotransmitters and neurotrophins, suppresses cellular apoptosis, modifies glial cell activity, causes cytokine expression, regulates activities of the hypothalamus-pituitary-adrenal axis and hypothalamus-pituitary-sex gland axes, causes changes in lymphocyte beta- receptors, heart rate variability, and electrical motor activity of the gut, and raises glial cell line- derived neurotrophic factor	needle, electrical or laser; once or twice a week	discomfort or slight bleeding at needle site
2. Mindfulness Meditation	improves attention; alters brain and immune function	8- week sessions	none apparent
3. Massage, Reiki, Yoga, Tai-Chi	PNS stimulation properties	varies; see references	muscle soreness, dizziness

* dosing data includes information from adult and physical health studies; maintenance doses may be much less than acute trial dosing

2 Recommended Daily Allowance (RDA)

** not inclusive; selected common or key risks presented

mental disorders, including depression and bipolar disorder during the 20th century, as evidenced by epidemiologic data showing lower rates of bipolar I, II, and NOS disorders in countries with higher seafood consumption.[7] In addition, genetic variants in fatty acid desaturases, which convert linoleic acid to arachidonic acid (AA) and alpha linolenic acid to EPA and DHA, can result in decreased EPA and increased linoleic acid (an omega-6), which might contribute to symptom expression.[8] No studies examining these variants and risk for mood symptoms or disorders were located.

Proposed mechanisms of LC-n-3PUFA treatment in both unipolar and bipolar depression include improving neural cell fluidity; suppressing neuronal signaling via second messenger generation, calcium channel and protein kinase C activity; lowering proinflammatory cytokines and oxidative stress; and reducing kindling.[9,10] Neuroimaging demonstrates lowered T2 whole-brain relaxation time values, consistent with increased membrane fluidity, in patients with bipolar disorder who take LC-n-3PUFA.[11] High-resolution structural magnetic resonance images (MRIs) show people with higher intake levels of LC-n-3PUFA have greater gray matter volume in the anterior cingulate cortex, the right hippocampus, and the right amygdala. These brain areas, involved in emotional arousal and regulation, are reduced in people with mood disorders.[12]

Evidence from open-label and controlled trials is best summarized in the first meta-analysis of omega-3 fatty acids specifically for bipolar disorder.[13] Six randomized controlled trials, including one pediatric trial, were found to have acceptable methodology for inclusion. The results support an effect for bipolar depression, but not manic symptoms, with effect sizes from $d = 0.34$ ($z = 2.118$; 95% CI, 0.035–0.641; $p = 0.029$) to 0.64 ($z = 3.303$; 95% CI, 0.261–1.023; $p = 0.001$, for analysis of the four adult studies all using the Hamilton Depression Rating Scale). The authors concluded that omega-3 fish oils are now recommended in the adjunctive treatment of bipolar disorder, especially for those with comorbid cardiovascular or metabolic conditions. They support currently accepted dosing recommendations of an EPA/DHA mix at about 1,000 mg/day, which can be increased gradually watching for emergence of increased cycling.[14] They also echo past calls for additional research to establish optimum formulations and dosage for LC-n-3PUFA treatment in bipolar disorder.

Whether LCn-3PUFAs help manic symptoms in CABD and whether differing dose ratios based on age result in differential response is not known, as there have been no randomized controlled trials (RCTs) of fish oil for CABD published to date. There is strong biologic plausibility to suspect that developing brains and bodies are more sensitive to or have differential effects when given treatment doses of LCn-3 PUFAs[15,16]; additionally, early-onset mood disorders may be more amenable to nutraceutical-based therapy, as total duration of illness and downstream effects of homeostatic "wear and tear" are possibly easier to reverse. There are four published pediatric pilot studies of LCn-3 PUFAs to date for depressive and bipolar illness.

Clayton et al.[17] documented that 6 weeks of open adjunctive omega-3 administration using a combination of EPA 360 mg and DHA 1,560 mg per day raised erythrocyte omega-3 levels in 18 adolescents with bipolar I or II disorder and was associated with reductions in both depressive and manic symptoms (p = 0002, p = 0.004) as well as improved global functioning (p < 0.001) and internalized and externalized symptoms via parent-ratings (p = 0.009, p = 0.014). Wozniak et al.[18] completed an 8-week open-label trial of combined EPA/DHA, starting at 1,125 mg EPA/165 mg DHA per day, with flexible combined EPA+DHA dosing between 1,290 and 4,300 mg/day, based on response, as monotherapy (stable stimulant dosing allowed) in 20 children and adolescents with bipolar I, II, or NOS and a Young Mania Rating Scale (YMRS) of >15. The total mean dose was 2,602.1 ± 1,013.5 mg/day at study end. An overall 8.9 ± 7.8 point YMRS reduction at study endpoint was noted, with 50% (n = 10) of subjects having a 30% reduction in baseline YMRS scores and 35% (n = 7) having a 50% reduction in baseline YMRS scores. Depressive scores also fell, as measured by the Child Depression Rating Scale (p = 0.002). Nemets et al.[19] gave 28 children with major depression EPA:DHA as a 2:1 ratio (380–400 mg EPA and 180–200 mg DHA) in a placebo-controlled randomized trial; highly significant effects were found: 40% of children treated with EPA + DHA met remission criteria. Additionally, 70% of those on active EPA + DHA responded, defined as a >50% reduction in depressive symptoms versus no responses in the placebo group. Most of the treatment response was noted by 12 weeks. Gracious et al.[20] conducted a pilot RCT of flax oil up to 12,000 mg/day in 51 children and adolescents with bipolar I and II disorder for up to 16 weeks. No difference was found for primary parent-informed mood measures, but moderate effects were present for clinician-rated global improvement and severity of overall illness in those with decreases in erythrocyte arachidonic acid and increases in alpha-linolenic acid and EPA. This study noted the importance of documenting meaningful physiologic change in fatty acid blood biomarkers as measures of compliance and outcome. Ongoing and future research of LCn-3 PUFAs should examine RBC changes as determinants of compliance and downstream metabolism in PUFA pathways, the latter likely influenced by genetic fatty acid desaturase (FADS) variants. Prospective studies should also determine whether dietary intake data can predict outcome, so that direct measures of dietary intake, as faster, more generally feasible, and potentially less costly than erythrocyte biomarkers, might also be used to personalize clinical care. Several studies are currently under way to further explore this intervention.

Omega-3 supplementation may also positively benefit concentration in the more than half of youth with CABD who also have comorbid ADHD. DHA supplementation in healthy boys has been found to increase activity in attention networks in the prefrontal cortex during sustained attention tasks.[21]

The side effect profile for LCn-3 PUFA administration is typically benign, with GI disturbance, including transient nausea or diarrhea, the most common concern, especially in younger children. Although typically well tolerated, rare cases of bleeding have been reported for concomitant use with aspirin and anticoagulants, especially when taken in exceptionally large doses.[22] Risk for bleeding may be in part due to reduced platelet activation.[23]

Limitations of these pediatric studies include small sample size, lack of controlled methodology, and lack of dietary intake and general diet quality data as potential predictors or confounds of response.

Amino Acids and Their Derivatives
Amino Acid Depletion Models

One experimental model of mania involves using amphetamines to release dopamine, resulting in psychostimulant effects.[24] Catecholamine synthesis can be reduced by lowering the availability of catecholamine precursors (tyrosine and phenylalanine). Cross-sectional studies in patients with bipolar disorder found correlations between plasma ratios of amino acids tyrosine and tryptophan and mood state and psychomotor activity, suggesting that alterations in ratios may be due to abnormalities in metabolism of neutral amino acids, and that these ratios could possibly serve as indicators of drug efficacy for individual response.[25,26] In rats given a tyrosine-free amino acid mixture, plasma tyrosine decreased, and decreased dopamine release occurred after amphetamine administration.[27] A similar study including healthy volunteers and adults with mania also demonstrated reduced effects of methamphetamine after administration of a tyrosine-free amino acid load.[28] The mixture was described as unpalatable. Scarna et al.[29] reported improvement in manic symptoms in 25 adults randomized to 1 week of daily branched-chain amino acids without tyrosine (BCAA, containing only leucine, isoleucine, and valine) versus placebo. BCAA intake correlated with lower manic symptoms within the first 6 hours of use, and this response continued for 1 week after the end of treatment. The presumed mechanism was that lowering tyrosine resulted in decreased dopamine release. Applebaum et al.[30] documented a similar therapeutic response, using an amino acid solution free of tryptophan in a 1-week double-blind placebo-controlled pilot trial in adults with mania, who were concurrently given sodium valproate, based on previous work that the intervention could rapidly lower plasma tryptophan by 80%.[31,32] Five of the 23 subjects withdrew after the first dose due to palatability and vomiting associated with the rapid tryptophan depletion (RTD); no patients became depressed or suicidal and no other side effects were noted. There are no reports for CABD.

L-tryptophan

L-tryptophan is the direct precursor amino acid in the synthesis of serotonin. Both antimanic and antidepressant effects have been described.[33,34] It was reported to cause manic symptoms when added to monoamine oxidase inhibitors,[35] yet also reported as improving manic symptoms in a small controlled trial in acutely manic adults.[36] We are not aware of amino acid supplementation in CABD, but Nemzer et al.[37] completed a double-blind sequential study in 14 children with attention-deficit disorder, administering for 1 week each of four conditions: tryptophan 100 mg/kg/day, d-amphetamine 5–10 mg/day, tyrosine 140 mg/kg/day, and placebo. Parents rated tryptophan as improving symptoms to the same extent as the stimulant, but teachers did not, possibly due to dosing (bid for tryptophan vs. once/day for stimulant). Side effects were reported as negligible except for one child who had excessive sleepiness related to tryptophan.

N-acetyl Cysteine

N-acetyl cysteine (NAC) is a dietary supplement and glutathione precursor. Its primary commercial use has been as a mucolytic and hepatoprotective agent after acetaminophen overdose. Major mental disorders, including bipolar disorder, have been linked to oxidative stress as a likely pathway by which symptoms may develop and progress.[38,39] Oxidative stress is mediated through dopamine and glutamate pathway imbalances, mitochondrial dysfunction, and proinflammatory cytokine receptor activation. Glutathione, as the chief antioxidant in the CNS, protects neurons from oxidative stress by scavenging free radicals in the brain. NAC has therefore been studied to determine its use as a metabolically neutral adjunctive or alternative treatment option. NAC might also work by modulating the glutamatergic system by increasing extracellular cysteine and synaptic vesicular release of glutamate, increasing the excitatory to inhibitory ratio.

Several preliminary RCTs found NAC beneficial in adults with schizophrenia and bipolar I and II disorder, including for both manic and depressive symptoms.[40-43] Acute effects in adults with bipolar disorder were safely maintained in a 2-month open follow-up extension study.[44] To date there are no studies of NAC in CABD, despite calls to expand research for NAC in bipolar disorders.[45,46] Two small RCTs using up to 2,700 mg/day of adjunctive NAC safely in children with autism showed reduction in irritability by 8 weeks as well as in repetitive movements.[47,48] Acute adverse effects are primarily gastrointestinal, although there is concern that long-term use, based on high-dose mouse studies, might increase cancer risk in smokers.

S-adenosyl Methionine

S-adenosyl methionine (SAM-e), found in all living cells, is an active endogenous methyl-donor compound synthesized from L-methionine. As a cofactor for numerous biochemical pathways, SAM-e leads to the production of hormones, neurotransmitters, nucleic acids, proteins, and phospholipids.[49] SAM-e is believed to augment CNS dopamine and norepinephrine levels, promote serotonin release, and also function as an antioxidant.[50] It has been found to enhance response to tricyclic, SSRI, and SNRI antidepressants in open and controlled clinical trials, and was shown to be more effective than imipramine in one study. Case reports and case series have reported benefit in children and adolescents with unipolar depression. SAM-e has not been sufficiently studied for bipolar disorder, due to a small open trial in which 9 of 11 patients with bipolar disorder switched to an elevated mood state.[51] It is unclear whether this was dose related. Due to its potential as a mitochondrial modulator, Nierenberg et al.[5] provided physiologic background to support study of SAM-e for bipolar disorder, as well as other potential mitochondrial modifiers, including N-acetyl cysteine (NAC), acetyl-L-carnitine (ALCAR), coenzyme Q10 (CoQ10), alpha-lipoic acid (ALA), creatine monohydrate (CM), and melatonin.

Acetyl-L-carnitine and Alpha-lipoic Acid

L-carnitine, obtained from diet or synthesized, is composed of lysine and methionine.[52] Carnitines shuttle fatty acids into mitochondria for oxidation and energy generation; they also scavenge reactive oxygen species.[53] Acetyl-L-carnitine (ALCAR) is reported to have better absorption and diffusion across the blood–brain barrier than other carnitines and to be neuroprotective.[54] There are at least nine placebo-controlled studies for ALCAR showing efficacy in depressive disorders, of which the most recent is Zanardi and Smeraldi.[55]

Alpha-lipoic acid, a mitochondrial coenzyme and potent antioxidant, increases cellular uptake of glucose for ATP synthesis.[56,57] Dietary sources include spinach, yeast, and red meats. Possible effects in bipolar disorder may be mediated by increasing recycling of other endogenous antioxidants, including CoQ10, vitamins C and E, and glutathione (GSH). Alpha-lipoic acid may also chelate heavy metals and promote antiapoptotic and neuroprotective effects against glutamate-induced intracellular calcium increases.[58] In a preliminary amphetamine mania model study in adult mice, alpha-lipoic acid was comparable to lithium in preventing and reversing increases in locomotor activity. As additional evidence to support human study, alpha-lipoic acid and lithium were also similar in preventing changes in superoxide dismutase, GSH, brain-derived neurotrophic factor (BDNF), and thiobarbituric acid reacting substances (TBARS).[59] Despite these basic data, a controlled pilot trial of acetyl-L-carnitine 1,000–3,000 mg/day and alpha-lipoic acid 600–1,800 mg/day for bipolar depression in adults (N = 40) did not show antidepressant effects using the Montgomery-Asberg Depression Rating Scale in both longitudinal (mean difference [95% confidence interval], –1.4 [–6.2 to 3.4], p = 0.58) and last-observation-carried-forward (–3.2 [–7.2 to 0.9], p = 0.12) analyses. The active treatment also did not enhance mitochondrial functioning via phosphorus magnetic resonance spectroscopy (N = 20) but did reduce phosphocreatine levels in the parieto-occipital cortex at week 12 (p = 0.002).[60]

Other Mitochondrial Modifiers
Coenzyme Q10

Proposed use of coenzyme Q10 (CoQ10) for bipolar disorder is based on its role as a lipid-soluble antioxidant within the ubiqinone system; it neutralizes free radicals directly and reduces vitamin E to absorbable α-tocopherol. CoQ10 is also present in the mitochondrial inner layer, where it generates an electrochemical gradient for electron transfer across mitochondrial electron transport chain complexes I to III.[5] CoQ10 is known to be helpful for hypertension and migraines. There is one study of 10 older adults with bipolar depression versus 7 healthy controls taking CoQ10 400–1,200 mg/day for 8 weeks. Imaging via 4 Tesla (31)Phosphorus magnetic resonance spectroscopy ((31)PMRS) scans was performed 8 weeks apart, using a novel magnetization transfer (MT) acquisition scheme to calculate the forward rate constant, k(for), of creatine kinase (CK). Depression severity decreased with CoQ10 treatment in the bipolar depressed group (F (3,7) = 4.87, p = .04), with significant reductions in the MADRS at weeks 2 (t (9) = –2.40, p = .04) and 4 (t (9) = –3.80, p = .004). A trend toward a lower k(for) of CK for those with bipolar depression versus healthy controls at baseline was noted. The authors concluded that RCTs exploring both high-energy phosphate metabolite alterations in geriatric bipolar depression and CoQ10 efficacy are warranted.[61]

Creatine Monohydrate

Creatine, found in meat and fish, is also synthesized by the liver and kidneys and is widely available as the dietary supplement creatine monohydrate. It is the precursor of phosphocreatine (PCr), which serves as a reservoir of inorganic phosphate for ATP production.[62] Creatine has antioxidant properties,[63] documented in neurodegenerative diseases. Reduced PCr concentrations were found in patients with mitochondrial disorders and in patients with bipolar disorder.[64] Clinical literature includes a case study documenting improved depressive and fibromyalgia symptoms[65] and an open-label study of treatment-resistant depression.[66] Dosing was intensive; 3 g/day for 1 week followed by 5 g/day for 3 weeks. The two bipolar depressed patients developed manic symptoms; those with unipolar illness had robust improvement in depression primarily within 1 week, although a U-shaped dose-response curve was suggested by two females who became more depressed at 5 g/day but again improved at 3 g/day. Adverse effects included transient nausea, flatus, and constipation. The authors expressed hope for larger controlled trials as monotherapy and as augmentation to standard antidepressants.

Melatonin

Melatonin and several metabolites are potent antioxidants, scavaging reactive oxygen and nitrogen species and increasing messenger ribonucleic acid (mRNA) expression of genes that produce glutathione peroxidase and superoxide dismutase.[67] Melatonin also stimulates GSH production[68] and boosts mitochondrial functioning, including through direct effects on mitochondrial deoxyribonucleic acid (mtDNA).[69] Agomelatine, a melatonergic agonist and 5-HT2c antagonist, is marketed in the United Kingdom and Australia as Valdoxan for treating major depression in adults. It was submitted for review by Novartis for review by the United States Food and Drug Administration. A preliminary open-label study found agomelatine 25 mg/day an effective and well-tolerated adjunct to valproate or lithium for acute depression in adults with bipolar II disorder.[70] Contraindications include renal or hepatic impairment; adverse effects include elevated liver function tests and potential for CYP450 drug-drug interactions.

Other Anti-Inflammatory Agents

Inflammation, repeatedly found in bipolar disorder and associated with higher rates of physical comorbidities, has generated hypotheses of immune function as a critical component of bipolar pathophysiology.[71] Therapeutic study of anti-inflammatory agents is under way; several readily available agents with known ease of use and strong safety profiles are provided next.

Minocycline and Aspirin (Acetylsalicylic Acid)

Minocycline, a tetracyclic antibiotic, has been proposed as an adjunct for bipolar disorder due to robust neuroprotective activities, including promotion of neurogenesis, antioxidant effects, and prevention of glutamate-induced excitotoxicity.[72] Additionally, minocycline may directly regulate pro-inflammatory cytokines. Adjunctive minocycline was helpful added to a probiotic in a mouse model of colitis[73]; no other studies of microbiome effects were found.

Miyaoka et al.[74] completed a 6-week open-label pilot study of adjunctive minocycline to selective serotonin reuptake inhibitor (SSRI) antidepressants in adults hospitalized with major depressive disorder (MDD) with psychotic features. A dose of 150 mg/day was associated with significant differences in both depressive and psychotic symptoms and was reported as well tolerated. Minocycline and low-dose acetylsalicylic acid (ASA) as adjunctive together or separately for bipolar depression in adults is currently being evaluated.[75] Minocycline is commonly prescribed for adolescents with acne, but no studies for mood disorder in youth have been published.

Low-dose aspirin inhibits prostaglandin (PG) H-synthase-1 (COX-1) in CNS microglia in basic science models; in higher doses, PGH-synthase 2 (COX-2) activity is inhibited, resulting in a peripheral anti-inflammatory effect in illnesses such as arthritis.[76] Similar to fluoxetine, ASA (10 mg/kg per day) given to adult mice reversed depressive behavior and oxidative stress created by chronic unpredictable stress.[77] Using a large Netherlands prescription database, a pharmacoepidemiologic study found low-dose aspirin added to lithium protected individuals with bipolar disorder, by reducing need for medication alteration. Other nonsteroidal anti-inflammatory agents and glucocorticoid exposure were not helpful and potentially harmful.[78] There is one published study of adjunctive ASA for adult MDD. Mendlewicz et al.[79] administered open-label adjunctive ASA 160 mg/day to 24 adults who had not responded to 4 weeks of an SSRI; a response rate of 52% was noted, with remission in 82% of the responders and 43% overall. Effects were noted within 1 week of the 4-week trial. A study examining ASA and NAC separately and in combination is underway (http://clinicaltrials.gov/ct2/show/NCT01797575; accessed 03/01/14).

No studies have been published to date on aspirin for CABD. An overview of its potential use in mental illness has been published.[80]

Cucurmin

Cucurmin is a polyphenol extract with potent anti-inflammatory effects. A study found reversal of depressive behavior from chronic mild stress in rats; cucurmin inhibited cytokine gene expression at both the mRNA and protein level, including reducing activation of nuclear factor kappa-light-chain-enhancer of activated B cells (NF-kB), a gateway of cytokine control.[81] A pilot study is under way for mental and physical health effects in CABD (Goldstein B, personal communication, 2013).

Other potential complementary or alternative treatments include novel calcium channel blockers, neurosteroids such as pregnenolone, and other hormonally based treatments, including tamoxifen. As these are in very early stages of exploration for adult mood disorders, it is beyond the scope of this chapter to review them for potential for use in CABD.

Vitamins and Minerals

Magnesium and Zinc

Low dietary magnesium and zinc intakes likely contribute to depression and anxiety. Greater dietary intake of magnesium lowered odds for MDD and dysthymia in women and older adults in population-based cohorts (for women, OR = 0.60, 95% CI 0.37–0.96).[82,83] Age, socioeconomic status, education, and other health behaviors did not alter the relationship. Each standard deviation increase in zinc intake also correlated with reduced odds for MDD and dysthymia (OR = 0.52, 95% confidence interval (CI) 0.31–0.88). Yary and Aazami[84] confirmed the association of dietary zinc intake with depression in postgraduate students. Patients with bipolar disorder with manic symptoms had higher zinc levels than levels from a healthy control group.[85]

Magnesium sulfate (300–400 mg/kg) acutely blocked methylphenidate-induced hyperlocomotion in a mouse model of mania.[86] Lower erythrocyte magnesium content was found at baseline in patients with severe major depression or with acute paranoid schizophrenia as compared to healthy controls; treatment with sertraline, haloperidol, carbamazepine, and sodium valproate treatment in those with depression, schizophrenia, and bipolar I disorder raised erythrocyte magnesium,[87] supporting change in diet intake, absorption, or utilization. Nine adults with severe rapid-cycling bipolar disorder were treated with magnesium aspartate hydrochloride 40 mEq/day in an open-label study for up to 32 weeks; four of nine were felt to respond equivalently to lithium.[88] In an open-label study, a continuous infusion of IV magnesium sulfate at 200 mg/hr was given to 10 adults with severe treatment-resistant mania for 7–23 days, in addition to concurrent lithium, haloperidol, and clonazepam; the authors felt conventional psychopharmacologic treatment doses were lower than otherwise typically used. Bradycardia via telemetry was a noted side effect but responded quickly to reducing the infusion rate.[89] A small RCT found verapamil + magnesium oxide was more effective than verapamil + placebo in reducing manic symptoms in bipolar adults.[90] To the best of our knowledge, there are no reports of magnesium treatment in CABD other than in combination multivitamin products.

Only one open study of zinc therapy was found for bipolar disorder.[91] The study assessed serum hepatocyte growth factor (HGF) and found low levels in bipolar patients versus similar controls, as well as a correlation between zinc and HGF in bipolar patients.

After receiving a minimum of 8 weeks of zinc picolinate 25 mg, subjects reported lower severity of bipolar symptoms. The mechanism postulated is that HGF modulates γ-aminobutyric acid (GABAergic) activity and enhances N-methyl-D-aspartic acid (NMDA) action in the hippocampus.[92,93]

Selenium

Dietary intake of selenium, a redox-active antioxidant mineral, was compared between young women participating in the Geelong Osteoporosis Study who developed episodes of MDD ($n = 18$) versus those who did not become depressed, on the hypothesis that redox alterations contribute to depression.[94] A low intake (defined as <8.9 µg/day) was associated with almost three times the likelihood of developing MDD (OR 2.95; 95% CI 1.00–8.72). Smoking, drinking alcohol, and low levels of physical activity were not related. The authors concluded that selenium warrants further investigation as a contributory factor for depression, as it may be a novel agent for prevention and intervention.

Chromium

Several small reports of improvement using chromium as an adjunct for unipolar depression resulted in a 2-year open-label continuation study of adjunctive chromium for rapid-cycling bipolar disorder.[95] After an initial add-on trial in 30 treatment-resistant predominantly depressed state adults, seven patients who took up to 800 µg/day of chromium for >1 year had a significant reduction in cycle number. One third had improvement in their depressive symptoms after 3 weeks of supplementation. The mean time to discontinuation was 204 ± 238 days (range, 12–736 days), with chromium overall well tolerated. Proposed mechanisms include facilitating monoamine neurotransmitter production and potentially sensitizing the hypothalamus to insulin. The authors concluded that further controlled study is warranted in a larger and less severely ill group, as it was not possible to show a group effect for the longer term administration. Chromium may therefore be useful as an adjunct acutely for bipolar depression in some individuals.

B Vitamins

B vitamins are necessary to synthesize neurotransmitters, including serotonin. Epidemiologic evidence correlates deficiency and low intake states with negative effects on youth mental health. A 17-year follow-up cross-sectional analysis of children born from 2,900 pregnancies in the West Australian Pregnancy Cohort (Raine) Study found reduced intake of vitamin B6 and folate correlated with higher internalizing behavior scores on the Youth Self Report.[96]

Folate/Folic Acid

Folate deficiency has been known as a medical cause of depression for over 50 years. Dihydrofolate is an essential vitamin derived from dietary sources of leafy greens, citrus fruits, liver, and yeast. Due to mandated food fortification of US grain products in 1998 to reduce incidence of neural tube defects, folate deficiency is less common but still found in about 20% of female adolescents and 23% of African American women (National Institutes of Health Office of Dietary Supplements Fact Sheet; http://ods.od.nih.gov/factsheets/Folate-HealthProfessional/#h3). Depressed adults are also more likely to have folate deficiency, possibly for genetic and epigenetic reasons, including dietary changes related to physical and economic consequences of depression.

Folic acid is the usual supplement, given in synthetic form due to improved bioavailability. It is converted to the active 5-methyl tetrahydrofolate (MTHF) by MTHF reductase (MTHFR), where it acts as a coenzyme or cosubstrate in single-carbon transfers in the synthesis of nucleic acids (DNA and RNA) and metabolism of amino acids, including to monoamine neurotransmitters. There are three known functional variants of the MTHFR enzyme. The most studied is the 677CT polymorphism, present in about 10% of the overall North American population, with ethnic differences in prevalence (Mediterranean/Hispanic >Caucasian >African-American).[97] The normal or wild-type genotype is 677CC; those who are homozygous for the T alleles (677TT) have a 70% reduced ability to metabolize folic acid to MTHF. This inability results in a relative increase in homocysteine, due to reduced conversion of homocysteine to methionine; the latter is the primary donor for DNA methylation and protein synthesis. Higher homocysteine levels are an independent risk factor for cardiovascular disease (CVD). Low dietary intake of folic acid contributes to mild hyperhomocysteinemia in only those with the 677TT genotype.[98] Individuals with the 158 VAL/MET polymorphism of the COMT gene also metabolize more methionine to homocysteine; those with both a functional 5-MTH reductase reduction and 158 VAL/MET polymorphism have a "double hit" resulting in the highest risk for hyperhomocysteinemia and subsequent CVD, including greater potential for blood clots.

Low folate levels were first linked to severity of depression,[9] and then to reduced response to antidepressants,[99,100] including SSRIs and nortriptyline.[101] An initial double-blind RCT of 500 μg/day of adjunctive folic acid added at the beginning of fluoxetine treatment in patients with MDD resulted in improvement in women but not men.[102] Other trials suggested positive effect,[103,104] but none excluded those with normal folate status. Serum B vitamin status may not matter unless low. A descriptive study in youth examined folate, B12, homocysteine, and MTHFR polymorphisms in those with schizophrenia ($n = 88$), mood disorders ($n = 22$), and healthy controls ($n = 94$).[105] Serum folate and B12 levels were all within normal limits, whereas mean homocysteine levels were almost twice as high in the mood and schizophrenic groups versus controls.

Studies of folate in mood-disordered individuals with deficiency include an RCT of adjunctive L-methylfolate at 15 mg/day added to antidepressant treatment in adults with MDD who had deficiency defined by RBC folate levels[106]; those in the L-methylfolate group showed greater improvement in depressive symptoms at 3 and 6 months.

Papakostas et al.[107] conducted an RCT with a novel trial design, a sequenced parallel comparison between two doses of adjunctive L-methyl folate in adults with persistent depression despite SSRI antidepressant treatment. For a dose of 15 mg/day of "medical food" branded Deplin, the response rate was about 1 in 3; 7.5 mg/day was helpful in several subjects but did not separate from placebo. Side effect profiles were equivalent between L-methyl folate and placebo. A longitudinal prevention study of folic acid supplementation in adolescents and young adults whose biologic parents have a history of depression or bipolar disorder is under analysis (http://www.clinicaltrials.gov).

An important clinical reason exists to consider a form of adjunctive folic acid or folate in youth with bipolar disorder. Sodium valproate, a commonly used mood stabilizer, potentially interferes with folate metabolism by inhibiting gut absorption as well as glutamate formyl transferase, an enzyme mediating production of folinic acid.[108] Three supplements, folic acid, vitamin C, and NAC, may be best to prevent valproate-induced teratogenicity, based on recent work describing more than one mechanism.[109]

Folic acid dosing has been considered safe up to doses of 15 mg/day; Morrell[110] stated that the US Food and Drug Administration restricted oral folic acid tablet doses to 1 mg due to now-disproven concerns that large amounts of folic acid could reduce the effectiveness of antiseizure medications.[111] It may also rarely mask B12 deficiency; therefore, these levels are often ordered together in clinical practice.

Vitamin B12

Vitamin B12 deficiency has been associated with case reports of manic symptoms. A 16-year-old male presenting with mixed mood symptoms, psychosis, and extrapyramidal symptoms was found to have vitamin B12 deficiency.[112] A 12-year-old boy with a similar presentation, including psychosis and extrapyramidal symptoms, responded to parenteral B12 therapy for deficiency.[113] An adult presenting with mania and found to have B12 deficiency also responded to intramuscular B12, and within 6 months had a normal mental status maintained by monthly B12 injections.[114] Irritability, however, is a known side effect of excessive B12.

Inositol

Inositol, sometimes referred to as vitamin B8, is a glucose isomer and a precursor for the intracellular phosphatidyl inositol (PI) second messenger system. Inositol is found in plants and animals, and is manufactured synthetically. A derivative, myoinositol, is active in serotonin pathways, helping to reverse desensitization of receptors. Reduced myoinositol levels from the cerebrospinal fluid of patients with mood disorders were first described in 1978.[115] Reduced frontal cortex levels were demonstrated in postmortem brain specimens from suicide victims and patients with bipolar disorder.[116] Levels may be state dependent: Lithium has been proposed to work in mania through lowering myoinositol.[117] Imaging studies have documented lower frontal myoinositol in unipolar and bipolar depressed patients, but higher frontal myoinositol in untreated manic patients;

myoinositol levels in children with bipolar disorder also decreased after 1 week of lithium treatment.[118–121]

Clinical trials include a study of open adjunctive inositol 12 grams per day for 4 weeks to antipsychotics in 11 treatment-resistant depressed adults. Mean Hamilton Depression Rating Scale scores declined by 15 points, nearly 50%.[122] A follow-up pilot RCT in unipolar or bipolar depressed adults confirmed improvement at 4 weeks compared to placebo, and again during an additional 6-week add-on study.[123,124] A trend to improvement was noted for inositol adjunctive to lithium or valproate, with calls made for larger adjunctive effectiveness studies.[125] Inositol 10–25 grams per day also decreased symptoms of treatment-resistant bipolar I or II depression in nearly 1 in 5 (17%) of adults in an NIMH Systematic Treatment Enhancement Program for Bipolar Disorder (STEP-BD) study, which compared risperidone, lamotrigine, and inositol as add-on treatments.[126] Rate of recovery for lamotrigine was 23% and risperidone 4.6%; although there was no significant difference between the three on primary analysis, secondary analyses favored lamotrigine. The authors felt, given the difficult clinical status and limited known options for treatment-resistant bipolar depression, that inositol "may have potential," possibly in those with irritability or anger. Inositol is considered generally safe for consumption, although headache can occur and large doses of over 12 g/day can cause mild gastrointestinal side effects such as nausea, diarrhea, and flatulence. Doses beyond this level, however, apparently do not cause increased severity of side effects.[127] Inositol may cause mania.[128]

Choline and Lecithin (Phosphatidyl Choline)

Phosphatidyl choline, one of three active forms of lecithin, is a lipotropic factor and a major component of cell membranes. It is formed from choline, an essential nutrient found in beef liver, chicken liver, eggs, beef steak, cod, broccoli, peanut butter, wheat germ, cauliflower, and milk (http://CholineInfo.org). Choline is commonly grouped with B vitamins as it is a necessary source of methyl groups for transfer; choline supplements may thus reduce homocysteine.[129] Choline increases synthesis and release of acetylcholine by neurons, increases membrane phospholipid synthesis, and also prevents fatty liver.

Data from the 2003–2004 National Health and Nutrition Examination Survey (NHANES) revealed that 90% of older American children, men, and women have mean choline intakes far below the daily adequate intake level (AI).[130] Actual dysfunction due to low choline intake varies, as many people have single-nucleotide polymorphisms (SNPs) that result in higher vulnerability if combined with low dietary intake. Large and impractical volumes of foods (noted earlier) are required to achieve the recommended daily intake, making it a common additive to vitamins.

Choline may impact mood via anti-inflammatory effects.[131] Senaratne et al.[132] found elevated choline compounds in the hippocampus and orbitofrontal cortex of euthymic bipolar patients via H1-MRS, indicating potential increases in membrane breakdown. Cholinergic genes were not associated with bipolar disorder or alcohol abuse or dependence in 474 samples from families.[133] Stoll et al.[134] reported elevated erythrocyte choline concentrations in patients with more severe bipolar illness and outcome.

Cohen et al.[135] presented an initial report of response in a preliminary open-label case series of adjunctive lecithin 15–30 mg/kg per day in eight manic inpatients; symptoms and rating scores worsened on discontinuation. He then conducted a double-blind placebo-controlled study in six bipolar adults using 30 mg/day with similar results.[136] Stoll et al.[137] described improvement in manic symptoms in five of six rapid-cycling bipolar adults given choline adjunctive to lithium; four of the six also had improvement in depressive symptoms. A single case reported that adding lecithin to lithium for mania in a 13-year-old was helpful initially, and as subsequent monotherapy; the adolescent took lecithin only for 2 years after the initial episode.[138] Lyoo et al.[139] performed a small adjunctive RCT of choline 50 mg/kg per day in eight lithium-treated bipolar patients. Choline supplementation decreased brain purine levels but did not change mood symptoms over 12 weeks. Results were interpreted as demonstrating that mitochondrial dysfunction creates an inability to meet the need for increased ATP production.

Vitamin D

There are no recent descriptive or trial publications on the relationship between vitamin D and bipolar disorder, but case series, epidemiologic studies, and several controlled trials document an association between vitamin D and overall mood, depression, psychosis, and suicide in varying cohorts. As these all relate to prominent features in bipolar illness, understanding vitamin D effects in the CNS provides rationale for studying whether and how normalizing serum vitamin D levels in D-deficient youth with BPSD might provide adjunct treatment or protection from illness progression and recurrent episodes.

Vitamin D is necessary for healthy neurodevelopment and brain functioning, but its role in the CNS is less appreciated and poorly understood compared to its role in bone metabolism. A review by Berk et al.[140] summarizes basic science findings that (1) vitamin D receptors (VDRs) and activating enzymes are prominent in the brain, especially in the hypothalamus and the substantia nigra; (2) maternal depletion in animal models produces offspring with abnormal brain shape, increased mitotic cells, and decreased nerve growth factor, neurotrophic factor, and neurotrophic factor receptors; (3) vitamin D is neuroprotective to hippocampal cells, through regulating calcium ion channels and activating protein kinase C and map Phosphokinase pathways; (4) VDRs help regulate glucocorticoid signaling in hippocampal cells; and (5) animal VDR knockout models show increased anxiety, decreased activity, and muscular and motor impairments, all phenotypic contributions to models of depression.

A correlation between low vitamin D and asthenia symptoms in depressed adult patients was described in 1974.[141] On the basis of rodent experiments, Stumpf and Privette[142] posited that vitamin D affected mood. A second associational study found that elderly individuals with vitamin D deficiency were more likely to have low mood and worse cognition.[143] Two RCTs with mood outcomes have been performed in adults. The first trial randomized adults with seasonal affective depression and vitamin D deficiency to broad-spectrum phototherapy versus vitamin D supplements; improvement in mood corresponded to changes in vitamin D levels despite group assignment.[144] In the second study, adults with depressive symptoms who were overweight or obese with comorbid vitamin D deficiency showed improvements in mood when given vitamin D supplementation versus placebo.[145] A cohort of psychiatric inpatient Parisian adolescents were also found to be largely vitamin D deficient (72.4%), with the mean 25-OHD value 15–16 ng/ml, lower in blacks and North Africans.[146] No differences in mean levels were found between those taking or not taking antipsychotics. Gracious et al.[147] found that adolescents admitted to acute mental health care services had over three times the odds of having psychotic features if they were vitamin D deficient; the sample was predominantly suffering from unipolar and bipolar depression. Race was no longer associated with psychosis when results were adjusted for vitamin D level, supporting a concern that vitamin D deficiency may contribute to disparity in health outcomes.

In an open-label treatment case series, Högberg et al.[148] described improvements in 54 depressed Swedish adolescents given supplemental vitamin D for insufficient or deficient levels. Levels of 25-OH vitamin D more than doubled and supplementation improved signs and symptoms via a rating scale developed by the authors specifically to measure those potentially associated with vitamin D deficiency, including depressed mood, irritability, tiredness, mood swings, sleep difficulties, weakness, and difficulty concentrating. Improvement in depression was also shown using a standardized rating scale, the Mood and Feelings Questionnaire (MFQ-S).

Suicide rates are highest in the spring, when serum levels of vitamin D are lowest; Umhau et al.[149] thus undertook a prospective, nested, case-control study and found that in deployed active duty military personnel, those with serum 25(OH)-D levels <15.5 ng/ml had the highest risk for suicide.

Vitamin D may influence mental functioning in bipolar disorder related to genotypic variances of the VDR. Ahmadi et al.[150] found in a case-control study that those with bipolar disorder had greater frequency of the FF genotype of the FOKI vitamin D receptor polymorphism, compared to those with schizophrenia and to healthy controls (odds ratio = 1.84, 95% CI; 0.81 to 4.17; relative risk = 1.31, CI 95%; 0.86 to 1.99). The FF genotype is associated with lower expression of the dopamine D1 receptor gene.

Parker and Brotchie[151] have called for rigorous study to determine whether vitamin D deficiency is antecedent and causal, a correlate, or a consequence of depression. Logically, vitamin D deficiency may relate with variable effect in all three ways, depending on dietary and solar intake and specific tissue concentrations, making study design and statistical analysis challenging. They noted "there is currently insufficient evidence to argue strongly for vitamin D supplementation in patients with depression, but such a strategy is worthy of consideration in depressed patients whose lifestyle and geographical residence may indicate a risk of vitamin D insufficiency—or where low vitamin D levels have been quantified." Studies are under way to further examine the use vitamin D supplementation in bipolar populations.

Vitamin E

In inflammatory and learned helplessness murine models of depression, α-tocopherol at doses of 10, 30, and 100 mg/kg orally reduced depressive behavior synergistically with antidepressants, with both acute and chronic antioxidant effects.[152,153] A cross-sectional study of fatty acid and vitamin E status in male software workers found that alpha-tocopherol may be protective against depressive symptoms.[154] No human studies were found for bipolar disorder.

Multinutrient Vitamin Preparations

Early publications and presentations on using multivitamin and mineral supplements for primary and adjunctive treatment in CABD were initially met with skepticism, due in part to lack of knowledge, including basic science studies of mechanisms of actions, as well as a nontraditional product development history. Successful use of micronutrient formulations for agitation syndromes in veterinary medicine were translated to direct clinical use of similar formulations in humans without controlled clinical trials, resulting in idiosyncratic patterns of use related to regional and Web-based influences, with both factors contributing to reluctance of traditional funding agencies to approve and support large-scale rigorous micronutrient compound studies for mental health conditions. A growing literature of case reports, case studies, replicated case series, and retrospective analyses, however, including reports of individuals tapered off conventional psychopharmacology due to apparent response, highlights need for RCTs to determine whether such compounds can stand alone as monotherapy, and how and to what extent they may be equivalent or possibly superior to conventional treatments. Small RCTs for other mental conditions (ADHD, acute stress) provide added justification.

Kaplan et al.[155] first published use of a "broad-based nutritional supplement of dietary nutrients, primarily chelated trace minerals and vitamins." Eleven adults aged 19–46 years with *DSM-IV* bipolar disorder took part in a 6-month open adjunctive trial. Symptom reductions of >50%, via the Hamilton Depression Scale, Brief Psychiatric Rating Scale, and Young Mania Rating Scale, were reported, with psychotropic medication reduced also by more than half. Effect sizes were large (>0.80) for each measure. The only side effect reported was nausea, which generally improved with taking the supplement with food. The authors noted that knowing whether any specific nutrient was "the important one" was less relevant than the fact that a combination of single or tandem micronutrient effects may be different among individuals, due to differing diet intakes and needs based on genetics. Case reports, small studies, and secondary analyses of clinical data of micronutrient use and effects in CABD, as well as theoretical mechanistic papers and a safety and tolerability review, have now been published.[156–160]

Frazier et al.[161] described 10 children aged 6–12 with bipolar spectrum disorders (BPSD) who were openly administered an updated version of the EMPowerplus™ micronutrient supplement for 8 weeks, EMPowerplus™ Advanced. After being tapered off psychotropic medication over 3 weeks, the children were given a dose of up to five capsules three times daily. Seven children completed the study, with overall adherence at 91%; three dropped out due to difficulty swallowing the capsules. Depression scores decreased 37% and mania scores decreased 45%, with side effects all reported as mild, including nausea, one episode of vomiting when taking the medication without food, and difficulty falling asleep. A subsequent publication[162] describes four of the tested serum vitamin concentrations increasing from pre- to postsupplementation: vitamin A-retinol; vitamin B6; vitamin E-α-tocopherol; and folate (all $p < 0.05$). Increases in serum 25-OH vitamin D approached significance ($p = 0.063$). No differences were found in dietary intake pre- to postsupplementation, suggesting blood nutrient level increases were due to EMP+. Side effects included transient insomnia and gastrointestinal upset. The authors concluded that RCTs of multinutrient supplements for BP spectrum disorders in youth are warranted.

To date, the multinutrient product most used in studies pertaining to mental health has been EMPowerplus™, manufactured by TrueHope (http://www.truehope.com). Barriers to greater use of such micronutrient products, in addition to lack of large-scale RCTs of efficacy and dissemination, include lack of coverage by most conventional and government health care insurances, cost (greater than most generic medications or copays, but cheaper than on-patent medications), and number of pills necessary per day (for EMPowerplus, initially 15 and most recently 8). Additionally, users may experience physical reactions when combined with conventional psychopharmacology, necessitating careful monitoring, titration, and tapering, depending on the psychotropic agents being taken. Multinutrient products offer potential, given the significant progress made in understanding basic and clinical mechanisms of effect for single and combined micronutrients, and RCTs should be pursued.

Lifestyle Modifications

Diet

Diet quality is linked to mental health in youth and adults, but no studies have yet examined diet in CABD, although there is a report in women with bipolar disorder. Evidence in youth is from cross-sectional population-based studies. In a Perth longitudinal cohort, internalizing (withdrawn/depressed) and externalizing (delinquent/aggressive) behaviors in 14-year-olds were associated with the Western dietary pattern, particularly for intake of takeout foods, sweets, and red meat. Higher intakes of green leafy vegetables and fresh fruit were associated with better behavioral scores.[163] Further analysis revealed the Western dietary pattern correlated with lower family income, more television viewing, and having a parent who smoked. Healthy eating was associated with female gender, greater maternal education, lower television exposure, better family functioning, and living in a two-parent household.[164] The same group also found that a high-quality breakfast of at least three food groups related to more favorable scores on the Child Behavior Checklist,[165] but only 11% of the adolescents ate at least three food groups at breakfast, and 7% did not eat any core food groups over a 3-day period. Of note for outcome and preventive work, eating meals together as a family during adolescence predicts higher quality diet (including greater intake of fruit and vegetables, especially dark-green and orange vegetables, and lower intake of soft drinks) at young adulthood.[166] A Canadian cohort study including adolescents found that across five waves roughly 2 years apart, greater fruit and vegetable intake was associated with lower odds of having had a major depressive episode in the previous 12 months (OR 0.72; 95% CI 0.71–0.75). Previous diagnosis of a mood or anxiety disorder also was related to lower fruit and vegetable intake (p < 0.05).[167] Another prospective cohort study of diet quality and depression in nearly 3,000 adolescents from East London found that those in the highest quintile of a predefined unhealthy diet score were about twice as likely to be symptomatic on the Strengths and Difficulties Questionnaire (SDQ) as those in the lowest quintile (OR 2.10, 95% CI 1.38–3.20).[168] An epidemiologic population-based study in adult women compared those with bipolar disorder and those without psychopathology; women with bipolar disorder had higher scores for a Western diet (p < 0.03) and trended toward higher glycemic loads; odds for bipolar disorder increased for each standard deviation increase in unfavorable "Western" (OR 1.88, 95% CI 1.33–2,65) and "modern" (OR 1.72, 95% CI 1.14–2.39) diet profiles, as well as glycemic load (OR 1.56, 95% CI 1.13–2.14).[169] A Western diet of processed or fried foods, refined grains, sugary products, and beer was also associated with a higher score on the 12-item General Health Questionnaire (GHQ-12) in over 1,000 women ages 20–93 years participating in the Geelong Osteoporosis Study, while a traditional diet of vegetables, fruit, meat, fish, and whole grains was associated with lower odds for major depression, dysthymia, and anxiety disorders. There were no confounds by age, socioeconomic status, education, or other health behaviors.[170] Other dietary studies are needed.

Ketogenic Diets

The ketogenic diet, historically used to impact severe seizure disorders, was proposed as a possibly useful strategy to alter bipolar illness symptoms by lowering CNS glucose and raising H^+ ions, reducing NMDA receptor activity,[171] and elevating GABA and other neurotransmitter levels.[172] El-Mallakh and Paskitti[173] described resurgence of and positive response to the ketogenic diet in two thirds of children with intractable epilepsy and stated that clinical trials, initially for relapse prevention in bipolar disorder, are warranted for the following: (1) some anticonvulsants are effective for bipolar disorder, (2) changes in brain energy use may reduce cerebral hypometabolism; and (3) the diet decreases intracellular sodium concentrations, a common property of all effective mood stabilizers. A single case study of a ketogenic diet for 2 weeks enhanced with medium chain triglycerides reported no effect; however, the patient did not display ketones in her urine.[174] Phelps et al.[175] documented successful treatment of two adults with bipolar II disorder who achieved and maintained a stable mood associated with 2- and 3-year periods of ketosis, with both able to discontinue pharmacologic treatments. Simple outpatient pharmacy-purchased urine test strips were used to document ongoing urinary ketones.

Close medical supervision is mandatory when using a ketotic diet, as side effects can include constipation, menstrual abnormalities, increased cholesterol and triglycerides, hemolytic anemia, elevated liver enzymes, renal and gallstones, and cardiac conduction changes predisposing to arrhythmia in susceptible individuals.

Probiotic Diets

Observing links between depression, anxiety, and acne, Stokes and Pillsbury[176] proposed that emotional states might alter normal intestinal microflora, increasing intestinal permeability and contributing to systemic inflammation. Newer understanding of gut microbiota and oral probiotics includes their influence on systemic inflammation, oxidative stress, glycemic control, tissue lipid content, and mood as well.[177] Pre- and probiotic and intestinal microbiota studies are under way, led by animal models demonstrating that probiotics such as lactobacillus and bifidobacteria influence behavior.[178] Mechanisms include changes in the production of local GABA and other neurotransmitters, and vagal nerve effects. As evidence builds, dietary bacterial manipulations may become a strategy for managing comorbid physical health risks and overall mood symptoms.

Light Therapy

Response rates for light therapy in adults with seasonal bipolar versus unipolar depression were initially reported as equivalent, with those with a bipolar I pattern of seasonal affective disorder (SAD) more likely to develop agitation as an adverse effect. Nonseasonally depressed bipolar patients were found to have better responses than unipolar depressed patients,[179] leading investigators to believe that bipolar patients may respond robustly to light interventions. Bright light is postulated to increase melatonin suppression as a potential mechanism of action. Adults with rapid-cycling bipolar disorder responded better to midday light compared to morning or evening.[180] Seven youth aged 16–22 years were treated for bipolar depression with full light therapy twice per day for persistent depressive symptoms; three showed a large response and two had a moderate response; no side effects were reported.[181]

Potential adverse effects of 10,000 lux UV-blocked white fluorescent light include headache, eyestrain, agitation, and nausea. More severely ill individuals with bipolar disorder have had light-induced worsening of depressive symptoms, ultrarapid cycling, mixed states, and suicidality[182]; full concurrent antimanic treatment may be needed. Sit et al.[183] described a case series of nine women with bipolar depression in which three of four given morning light developed mixed states. Changing the timing of light to midday and lowering the duration to 15 minutes was subsequently advised, with some women additionally gaining full response.

Exercise

Lower levels of physical activity in childhood predict adult depression.[184] Preliminary evidence supports use of a combination of healthy lifestyle practices for depression in adults. Garcia-Toro et al.[185] performed a controlled trial of diet modification, exercise, sunlight exposure, and regular sleep patterns in 80 non–seasonally depressed outpatients as adjunctive to antidepressant treatment. Greater improvement in depressive symptoms, with a higher number of responders and remitters, and lower psychopharmacology use was found in the active group. Murray et al.[186] described exercise as part of what high-functioning individuals do within a larger self-management strategy to help maintain stable mood and health. Yet there are a sufficient number of negative studies of exercise for depression, possibly related to methodologic issues. A large controlled trial of coached exercise in adults with mild or greater depression, excluding psychosis and bipolar disorder, did not show effects on self-reported depressive symptoms or reduced use of medication (Chaulder et al. 2013). The exercise dose or types, however, were not standardized. Cooney et al.[187] in a Cochran meta-analysis, stated "exercise is moderately more effective than a control intervention for reducing symptoms of depression, but analysis of methodologically robust trials only shows a smaller effect in favour of exercise." The authors state exercise is as effective as proven psychological or pharmacologic therapies, but note conclusions are based on only several small trials and that the likelihood of bias is high due to methodologic issues of blinding and self-reported ratings.

Exercise as a useful complementary technique in bipolar disorder was examined using self-reports from adults with bipolar disorder who were taking part in a conventional comparative effectiveness study; depression was associated with less exercise and mania with more exercise.[188] Causation, let alone its direction, was not established, but it seems plausible that the amount of exercise resulted from the mood symptoms rather than vice versa. An earlier epidemiologic study in over 20,000 people had similar findings; diagnoses in those who exercised the most were likely to have alcohol dependence and bipolar II disorder.[189] The therapeutic potential of exercise for bipolar disorder is of great importance for mood, neurocognition,[190] and physical health effects, but added difficulties for studies to address include confounding and adherence concerns, need for individualized dose titration depending on conditioning and baseline mood state, and complicated statistical models to incorporate mood state and severity prior to prescribed exercise as an a priori condition. In a study of youth at high risk for bipolar disorder, cerebellar functioning abnormalities were present as compared with controls, indicating balance may be a baseline concern that might improve with exercise but might also require careful planning to minimize risk for harm.[191] Yet the value of exercise to overall health is straightforward, unless individuals are in an uncontrolled state increasing risk taking or decreasing regard for self-harm.

Trigger Identification

Identifying mood episode triggers may be useful to obtain early support and personalized intervention to minimize or prevent episodes. Proudfoot et al.[192] gave 198 young adults with bipolar disorder an online survey to capture unique and common triggers for mania and hypomania, depression, or both. Precipitating situations and behaviors were rated for frequency; in-depth interviews in 11 participants provided validity. Triggers associated with manic or hypomanic episodes included the following: "falling in love, recreational stimulant use, starting a creative project, late night partying, going on vacation and listening to loud music." Depressive episode triggers included the following: "stressful life events, general stress, fatigue, sleep deprivation, physical injury or illness, menstruation, and decreases in physical exercise."

Smoking Cessation

Tobacco smoking, a potentially modifiable lifestyle habit, raises risk for major depression in women, in both case-control and retrospective cohort study designs.[193] As smoking is a risk for systemic inflammation, prevention and early intervention in youth with bipolar disorder may lessen future mental and physical health burden. Monitoring, motivating for cessation, and offering tips for reducing use are important tasks that should be part of routine care visits. State resources specifically targeting adolescent smokers, such as quit lines, are often available.

Healing Arts

Acupuncture

Abstracts from the Chinese literature indicate multiple potential mechanisms for the effects of acupuncture in depression. These include upregulating neurotransmitters and neurotrophins, suppressing cellular apoptosis, modifying glial cell activity and cytokine expression, regulating the activities of the hypothalamus-pituitary-adrenal and hypothalamus-pituitary-gonad axes, and changing lymphocyte beta-receptors, heart rate variability, and electrical motor activity of the gut.[194,195] A pilot RCT showed that electroacupuncture for depression raises glial cell line-derived neurotrophic factor (GDNF).[196] Literature on acupuncture is now being published in English language journals, with overall study quality improving. Luo initially reported positive effects of electroacupuncture, similar to that of amitriptyline and amitriptyline and acupuncture combined, in a randomized trial in depressed adults.[197] Röschke et al.[198] did not find a difference in a single-blind study for acupuncture in depressed adults between verum acupuncture, placebo acupuncture, and a control group, but all subjects were concomitantly treated with mianserin. Two randomized trials of acupuncture across 8 and 12 weeks, respectively, for depressive and hypomanic symptoms in 46 adults, showed improvement in all groups, despite control conditions of points off the acupuncture meridian or at general illness sites.[199] A similar response was found in a study of a wide age range of adults with depression; those randomized to 12 thirty- minute sessions across 6–8 weeks of two-point electroacupuncture protocol (verum acupuncture) and those who received needling at nonchannel scalp points with sham electrostimulation (control acupuncture) had similar decreases in depressive symptoms, corresponding to an overall improvement of 38%–40% in both groups.[200] Other recent publications document acupuncture as effective for depression in adults, including as an adjuvant to SSRI treatments; these studies have improved methodologies, including rigorous sham conditions.[201–203] Laser acupuncture for depression has also been shown to improve depression in an Australian cohort taking part in a double-blind RCT.[204] A small pilot US study in adult MDD confirmed by structured interview compared twice-weekly to once-weekly electroacupuncture as augmentation; both groups showed significant improvement in HAM-D scores.[205] A large comparative effectiveness RCT of acupuncture to standardized general counseling or usual care in the United Kingdom, including possible antidepressant treatment in all groups, found positive effect for acupuncture, equal to or better than counseling, and to usual care.[206] The authors note that to date, acupuncture is only covered by the National Health Service for chronic pain treatment.

Although there are no publications about acupuncture as a CAM treatment for CABD, adult studies appear promising, with expanding confirmatory literature for depression and suggestive literature for manic or hypomanic symptoms emerging. Acceptance, availability, tolerability, cost, and durability of effect will be factors to consider in future studies of its use in CABD.

Mindfulness Meditation

Attentional dysfunction has been described as an intermediate phenotype in BD due to its consistency as a neuropsychological finding, with asymmetric activity at rest and during activation noted on electroencephalogram (EEG).[207,208] Howells et al.[209] performed EEGs during resting states and during completion of a continuous performance test before and after an 8-week mindfulness-based cognitive therapy (MBCT) intervention in 12 euthymic adults with bipolar disorder and 9 control participants. MBCT was chosen due to the aim of meditative practices as to "reduce or eliminate irrelevant thought processes through training of internalized attention."[210] The mindfulness intervention was related to improvements in attentional readiness and reduced activation in response to nonrelevant information processing. Also important to the pathophysiology of bipolar disorder, 8 weeks of training in mindfulness meditation has been shown to alter brain and immune function 4 months later, including left-sided anterior activation (associated with positive affect), and a rise in antibody titers to influenza vaccine; the two changes were positively correlated.[211] No published reports of strict MBCT studies for youth with bipolar disorder were located, but components are commonly added to skills groups used in clinical practice with children and adolescents, and are under study, including for sleep issues related to bipolar disorder.

Massage, Reiki, Yoga, and Tai-Chi

Pediatric providers may find patients and families with mood concerns using an integrative approach, especially including Tai-chi and yoga.[212] Qureshi and Al-Bedah[213] review the use of ayurvedic medicine, homeopathy, and yoga as CAM for mood disorders, including some techniques which have been found to be helpful for depression, with certain studies showing increases in serum BDNF. There are no published studies for CABD, although the potential for benefit, especially with yoga and Tai-chi due to deep breathing, guided meditation, and overall peripheral nervous system (PNS) stimulation properties, seems intuitive. The literature to date has generally focused on using these techniques in individuals, including children, with mood symptoms related to chronic pain, aging, or cancer. Insufficient evidence is available to evaluate their use for CABD.

Conclusions

Information on CAM strategies to improve mood disorders, especially those based on emerging pathophysiologic mechanisms of oxidative stress, mitochondrial dysfunction, and inflammation, is expanding at a fast pace due to global interest. The rich literature developing includes cell and animal models, epidemiologic, pharmacogenetic and genomic studies, and clinical trials with peripheral and CNS biomarkers, which together may ultimately justify specific CAM uses as primary or adjunctive for bipolar symptom prevention and intervention. Combining CAM approaches may be especially powerful, and when personalized for nutritional deficiency and lifestyle, synergism, and genetic and metabolic factors, will offer a tailored approach potentially more acceptable than traditional psychopharmacology to youth and their families. Although much research into CAM for CABD is needed, particularly to determine biomarkers of response, dosing, efficacy, and safety, common uses and signals of safety and efficacy from adult studies may warrant a "phase IV" approach, as many CAM techniques are historical and actively used outside traditional psychiatric practice. Sufficient funding opportunities in youth are necessary to ensure that study of promising strategies are realized, to establish those of most help for the vulnerable group of youth at risk for or already presenting with signs and symptoms of CABD.

Author Disclosures

Dr. Gracious has no conflicts to disclose. She currently receives funding from Nationwide Children's Hospital and The Ohio State University, through the Department of Psychiatry Jeffrey Research Fellowship, The Research Institute at Nationwide Children's Hospital, the OSU Food Innovation Center, and the National Institute of Mental Health (NIMH R01 MH073801-07; Fristad, Site PI).

References

1. Arnold LE. Fish oil is not snake oil. *J Am Acad Child Adolesc Psychiatry*. 2011;50(10):969–71.
2. Sylvia LG, Peters AT, Deckersbach T, Nierenberg AA. Nutrient-based therapies for bipolar disorder: a systematic review. *Psychother Psychosom*. 2013;82(1):10–19.
3. Sarris J, Mischoulon D, Schweitzer I. Adjunctive nutraceuticals with standard pharmacotherapies in bipolar disorder: a systematic review of clinical trials. *Bipolar Disord*. 2011;13(5–6):454–65.

4. Sarris J, Lake J, Hoenders R. Bipolar disorder and complementary medicine: current evidence, safety issues and clinical considerations. *J Altern Complement Med.* 2011;17(10):881–90.

5. Nierenberg AA, Kansky C, Brennan BP, Shelton RC, Perlis R, Iosifescu DV. Mitochondrial modulators for bipolar disorder: a pathophysiologically informed paradigm for new drug development. *Aust NZ J Psychiatry.* 2013;47(1):26–42.

6. Hibbeln JR, Nieminen LR, Blasbalg TL, Riggs JA, Lands WE. Healthy intakes of n-3 and n-6 fatty acids: estimations considering worldwide diversity. *Am J Clin Nutri.* 2006;83:1483S–93S.

7. Noaghial S, Hibbeln JR. Cross-national comparisons of seafood consumption and rates of bipolar disorders. *Am J Psychiatry.* 2003;160:2222–7.

8. Schaeffer L, Gohlke H, Muller M, et al. Common genetic variants of the FDAS1 FADS2 gene cluster and their reconstructed haplotypes are associated with the fatty acid composition in phospholipids. *Hum Mol Genet.* 2006;15:1745–56.

9. Salem N Jr, Litman B, Kim HY, Gawrisch K. Mechanisms of action of docosahexaenoic acid in the nervous system. *Lipids.* 2001;36:945–59.

10. Stahl LA, Begg DP, Weisinger RS, Sinclair AJ. The role of omega-3 fatty acids in mood disorders. *Curr Opin Investig Drugs.* 2008;9:57–64.

11. Hirashima F, Parrow AM, Stoll AL, et al. Omega-3 fatty acid treatment and T_2 whole brain relaxation times in bipolar disorder. *Am J Psychiatry.* 2004;16:1922–4.

12. Conklin BR. New tools to build synthetic hormonal pathways. *Proc Natl Acad Sci USA.* 2007;104(12): 4777–8.

13. Sarris J, Mischoulon D, Schweitzer I. Omega-3 for bipolar disorder: meta-analyses of use in mania and bipolar depression. *J Clin Psychiatry.* 2012;73(1):81–6.

14. Freeman MP, Fava M, Lake J, et al. Complementary and alternative medicine in major depressive disorder: the American Psychiatric Association Task Force report. *J Clin Psychiatry.* 2010;71(6):669–81.

15. Montgomery P, Burton JR, Swell RP, Spreckelsen TF, Richardson AJ. Low blood long chain omega-3 fatty acids in UK children are associated with poor cognitive performance and behavior: a cross-sectional analysis from the DOLAB study. *PLos One.* 2013;8:6:e66697.

16. Kuratko CN, Barrett EC, Nelson EB, Salem N Jr. The relationship of docosahexaenoic acid (DHA) with learning and behavior in healthy children: a review. *Nutrients.* 2013;5(7):T2777–810.

17. Clayton EH, Hanstock TL, Hirneth SJ, Kable CJ, Garg ML, Hazell PL. Reduced mania and depression in juvenile bipolar disorder associated with long-chain omega-3 polyunsaturated fatty acid supplementation. *Eur J Clin Nutr.* 2009;63(8):1037–40.

18. Wozniak J, Biederman J, Mick E, Waxmonsky J, Hantsoo L, Best C, Cluette-Brown JE, Laposata M. Omega-3 fatty acid monotherapy for pediatric bipolar disorder: A prospective open-label trial. *European Neuropsychopharmacology* 2007; 17(6–7):440–7.

19. Nemets H, Nemets B, Apter A, Bracha Z, Belmaker RH. Omega-3 treatment of childhood depression: a controlled, double blind pilot study. *Am J Psychiatry.* 2006;163(6):1098–100.

20. Gracious BL, Chirieac MC, Costescu S, Finucane TL, Youngstrom EA, Hibbeln JR. Randomized, placebo-controlled trial of flax oil in pediatric bipolar disorder. *Bipolar Disord.* 2010;12(2):142–54.

21. McNamara RK, Able J, Jandacek R, et al. Docosahexaenoic acid supplementation increases prefrontal cortex activiation during sustained attention in healthy boys: a placebo-controlled, dose-ranging, functional magnetic resonance imaging study. *Am J Clin Nutr.* 2010; 91(4):1060–7.

22. Stanger MJ, Thompson LA, Young AJ, Lieberman HR. Anticoagulant activity of select dietary supplements. *Nutr Rev.* 2012;70(2):107–17.

23. Cohen MG, Rossi JS, Garbarino J, et al. Insights into the inhibition of platelet activation by omega-3 polyunsaturated fatty acids: beyond aspirin and clopidogrel. *Thromb Res.* 2011;128(4):335–40.

24. Jacobs D, Silverstone T. Dextroamphetamine-induced arousal in human subjects as a model for mania. *Psychol Med.* 198;16:323–9.

25. Kaneko M, Watanabe K, Kumashiro H. Plasma ratios of tryptophan and tyrosine to other large neutral amino acids in manic-depressive patients. *Jpn J Psychiatry Neurol.* 1992;46(3):711–20.

26. Watamabe K. Analysis of plasma amino acids-tryptophan and tyrosine ratios to other large neutral amino acids in manic-depressive illness. *Nihon Rinsho.* 1994;52(5):1152–8.

27. McTavish SFB, Cowen PJ. Effect of a tyrosine-free amino acid mixture on regional brain catecholamine synthesis and release. *Psychopharmacology*. 1999;141:182–8.

28. McTavish SFB, McPherson MH, Harmer CJ, et al. Antidopaminergic effects of dietary tyrosine depletion in healthy subjects and patients with manic illness. *Br J Psychiatry*. 2001;179:356–60.

29. Scarna A, Gijsman HJ, McTavish SF, Harmer CJ, Cowen PJ, Goodwin GM. Effects of a branched-chain amino acid drink in mania. *Br J Psychiatry*. 2003;182:210–3.

30. Applebaum J, Bersudsky Y, Klein E. Rapid tryptophan depletion as a treatment for acute mania: a double-blind, pilot-controlled study. *Bipolar Disord*. 2007;;9(8):884–7.

31. Delgado PL, Charney DS, Price LH, Landis H, Heninger GR. Neuroendocrine and behavioral effects of dietary tryptophan restriction in healthy subjects. *Life Sci*. 1989;45:2323–32.

32. Harper AE, Benevenga NJ, Wohlhueter RM. Effects of ingestion of disproportionate amounts of amino acids. *Physiol Rev*. 1970;50:428–558.

33. Moreno FA, Heninger GR, McGahuey CA, Delgado PL. Tryptophan depletion and risk of depression relapse: a prospective study of tryptophan depletion as a potential predictor of depressive episodes. *Biol Psychiatry*. 2000;48:327–9.

34. Murphy DL, Baker M, Goodwin FK, Miller H, Kotin J, Bunney WE. L-tryptophan in affective disorders: Indoleamine changes and differential clinical effects. *Psychopharmacologia*. 1974;34:11–20.

35. Goff DC. Two cases of hypomania following the addition of L-tryptophan to a monoamine oxidase inhibitor. *Am J Psychiatry*. 1985;142(12):1487–8.

36. Chouinard G, Young SN, Annable L. A controlled clinical trial of L-tryptophan in acute mania. *Biol Psychiatry*. 1985; 20(5):546–57.

37. Nemzer ED, Arnold LE, Votolato NA, McConnell H. Amino acid supplementation as therapy for attention deficit disorder. *J Am Academy Child Adolesc Psychiatry*. 1986; 4:509–13.

38. Gawryluk JW, Wang JF, Andreazza AC, et al. Decreased levels of glutathione, the major brain antioxidant, in post-mortem prefrontal cortex from patients with psychiatric disorders. *Int J Neuropsychopharmacol*. 2011;14:123–30.

39. Dean O, Giorlando F, Berk M. N-acetylcysteine in psychiatry: current therapeutic evidence and potential mechanisms of action. *J Psychiatry Neurosci*. 2011;36:78–86.

40. Berk M, Copolov D, Dean O, et al. N-acetyl cysteine as a glutathione precursor for schizophrenia—a double-blind, randomized, placebo-controlled trial. *Biol Psychiatry*. 2008;64:361–8.

41. Berk M, Copolov DL, Dean O, et al. N-acetyl cysteine for depressive symptoms in bipolar disorder—a double-blind randomized placebo-controlled trial. *Biol Psychiatry*. 2008;64:468–75.

42. Magalhães PV, Dean OM, Bush AI, et al. A preliminary investigation on the efficacy of N-acetyl cysteine for mania or hypomania. *Aust NZ J Psychiatry*. 2013;47(6):564–8.

43. Magalhaes PV, Dean OM, Bush AI, et al. N-acetyl cysteine add-on treatment for bipolar II disorder: a subgroup analysis of a randomized placebo-controlled trial. *J Affect Disord*. 2011;129:317–20.

44. Berk M, Dean OM, Cotton SM, et al. Maintenance N-acetyl cysteine treatment for bipolar disorder: a double-blind randomized placebo controlled trial. *BMC Med*. 2012;10:91.

45. Berk M, Malhi GS, Gray LJ, Dean OM. The promise of N-acetylcysteine in neuropsychiatry. *Trends Pharmacol Sci* 2013;34(3):167–77.

46. Goldstein BI. In this issue/abstract thinking: NAC attack: is N-acetylcysteine ready for prime time in child and adolescent psychiatry? *J Am Acad Child Adolesc Psychiatry*. 2013;52(2):111–2.

47. Hardan AY, Fung LK, Libove RA, et al. A randomized controlled pilot trial of oral N-acetylcysteine in children with autism. *Biol Psychiatry*. 2012;71(11):956–61.

48. Ghanizadeh A, Moghimi-Sarani E. A randomized double blind placebo controlled clinical trial of N-Acetylcysteine added to risperidone for treating autistic disorders. *BMC Psychiatry*. 2013;13:196.

49. Papakostas GI, Alpert JE, Fava M. S-adenosyl-methione in depression: a comprehensive review of the literature. *Curr Psychiatry Reports*. 2003;5(6):460–6.

50. Brown JM, Ball JG, Wright MS, Van Meter S, Valentovic MA. Novel protective mechanisms for S-adenosyl-L-methionine against acetaminophen hepatotoxicity: improvement of key antioxidant enzymatic function. *Toxicol Lett*. 2012;212(3):320–8.

51. Carney MW, Chary TK, Bottiglieri T, et al. The switch mechanism and the bipolar/unipolar dichotomy. *British J Psychiatry*. 1989;154:48–51.

52. Hoppel C. The role of carnitine in normal and altered fatty acid metabolism. *Am J Kidney* Dis. 2003;41:S4–12.

53. Al-Majed AA, Sayed-Ahmed MM, Al-Omar FA, et al. Carnitine esters prevent oxidative stress damage and energy depletion following transient forbrain ischemia in the rat hippocampus. *Clin Exp Pharmacol* Physiol. 2006;33:725–33.

54. Ames BN, Liu J. Delaying the mitochondrial decay of aging with acetylcarnitine. *Ann NY Acad Sci.* 2004;1033:108–16.

55. Zanardi R, Smeraldi E. A double-blind, randomized, controlled clinical trial of acetyl-L-carnitine vs. amisulpride in the treatment of dysthymia. *Eur Neuropsychopharmacol.* 2006;16:281–7.

56. Packer L, Witt EH, Tritschler HJ. Alpha-lipoic acid as a biological antioxidant. *Free Radical Biol Med.* 1995;19:227–50.

57. Estrada DE, Weart HS, Tsakiridis T, et al. Stimulation of glucose uptake by the natural coenzyme alpha-lipoic acid/thioctic acid: participation of elements of the insulin signaling pathway. *Diabetes.* 1996;45:1798–804.

58. Liu J. The effects and mechanisms of mitochondrial nutrient alpha-lipoic acid on improving age-associated mitochondrial and cognitive dysfunction: an overview. *Neurochem Res.* 2008;33:194–203.

59. Macêdo DS, Medeiros CD, Cordeiro RC, et al. Effects of alpha-lipoic acid in an animal model of mania induced by D-amphetamine. *Bipolar Disord.* 2012;14(7):707–18.

60. Brennan BP, Jensen JE, Hudson JI, et al. A placebo-controlled trial of acetyl-L-carnitine and alpha-lipoic acid in the treatment of bipolar depression. *J Clin Psychopharmacol.* 2013;33(5):627–35.

61. Forester BP, Zuo CS, Ravichandran C, et al. Coenzyme Q10 effects on creatine kinase activity and mood in geriatric bipolar depression. *J Geriatr Psychiatry Neurol.* 2012;25(1):43–50.

62. Ames A III. CNS energy metabolism as related to function. *Brain Res Brain Res Rev.* 2000;34:42–68.

63. Tarnopolsky MA. The mitochondrial cocktail: rationale for combined nutraceutical therapy in mitochondrial cytopathies. *Adv Drug Delivery Rev.* 2008;60:1561–7.

64. Stork C, Renshaw PF. Mitochondrial dysfunction in bipolar disorder: evidence from magnetic resonance spectroscopy research. *Mol Psychiatry.* 2005;10:900–19.

65. Amital Dt, Vishne T, Roitman S, et al. Observed effects of creatine monohydrate in a patient with treatment-resistant depression and fibromyalgia. *Am J Psychiatry.* 2006;163:1840–1.

66. Roitman S, Green T, Osher Y, Karni N, Levine J. Creatinine monohydrate in resistant depression: a preliminary study. *Bipolar Disord.* 2007;9:754–8.

67. Acuna-Castroviejo D, Escames G, Rodriguez MI et al. Melatonin role in the mitochondrial function. *Frontiers* Biosci. 2007;12:947–63.

68. Albarran MT, Lopez-Burillo S, Pablos MI, et al. Endogenous rhythms of melatonin, total antioxidant status and superoxide dismutase activity in several tissues of chick and their inhibition by light. *J Pineal* Res. 2001;30:227–33.

69. Acuna-Castroviejo D, Escames G, Lopez LC, et al. Melatonin and nitric oxide: two required antagonists for mitochondrial homeostasis. *Endocrine.* 2005;27:159–68.

70. Fornaro M1, McCarthy MJ, De Berardis D, et al. Adjunctive agomelatine therapy in the treatment of acute bipolar II depression: a preliminary open label study. Neuropsychiatr Dis Treat. 2013;9:243–51.

71. Hamdani N, Doukhan R, Kurtlucan O, Tamouza R, Leboyer M. Immunity, inflammation, and bipolar disorder: diagnostic and therapeutic implications. *Curr Psychiatry Rep.* 2013;15(9):387.

72. Torrey EF, Davis JM. Adjunct treatments for schizophrenia and bipolar disorder: what to try when you are out of ideas. *Clin Schizophr Relat Psychoses.* 2012;5(4):208–16.

73. Garrido-Mesa N, Utrilla P, Comalada M, et al. The association of minocycline and the probiotic Escherichia coli Nissle 1917 results in an additive beneficial effect in a DSS model of reactivated colitis in mice. *Biochem Pharmacol.* 2011;82(12):1891–900.

74. Miyaoka T, Wake R, Furuya M, et al. Minocycline as adjunctive therapy for patients with unipolar psychotic depression: an open-label study. *Prog Neuropsychopharmacol Biol Psychiatry.* 2012;37(2):222–6.

75. Savitz J, Preskorn S, Teague TK, Drevets D, Yates W, Drevets W. Minocycline and aspirin in the treatment of bipolar depression: a protocol for a proof-of-concept, randomised, double-blind, placebo-controlled, 2x2 clinical trial. *BMJ Open.* 2012;2(1):e000643.

76. Choi SH, Aid S, Choi U, et al. Cyclooxygenases-1 and -2 differentially modulate leukocyte recruitment into the inflamed brain. *Pharmacogenomics J.* 2010;10:448e57.

77. Moretti M, Colla A, de Oliveira Belan G, et al. Ascorbic acid treatment, similar to fluoxetine, reverses depressive-like behavior and brain oxidative damage induced by chronic unpredictable stress. *J Psychiatric Res.* 2012;46:331–40.

78. Stolk P, Souverein PC, Wilting I, et al. Is aspirin useful in patients on lithium? A pharmacoepidemiological study related to bipolar disorder. *Prostaglandins Leukot Essent Fatty Acids.* 2010;82:9e14.

79. Mendlewicz J, Kriwin P, Oswald P, et al. Shortened onset of action of antidepressants in major depression using acetylsalicylic acid augmentation: a pilot open-label study. *Int Clin Psychopharmacol.* 2006;21:227e31.

80. Berk M, Dean O, Drexhage H, et al. Aspirin: a review of its neurobiological properties and therapeutic potential for mental illness. *BMC Med.* 2013;11:74.

81. Jiang H, Wang Z, Wang Y, et al. Antidepressant-like effects of curcumin in chronic mild stress of rats: involvement of its anti-inflammatory action. *Prog Neuropsychopharmacol Biol Psychiatry.* 2013;47C:33–9.

82. Jacka FN, Overland S, Stewart R, Tell GS, Bjelland I, Mykletun A. Association between magnesium intake and depression and anxiety in community-dwelling adults: the Hordaland Health Study. *Aust NZ J Psychiatry.* 2009;43(1):45–52.

83. Jacka FN, Maes M, Pasco JA, Williams LF, Berk M. Nutrient intakes and the common mental disorders in women. *J Affect Disord.* 2012;141(1):79–85.

84. Yary T, Aazami S. Dietary intake of zinc was inversely associated with depression. *Biol Trace Elem Res.* 2012;145(3):286–90.

85. Gonzáles-Estecha M, Trasobares EM, Tajima K, et al. Trace elements in bipolar disorder. *J Trace Elem Med Biol.* 2011;S1:S78–83.

86. Barbosa FJ, Hesse B, de Almeida RB, Baretta IP, Boemgen-Lacerda R, Andreatini R. Magnesium sulfate and sodium valproate block methylphenidate-induced hyperlocomotion, an animal model of mania. *Pharmacol Rep.* 2011;63(1):64–70.

87. Nechifor M. Interactions between magnesium and psychotropic drugs. *Magnes Res.* 2008;21(2):97–100.

88. Chouinard G, Beauclair L, Geiser R, Etienne P. A pilot study of magnesium aspartate hydrochloride (Magnesiocard) as a mood stabilizer for rapid cycling bipolar affective disorder patients. *Prog Neuropsychopharmacol Biol Psychiatry.* 1990;14(2):171–80.

89. Heiden A, Frey R, Presslich O, Blasbichler T, Smetana R, Kasper S. Treatment of severe mania with intravenous magnesium sulphate as a supplementary therapy. *Psychiatry Res.* 1999;89(3):239–46.

90. Giannini AJ, Nakoneczie AM, Melemis SM, Ventresco J, Condon M. Magnesium oxide augmentation of verapamil maintenance therapy in mania. *Psychiatry Res.* 2000;93(1):83–7.

91. Russo AJ. Decreased serum hepatocyte growth factor (HGF) in individuals with bipolar disorder normalizes after zinc and anti-oxidant therapy. *Nutr Metab Insights.* 2010;3:49–55.

92. Bae MH, Bissonette GB, Mars WM, et al. Hepatocyte growth factor (HGF) modulates GABAergic inhibition and seizure susceptibility. *Exp Neurol* 2010;221:129–35.

93. Akimoto M, Baba A, Ideda-Matsuo Y, et al. Hepatocyte growth factor as an enhancer of nmda currents and synaptic plasticity in the hippocampus. *Neuroscience.* 2004;128(1):155–62.

94. Pasco JA, Jacka FN, Williams LJ, et al. Dietary selenium and major depression: a nested case-control study. *Complement Therap Med.* 2012;20(3):119–23.

95. Amann BL, Mergl R, Vieta E, et al. A 2-year, open-label pilot study of adjunctive chromium in patients with treatment-resistant rapid-cycling bipolar disorder. *J Clin Psychopharmacol.* 2007;27(1):104–6.

96. Herbison CE, Hickling S, Allen KL, et al. Low intake of B-vitamins is associated with poor adolescent mental health and behavior. *Prev Med.* 2012;55(6):634–8.

97. Schneider JA, Rees DC, Liu YT, Clegg JB. Worldwide distribution of a common methylenetetrahydrofolate reductase mutation. *Am J Hum Genet.* 1998;62(5):1258–60.

98. Jacques PF, Bostom AG, Williams RR, et al. Relation between folate status, a common mutation in methylenetetrahydrofolate reductase, and plasma homocysteine concentrations. *Circulation.* 1996;93(1):7–9.

99. Reynolds EH, Preece JM, Bailey J, Coppen A. Folate deficiency in depressive illness. *Br J Psychiatry.* 1970;117:287–92.

100. Fava M, Borus JS, Alpert JE, et al. Folate, B12, and homocysteine in major depressive disorder. *Am J Psychiatry.* 1997;154:426–8.

101. Alpert M, Silva R, Pouget E. Folate as a predictor of response to sertraline or nortriptyline in geriatric depression. Paper presented at: 36th Annual Meeting of the NCDEU; May 28–31, 1996; Boca Raton, FL.

102. Coppen A, Bailey J. Enhancement of the antidepressant action of fluoxetine by folic acid: a randomized, placebo controlled trial. *J Affect Disord.* 2000;60:121–30.

103. Resler Gl, Lavie R, Campos J, et al. Effect of folic acid combined with fluoxetine in patients with major depression on plasma homocysteine and vitamin B12, and serotonin levels in lymphocytes. *Neuroimmunomodulation.* 2008;15(3):145–52.

104. Alpert JE, Mischoulon D, Rubenstein GE, Bottonari K, Nierenberg AA, Fava M. Folinic acid (Lecovorin) as an adjunctive treatment for SSRI-refractory depression. *Ann Clin Psychiatry.* 2002;14:33–8.

105. Kevere L, Purvina S, Bauze D, et al. Elevated serum levels of homocysteine as an early prognostic factor of psychiatric disorders in children and adolescents. *Schizophr Res Treat.* 2012;2012:373261.

106. Godfrey PS, Toone BK, Carney MW, et al. Enhancement of recovery from psychiatric illness by methylfolate. *Lancet.* 1990;336:392–5.

107. Papakostas GI, Shelton RC, Zajecka JM, et al. l-Methylfolate as adjunctive therapy for SSRI-resistant major depression: results of two randomized, double-blind, parallel-sequential trials. *Am J Psychiatry.* 2012;169:1267–74.

108. Wegner C, Nau H. Alteration of embryonic folate metabolism by valproic acid during organogenesis: implications for mechanism of teratogenesis. *Neurology.* 1992;42:17–24.

109. Hsieh CL, Wang HE, Tsai WJ, Chiung CP, Peng RY. Multiple point action mechanism of valproic acid-teratogenicity alleviated by folic acid, vitamin C, and N-acetylcysteine in chicken embryo model. *Toxicology.* 2012;291(1–3):32–42.

110. Morrell MJ. Folic acid and epilepsy. *Epilepsy Curr.* 2002;2(2):31–4.

111. Reynolds EH. Mental effects of anticonvulsants and folic acid metabolism. *Brain* 1968;91:197–214.

112. Tufan AE, Bilici R, Usta G, Erdogan A. Mood disorder with mixed, psychotic features due to vitamin b12 deficiency in an adolescent: case report. *Child Adolesc Psychiatry Ment Health.* 2012;6(1):6–25.

113. Dogan M, Ozdemir O, Sal EA, Dogan SZ, Ozdemir P, Cesur Y, Caksen H. Psychotic disorder and extrapyramidal symptoms associated with vitamin B12 and folate deficiency. *J Trop Pediatr.* 2009;5(3):205–7.

114. Goggans FC. A case of mania secondary to vitamin B12 deficiency. *Am J Psychiatry.* 1984;141(2):300–1.

115. Barkai A, Dunner DL, Gross HA, Mayo P, Fieve RR. Reduced myo-inositol levels in cerebrospinal fluid from patients with affective disorders. *Biol Psychiatry.* 1978;13:65–72.

116. Shimon H, Agam G, Belmaker RH, Hyde TM, Kleinman JE. Reduced frontal cortex inositol levels in postmortem brain of suicide victims and patients with bipolar disorder. *Am J Psychiatry.* 1997;154:1148–50.

117. Atack JR. Inositol monophosphatase, the putative therapeutic target for lithium. *Brain Res Rev.* 1996;22:183–90.

118. Frey R, Metzler D, Fischer P, et al. Myo-inositol in depressive and healthy subjects determined by frontal 1H-magnetic resonance spectroscopy at 1.5 tesla. *J Psychiatr Res.* 1998;32:411–20.

119. Moore GJ, Bebchuk JM, Parrish JK, et al. Temporal dissociation between lithium-induced changes in frontal lobe myoinositol and clinical response in manic-depressive illness. *Am J Psychiatry.* 1999;156:1902–8.

120. Davanzo P, Thomas MA, Yue K, et al. Decreased anterior cingulated myoinositol/creatine spectroscopy resonance with lithium treatment in children with bipolar disorder. *Neuropsychopharmacol.* 2001;24:359–9.

121. Davanzo P, Yue K, Thomas MA, et al. Proton magnetic resonance spectroscopy of bipolar disorder *versus* intermittent explosive disorder in children and adolescents. *Am J Psychiat.* 2003;160:1442–52.

122. Levine J, Gonsalves M, Babur I, et al. Inositol 6 g may be effective in depression but not in schizophrenia. *Hum Psychopharmacol.* 1993;8:49–53.

123. Levine J, Barak Y, Gonzalues M, et al. Double-blind, controlled-trial of inositol treatment of depression. *Am J Psychiatry.* 1995;152:792–4.

124. Chengappa KN, Levine J, Gershon S, et al. Inositol as an add-on treatment for bipolar depression. *Bipolar Disord.* 2000;2:47–55.

125. Eden Evins A, Demopulos C, Yovel I, et al. Inositol augmentation of lithium or valproate for bipolar depression. *Bipolar Disord.* 2006;8(2):168–74.

126. Nierenberg AA, Ostacher MJ, Calabrese JR, et al. Treatment-resistant bipolar depression: a STEP-BD equipoise randomized effectiveness trial of antidepressant augmentation with lamotrigine, inositol, or risperidone. *Am J Psychiatry.* 2006;163(2):210–6.

127. Carlomagno G, Unfer V. Inositol safety: clinical evidences. *Eur Rev Med Pharmacol Sci.* 2011;15(8):931–6.

128. Levine J, Witztum E, Greenberg BD, et al. Inositol-induced mania? [letter]. *Am J Psychiatry.* 1996;153:839.

129. Ueland PM. Choline and betaine in health and disease. *J Inherit Metab Dis.* 2010;34(1):3–15.

130. Zeisel SH, da Costa KA. Choline: an essential nutrient for public health. *Nutr Rev.* 2009;(11):615–23.

131. Detopoulou P, Panagiotakos DB, Antonopoulou S, Pitsavos C, Stefanadis C. Dietary choline and beta-ine intakes in relation to concentrations of inflammatory markers in healthy adults: the ATTICA study. *Am J Clin Nutr.* 2008;87(2):424–30.

132. Senaratne R, Milne AM, MacQueen GM, Hall GB. Increased choline-containing compounds in the orbitofrontal cortex and hippocampus in euthymic patients with bipolar disorder: a proton magnetic reseonance spectroscopy study. *Psychiatry Res.* 2009;172(3):205–9.

133. Shi J, Hattori E, Zou H, et al. No evidence for association between 19 cholinergic genes and bipolar disorder. *Am J Med Genet B Neuropsychiatr Genet.* 2007;144B(6):715–23.

134. Stoll AL, Cohen BM, Snyder MB, Hanin I. Erythrocyte choline concentration in bipolar disorder: a predictor of clinical course and medication response. *Biol Psychiatry.* 1991;29(12):1171–80.

135. Cohen BM, Miller AL, Lipinski JF, Pope HG. Lecithin in mania: a preliminary report. *Am J Psychiatry.* 1980;137(2):242–3.

136. Cohen BM, Lipinski JF, Altesman RI. Lecithin in the treatment of mania: double-blind, placebo-controlled trials. Am J Psychiatry. 1982 Sep;139(9):1162–4.

137. Stoll AL, Sachs GS, Cohen BM, Lafer B, Christensen JD, Renshaw PF. Choline in the treatment of rapid-cycling bipolar disorder: clinical and neurochemical findings in lithium-treated patients. *Biol Psychiatry.* 1996;40(5):382–8.

138. Schreier HA. Mania responsive to lecithin in a 13-year old girl. *Am J Psychiatry.* 1982;139:108–10.

139. Lyoo IK, Demopulos CM, Hirashima F, Ahn KH, Renshaw PF. Oral choline decreases brain purine levels in lithium-treated subjects with rapid-cycling bipolar disorder: a double-blind trial using proton and lithium magnetic resonance spectroscopy. *Bipolar Disord.* 2003;5(4):300–6.

140. Berk M, Sanders KM, Pasco JA, et al. Vitamin D deficiency may play a role in depression. *Med Hypotheses.* 2007;69:1316–9.

141. Bech P, Hey H. Depression or asthenia related to metabolic disturbances in obese patients after intestinal bypass surgery. *Acta Psychiatr Scand.* 1979;59:462–70.

142. Stumpf WE, Privette TH. Light, vitamin D and psychiatry. Role of 1,25 dihydroxyvitamin D3 (soltriol) in etiology and therapy of seasonal affective disorder and other mental processes. *J Psychopharmacol.* 1989;97:285–94.

143. Wilkins C, Sheline Y, Roe C, Birge S, Morris J. Vitamin D deficiency is associated with low mood and worse cognitive performance in older adults. *Am J Geriatr Psychiatry.* 2006;14:1032–40.

144. Gloth FM 3rd, Alam W, Hillis B. Vitamin D vs broad spectrum phototherapy in the treatment of seasonal affective disorder. *J Nutr Health Aging.* 1999;3(1):5–7.

145. Jorde R, Sneve M, Figenschau Y, Svartberg J, Waterloo K. Effects of vitamin D supplementation on symptoms of depression in overweight and obese subjects: randomized double blind trial. *J Intern Med.* 2008;264(6):599–609.

146. Bonnot O, Inaoui R, Raffin-Viard M, Bodeau N, Coussieu C, Cohen D. Children and adolescents with severe mental illness need Vitamin D supplementation regardless of disease or treatment. *J Child Adolesc Psychopharmacol.* 2011;21(2):157–61.

147. Gracious BL, Finucane TL, Friedman-Campbell M, Messing S, Parkhurst MN. Vitamin-D deficiency and psychotic features in mentally ill adolescents: a cross-sectional study. *BMC Psychiatry.* 2012;12:38.

148. Högberg G, Gustafsson SA, Hallstom T, Gustafsson T, Klawitter B, Petersson M. Depressed adolescents in a case-series were low in vitamin D and depression was ameliorated by vitamin D supplementation. *Acta Paediatr*. 2012;101(7):779–83.

149. Umhau JC, George DT, Heaney RP, et al. Low vitamin D status and suicide: a case-control study of active duty military service members. *PLoS One*. 2013;8(1):e51543.

150. Ahmadi S, Mirzaei K, Hossein-Nezhad A, Shariati G. Vitamin D receptor FokI genotype may modify the susceptibility to schizophrenia and bipolar mood disorder by regulation of dopamine D1 receptor gene expression. *Minerva Med*. 2012;103(5):383–91.

151. Parker G, Brotchie H. D' for depression: any role for vitamin D? 'Food for Thought' II. *Acta Psychiatr Scand*. 2011;124(4):243–9.

152. Lobato KR, Cardoso CC, Binfaré RW, et al. alpha-Tocopherol administration produces an antidepressant-like effect in predictive animal models of depression. *Behav Brain Res*. 2010; 209(2):249–59.

153. Manosso LM, Neis VB, Moretti M, et al. Antidepressant-like effect of α-tocopherol in a mouse model of depressive-like behavior induced by TNF-α. *Prog Neuropsychopharmacol Biol Psychiatry*. 2013;46C:48–57.

154. Tsuboi H, Watanabe M, Kobayashi F, Kimura K, Kinae N. Associations of depressive symptoms with serum proportions of palmitic and arachidonic acids, and α-tocopherol effects among male population—a preliminary study. *Clin Nutr*. 2013;32(2):289–93.

155. Kaplan BJ, Simpson JSA, Ferre RC, Gorman C, McMullen D, Crawford SG. Effective mood stabilization in bipolar disorder with a chelated mineral supplement. *J Clin Psychiatry*. 2001;62:936–44.

156. Kaplan BJ, Crawford SG, Gardner B, Farrelly G. Treatment of mood lability and explosive rage with minerals and vitamins: two case studies in children. *J Child Adolesc Psychopharmacol*. 2002;12(3):205–19.

157. Kaplan BJ, Crawford SG, Field CJ, Simpson JS. Vitamins, minerals, and mood. *Psychol Bull*. 2007;133(5):747–60.

158. Kaplan BJ, Crawford SG, Field CJ, Kolb B. Improved mood and behavior during treatment with a mineral-vitamin supplement: an open-label case series of children. *J Child Adolesc Psychopharmacol*. 2004;14(1):115–22.

159. Rucklidge JJ, Gately D, Kaplan BJ. Database analysis of children and adolescents with bipolar disorder consuming a micronutrient formula. *BMC Psychiatry*. 2010;10:74.

160. Simpson JS, Crawford SG, Goldsterin ET, Field C, Burgess E, Kaplan BJ. Systematic review of safety and tolerability of a complex micronutrient formula used in mental health. *BMC Psychiatry*. 2011;11:62.

161. Frazier EA, Fristad MA, Arnold LE. Feasibility of a nutritional supplement as treatment for pediatric bipolar spectrum disorders. *J Altern Complement Med*. 2012;18(7):678–85.

162. Frazier EA, Gracious BL, Arnold LE, et al. Nutritional and safety outcomes from an open-label micronutrient intervention for pediatric bipolar spectrum disorders. *J Child Adolesc Psychopharmacol*. 2013;23(8)558–67.

163. Oddy WH, Robinson M, Ambrosini GL, et al. The association between dietary patterns and mental health in early adolescence. *Prev Med*. 2009;49(1):39–44.

164. Ambrosini GL, Oddy WH, Robinson M, et al. Adolescent dietary patterns are associated with lifestyle and family psycho-social factors. *Pub Health Nutr*. 2009;12(10):1807–15.

165. O'Sullivan TA, Robinson M, Kendall GE, et al. A good-quality breakfast is associated with better mental health in adolescence. *Pub Health Nutr*. 2009;12(2):249–58.

166. Larson NI, Neumark-Szlainer D, Hannan PJ, Story M. Family meals during adolescence are associated with higher diet quality and healthful meal patterns during young adulthood. *J Am Diet Assoc*. 2007;107(9):1502–10.

167. McMartin SE, Jacka FN, Colman I. The association between fruit and vegetable consumption and mental health disorders: evidence from five waves of a national survey of Canadians. *Prev Med*. 2013;56(3–4):225–30.

168. Jacka FN, Rothon C, Taylor S, Berk M, Stansfield SA. Diet quality and mental health problems in adolescents from East London: a prospective study. *Soc Psychiatry Psychiatr Epidemiol*. 2013;48(8):1297–306.

169. Jacka FN, Pasco HA, Mykletun A, et al. Diet quality in bipolar disorder in a population-based sample of women. *J Affect Disord*. 2011;129(1–3):332–7.

170. Jacka FN, Pasco Ja, Mykletun A, et al. Association of Western and traditional diets with depression and anxiety in women. *Am J Psychiatry*. 2010;167(3):305–11.

171. Traynelis SF, Cull-Candy SG. Proton inhibition of N-methyl-D-aspartate receptors in cerebellar neurons. *Nature*. 1990;345(6273):347–50.

172. Dahlin M, Elfving A, Ungerstedt U, Amark P. The ketogenic diet is known to modulate levels of excitatory and inhibitory amino acids in the CSF in children with refractory epilepsy. *Epilepsy Res*. 2005;64(3):115–25.

173. El-Mallakh RS, Paskitti ME. The ketogenic diet may have mood-stabilizing properties. *Med Hypotheses*. 2001;57(6):724–6.

174. Yaroslavsky Y, Stahl Z, Belmaker RH. Ketogenic diet in bipolar illness. *Bipolar Disord*. 2002;4(1):75.

175. Phelps JR, Siemers SV, El-Mallakh RS. The ketogenic diet for type II bipolar disorder. *Neurocase*. 2012 Oct 3. Epub ahead of print.

176. Stokes JH, Pillsbury DH. The effect on the skin of emotional and nervous states: theoretical and practical consideration of a gastrointestinal mechanism. *Arch Dermatol Syphilol*. 1930;22:962–93.

177. Bowe WP, Patel NB, Logan AC. Acne vulgaris, probiotics and the gut-brain-skin axis: from anecdote to translational medicine. *Benef Microbes*. 2013:1–15. Epub ahead of print.

178. Bested AC, Logan AC, Selhub EM. Intestinal microbiota, probiotics and mental health: from Metchnikoff to modern advances: part III- convergence toward clinical trials. *Gut Pathog*. 2013;5(1):4.

179. Deltito JA1, Moline M, Pollak C, Martin LY, Maremmani I. Effects of phototherapy on non-seasonal unipolar and bipolar depressive spectrum disorders. *J Affect Disord*. 1991 Dec;23(4):231–7.

180. Leibenluft E, Turner EH, Feldman-Naim S, Schwartz PJ, Wehr RA, Rosenthal NE. Light therapy in patients with rapid-cycling bipolar disorder: preliminary results. *Psychopharmacol Bull*. 1995;31:705–10.

181. Papatheodorou G, Kutcher S. The effect of adjunctive light therapy on ameliorating breakthrough depressive symptoms in adolescent-onset bipolar disorder. *J Psychiatry Neurosci*. 1995;20(3):226–32.

182. Praschak-Reider N, Neumeister A, Hesselman B, Willeit M, Barnas C, Kasper S. Suicidal tendancies as a complication of light therapy for seasonal affective disorder: a report of three cases. *J Clin Psychiatry*. 1997;58:389–92.

183. Sit D, Wisner KL, Hanusa BH, Stull S, Terman M. Light therapy for bipolar disorder: a case series in women. *Bipolar Disord* 2007;9:918–27.

184. Jacka FN, Pasco JA, Dodd S, Williams LJ, Nicholson GC, Berk M. Lower levels of physical activity in childhood predict adult depression. *J Affec Disorders*. 2008;107(Suppl. 1):S58–9.

185. Garcia-Toro M, Ibarra O, Gili M, et al. Four hygienic-dietary recommendations as add-on treatment in depression: a randomized-controlled trial. *J Affect Disord*. 2012;140(2):200–3.

186. Murray G, Suto M, Hole R, Hale S, Amari E, Michalak EE. Self-management strategies used by 'high functioning' individuals with bipolar disorder: from research to clinical practice. *Clin Psychol Psychother*. 2011;18(2):95–109.

187. Cooney GM, Dwan K, Greig CA, et al. Exercise for depression. *Cochrane Database Sys Rev*. 2013;9:CD004366. doi: 10.1002/14651858.CD004366.pub6

188. Sylvia LG, Friedman ES, Kocsis JH, et al. Association of exercise with quality of life and mood symptoms in a comparative effectiveness study of bipolar disorder. *J Affect Disord*. 2013;151(2):722–7.

189. Dakwar E, Blanco C, Lin KH, et al. Exercise and mental illness: results from the National Epidemiologic Survey on Alcohol and Related Conditions (NESARC). *J Clin Psychiatry*. 2012;73(7):960–6.

190. Kucyi A, Alsuwaidan MT, Liauw SS, McIntyre RS. Aerobic physical exercise as a possible treatment for neurocognitive dysfunction in bipolar disorder. *Postgrad Med*. 2010;122(6):107–16.

191. Giles LL, DelBello MP, Gilbert DL, Stanford KE, Shear PK, Strakowski SM. Cerebellar ataxia in youths at risk for bipolar disorder. *Bipolar Disord*. 2008;10(6):733–7.

192. Proudfoot J, Whitton A, Parker G, Doran J, Manicavasagar V, Delmas K. Triggers of mania and depression in young adults with bipolar disorder. *J Affect Disord*. 2012;143(1–3):196–202.

193. Pasco JA, Williams LJ, Jacka FN, et al. Tobacco smoking as a risk factor for major depressive disorder: population-based study. *Br J Psychiatry*. 2008;193(4):322–6.

194. Hu L, Liang J, Jin SY, Han YJ, Lu J, Tu Y. [Progress of researches on mechanisms of acupuncture underlying improvement of depression in the past five years]. [Article in Chinese] *Zhen Ci Yan Jiu*. 2013;38(3):253–8.

195. Litscher G, Cheng G, Wang L, et al. Biomedical teleacupuncture between China and Austria using heart rate variability-part2: patients with depression. *Evid Based Complement Alternat Med.* 2012;2012:145904. doi: 10.1155/2012/145904.

196. Sun H, Zhao H, Ma C, et al. Effects of electroacupuncture on depression and the production of glial cell line-derived neurotrophic factor compared with fluoxetine: a randomized controlled pilot study. *J Altern Complement Med.* 2013;19(9):733–9.

197. Luo H, Meng F, Jia Y, Zhao X. Clinical research on the therapeutic effect of the electro-acupuncture treatment in patients with depression. *Psychiatry Clin Neurosci.* 1998;52:S338–40.

198. Röschke J, Wolf Ch, Müller MJ, et al. The benefit from whole body acupuncture in major depression. *J Affect Disord.* 2000;57:73–81.

199. Dennehy EB, Schnyer R, Bernstein IH, et al. The safety, acceptability, and effectiveness of acupuncture as an adjunctive treatment for acute symptoms in bipolar disorder. *J Clin Psychiatry.* 2009; 70(6):897–905.

200. Andreescu C, Glick RM, Emeremni CA, Houck PR, Mulsant BH. Acupuncture for the treatment of major depressive disorder: a randomized controlled trial. *J Clin Psychiatry.* 2011;72(8):1129–35.

201. Zhang WJ, Yang XB, Zhong BL. Combination of acupuncture and fluoxetine for depression: a randomized, double-blind, sham-controlled trial. *J Altern Complement Med.* 2009;15(8):837–44.

202. Zhang ZJ, Chen HY, Yip KC, Ng R, Wong VT. The effectiveness and safety of acupuncture therapy in depressive disorders: systematic review and meta-analysis. *J Affect Disord.* 2010;124(1–2):9–21.

203. Qu SS, Huang Y, Zhang ZJ, et al. A 6-week randomized controlled trial with 4-week follow-up of acupuncture combined with paroxetine in patients with major depressive disorder. *J Psychiatr Res.* 2013;47(6):726–32.

204. Quah-Smith I, Smith C, Crawford JD, Russell J. Laser acupuncture for depression: a randomized double blind controlled trial using low intensity laser intervention. *J Affect Disord.* 2013;148(2–3):179–87.

205. Mischoulon D, Brill CD, Ameral VE, Fava M, Yeung AS. A pilot study of acupuncture monotherapy in patients with major depressive disorder. *J Affect Disord.* 2012;141(2–3):469–73.

206. MacPherson H, Richmond S, Bland M, et al. Acupuncture and counselling for depression in primary care: a randomised controlled trial. *PLoS Med.* 2013;10(9):e1001518.

207. Kolur US, Reddy YC, John JP, Kandavel T, Jain S. Sustained attention and executive functions in euthymic young people with bipolar disorder. *Br J Psychiatry.* 2006;189:453–8.

208. Strakowski SM, Adler CM, Holland SK, Mills N, DelBello MP. A preliminary fMRI study of sustained attention in euthymic, unmedicated bipolar disorder. *Neuropsychopharmacology.* 2004;29(9):1734–40.

209. Howells FM, Ives-Deliperi VL, Horn NR, Stein DJ. Mindfulness based cognitive therapy improves frontal control in bipolar disorder: a pilot EEG study. *BMC Psychiatry.* 2012;12:1–8.

210. Rubia K. The neurobiology of meditation and its clinical effectiveness in psychiatric disorders. *Biol Psychol.* 2009;82(1):1–11.

211. Davidson RJ, Kabat-Zinn J, Schumacher J, et al. Alterations in brain and immune function produced by mindfulness meditation. *Psychosom Med.* 2003;65:564–70.

212. Banasiewicz B, Kemper KJ. Integrative care for adolescent mood problems: brief report from a Pediatric Second Opinion Clinic. *Clin Pediatr (Phila).* 2013;52(1):89–91.

213. Qureshi NA, Al-Bedah AM. Mood disorders and complementary and alternative medicine: a literature review. *Neuropsychiatr Dis Treat* 2013;9:639–58.

Neurobiology of Bipolar Disorder

Section Editor: Stephen M. Strakowski

Neurobiology of Developing Bipolar Disorder

Jillian M. Russo, Sonja M. C. de Zwarte,
and Hilary P. Blumberg

Overview

Bipolar disorder is increasingly recognized to have a peak in onset during the adolescent years,[1,2] when dynamic maturational changes in neural systems involved in the disorder are also occurring, implicating shifts from healthy neurodevelopmental trajectories during adolescence in the disorder.[3] Support is provided by preliminary neuroimaging work that shows some brain differences that appear to be present in youths with bipolar disorder, and other differences that appear to progress during adolescence and young adulthood.

This chapter will examine neuroimaging data that support a developmental neurobiology that may contribute to the development of bipolar disorder. Brain regions implicated in bipolar disorder are discussed with regard to their developmental trajectories and evidence for alterations in their trajectories. The review will focus on neural systems that subserve regulation of emotional and motivational behaviors, as abnormalities in the regulation of these behaviors are the hallmark of bipolar disorder. This chapter will focus on three brain structures that are key in these systems and behaviors: the amygdala, ventral striatum, and ventral prefrontal cortex. In addition to evidence for abnormalities within these structures in mood disorders, increasing evidence suggests that abnormalities in the connections between these brain structures may be important in bipolar disorder, and thus the connections will also be a focus of this review.

Structural magnetic resonance imaging (sMRI), functional magnetic resonance imaging (fMRI), and diffusion tensor imaging (DTI) studies will be discussed in order to elucidate morphological, functional, and connectivity abnormalities implicated in the development of bipolar disorder in adolescence and the progression into adulthood. Additionally, the chapter will discuss data on individuals who have not yet developed bipolar disorder but who are at genetic risk owing to first-degree family members with bipolar disorder, as they may inform understanding of the relationship between brain abnormalities and vulnerability to developing the disorder. Data in individuals with bipolar disorder will also be compared to those in individuals with major depressive disorder, to discuss issues regarding specificity and diagnostic boundaries between mood disorders that may help to distinguish bipolar disorder from other disorders. Distinguishing bipolar disorder from major depressive disorder, especially early in the course of illness, is often difficult and is important in choosing appropriate interventions. Depressive episodes are often the presenting episodes of bipolar disorder in adolescence,[4] and misdiagnosis can lead to interventions that have the potential to worsen the course of bipolar disorder.[5-7] However, there is currently no marker to help to distinguish depressive episodes of bipolar disorder from depressive episodes of major depressive disorder.

Development of Brain Systems Implicated in Bipolar Disorder

The corticolimbic neural systems implicated in bipolar disorder undergo dynamic maturational changes during adolescence. As this coincides with a peak in the emergence of bipolar disorder, it implicates abnormalities in the developmental trajectories in these systems during adolescence in the development of bipolar disorder. Unfortunately, there is a paucity of data on the development of these systems in humans. Assumptions about development are often extrapolated from animal models and from findings in neighboring structures. For example, there has been more developmental research performed in the dorsolateral prefrontal cortex than in the ventral prefrontal cortex. Thus, prefrontal cortex developmental processes are inferred from those in dorsal regions, although how similar the processes are in the ventral prefrontal cortex is unclear. The little data that are available suggest that there are sequential aspects to neurodevelopment. Relative to subcortical structures, anterior cortical structures show more pronounced developmental changes later into development, as they continue to show very dynamic maturational changes during adolescence and early adulthood.

Studies of brain structure suggest that maturation progresses from more primitive subcortical brain structures to later evolving anterior cortical structures, subserving the development of higher executive control of behavior.[8,9] Maturation during adolescence includes the pruning of synaptic processes in the prefrontal cortex, resulting in the development of more refined and mature behavioral responses.[8] Chugani[10] and others[11] have also reported data supporting regional sequences of functional development consistent with this pattern: The ontogeny of regional brain activity follows phylogeny, with behavior increasingly dependent on prefrontal cortex activity and decreasingly on activity in the subcortical amygdala and ventral striatum. Thus, behavioral maturation shows increases in higher order adaptive control of emotions and impulses.

The sequential development within corticolimbic neural systems could influence when differences in specific brain regions, and behaviors associated with them, become evident in the progression of bipolar disorder. For example, the amygdala processes information about visual stimuli received from posterior visual cortices, associates the stimuli with emotional and motivational valence, and provides basic information to help decide whether to avoid a stimulus, if dangerous, or to approach it.[12-15] Additionally, the amygdala has specific cells that respond to emotional faces, stimuli critical to interpret early in development.[16] This function suggests disorders that display abnormalities in the processing of emotional stimuli, and particularly faces, may be indicative of abnormalities in the amygdala. As the amygdala is a subcortical structure, which processes basic aspects of the emotional stimuli, it is possible that amygdala abnormalities may be apparent relatively early in bipolar disorder.

The prefrontal cortex integrates information not only from the amygdala but also from posterior association, limbic, and anterior brain structures that provide experiential information about the emotional and motivational relevance of stimuli, and information about internal and external milieus, synthesized in the prefrontal cortex to provide more mature and adaptive executive feedback to regulate subcortical responses.[17,18] The prefrontal cortex and its executive functions continue to develop through adolescence and into early adulthood. Neuroimaging studies in humans are consistent with this pattern of sequential development. For example, sMRI studies have demonstrated predicted gray matter changes during adolescence and young adulthood.[19-21] FMRI studies have demonstrated an increase over adolescence and young adulthood in reliance on focused prefrontal cortex activity compared to subcortical activity, during emotion and motivation regulation, and goal-directed behavior.[3,22] These continued dynamic maturational changes during adolescence and young adulthood suggest that abnormalities in prefrontal cortex in bipolar disorder may not be fully expressed until this cortex has passed through these developmental stages. Therefore, differences in prefrontal cortex development between individuals with and without bipolar disorder may progress into late adolescence and early adulthood.

The prefrontal cortex shares substantial inhibitory connections with the amygdala and the ventral striatum, which can help the prefrontal cortex to apply "the brakes" to behaviors when they are not adaptive.[23] Although the basics of the internal structure and chemistry for these connections are completed before birth, connections between subcortical structures and the prefrontal cortex continue to develop through childhood and into adolescence and young adulthood, and may be influenced by postnatal experiences and activity within the connected regions.[24,25] Animal models have demonstrated continued sprouting of connections from the amygdala to prefrontal cortex throughout adolescence.[26] Human postmortem and neuroimaging studies have shown that the myelination of these connections continues through adolescence and into young adulthood, further into adulthood than the gray matter changes.[27–31] The substantial developmental changes in the connections over adolescence and young adulthood also suggest that if white matter connections are involved in the pathophysiology of bipolar disorder, they may particularly show changes in their expression during these epochs in the disorder.[20,21,26,32]

Summary

A peak in the emergence of bipolar disorder in adolescence coincides with the dynamic maturation of the prefrontal cortex and its connections during this period. Maturation of prefrontal cortex and subcortical-cortical connections is thought to continue after subcortical structures have passed through their major development phases. This pattern of development suggests that abnormalities within the subcortical, cortical, and connecting structures may become evident at different times in the progression of development of bipolar disorder from childhood to early adulthood. Neuroimaging findings in bipolar disorder will be reviewed later in the chapter, with particular attention to findings that may support these neurodevelopmental patterns in the disorder.

Neuroimaging Data in Developing Bipolar Disorder

This section will discuss neuroimaging data in bipolar disorder. Data from sMRI, fMRI, and then DTI will be reviewed. Findings in adults with bipolar disorder will be briefly reviewed first, followed by findings in youth that show continuities and discontinuities with the adult findings. Some brain circuitry characteristics appear to continue to progress into adulthood in bipolar disorder and seem to not emerge until later in the disorder, implicating developmental changes. Findings in adolescents at risk for bipolar disorder, and, finally, findings of similarities and differences with adolescents diagnosed with major depressive disorder will be presented. For each neuroimaging modality, first amygdala and ventral striatum findings that are seen more consistently early in the disorder will be reviewed, followed by findings in the prefrontal cortex that show more evidence for progression during adolescence and young adulthood in the disorder.

Structural Magnetic Resonance Imaging
Amygdala
Findings in Adults

Owing to its central role in processing emotional stimuli, the amygdala is one of the most studied brain structures in bipolar disorder. Although differences in amygdala structure in adults with bipolar disorder are widely reported, the direction of findings differs across studies. While smaller volumes in adults with bipolar disorder compared to healthy adults have been shown,[33,34] other studies have indicated an increase in amygdala volume.[35–37] One factor that might contribute to these discrepancies may be exposures to different medications and medications that research participants are taking at the time of scanning. For example, Savitz and colleagues[38] investigated amygdala structure in adults who were medicated and unmedicated. Compared to healthy comparison adults, unmedicated adults with bipolar disorder had significantly smaller amygdala, while medicated adults with bipolar disorder trended toward having larger amygdala. Inconsistencies in findings in amygdala in adults with bipolar disorder could also be due to additional heterogeneities in subject samples, such as in clinical subtypes, number of mood episodes, and/or in MRI methodologies.

Findings in Adolescents

In a study of adolescents and adults with bipolar disorder, both age groups showed decreased amygdala gray matter volume.[34] Factors underlying differences between the findings for adults in this study from previous reports are not clear. However, one difference among studies is that this study has fewer subjects who had experienced psychotic symptoms than some of the studies that found increases in amygdala volume.

In contrast to the variable findings in adults with bipolar disorder, the decreased amygdala volume found in adolescents with bipolar disorder is one of the most replicated findings in studies of the disorder.[34,39–42] This decrease in amygdala volume has been demonstrated across different mood states at time of scanning.[34,39,40] It is possible that early-onset bipolar disorder has morphological features in the amygdala that differ from those in later onset, and that inclusion of varying proportions of early- and later onset bipolar disorder across the studies might be contributing to variability among findings in adults.[43]

Although the observation of amygdala findings in adolescents with bipolar disorder suggests that a difference in amygdala structure may be a relatively early abnormality in bipolar disorder, the decreases were observed in adolescents who had already experienced an episode of the disorder. Therefore, it is not clear whether structural abnormalities in amygdala are related to vulnerability to developing bipolar disorder or are a result of episodes. Some studies suggest that amygdala volume abnormalities may continue to progress after illness onset with repeated episodes, resulting in decreased volume after the initial presentation of manic symptoms.[44] For example, Bitter et al.[45] studied adolescents during a first manic or mixed episode and again 1 year later. Initially, there was no difference in amygdala volume among subjects with bipolar disorder, attention-deficit/hyperactivity disorder, and healthy comparison adolescents. However, at 1-year follow up, subjects with bipolar disorder had a significant bilateral decrease and/or failure to display a developmentally appropriate increase in volume, as suggested by comparisons to the other two groups.[45] Geller et al.[46] also found decreasing amygdala volume with age in adolescents with bipolar disorder, relative to volume in healthy comparison adolescents. This finding suggests that there may be progression in amygdala abnormalities following manic episodes. A small longitudinal study, conducted over a 2-year period, suggested that amygdala volume decreases in bipolar disorder are retained once the size decrease is established.[47] The longitudinal studies taken together suggest that amygdala volume loss may occur during early episodes, perhaps corresponding to interepisode shortening that can occur during the first five to ten episodes. More study is needed to clarify the extent to which amygdala volume differences in adolescence remain consistent or progresses over development, particularly early in the course of the disorder.

There is also suggestion that mood-stabilizing medications may have potential to reverse structural abnormalities in the amygdala in youths. For example, Chang et al.[40] noted that children and adolescents with bipolar disorder had smaller amygdala gray matter volume than youths without the disorder; however, the volumes were larger if the youths with bipolar disorder had past lithium or valproate exposure. This observation raises the possibility that certain mood-stabilizing medications may protect against structural atrophy. It also suggests that medications may contribute to variable findings in adolescents. However, one study of children at risk for bipolar disorder with subdiagnostic mood symptoms, treated with divalproex monotherapy for 12 weeks did not demonstrate any changes in amygdala volume.[48] It is unclear whether this is related to dosing or duration of treatment and/or youths studied not yet having developed the disorder.

Evidence suggests a relationship between amygdala volume decreases and amygdala dysfunction in bipolar disorder. Kalmar et al.[42] showed that amygdala volumes in adolescents with bipolar disorder were significantly smaller when compared to healthy control adolescents. Furthermore, the study revealed an inverse relationship between volume and activity such that adolescents with the smallest volumes showed the most excessive responses to emotional stimuli. This finding suggests possible pathological processes that could result in this association, such as decreases in inhibitory neurons or excessive glutamatergic inputs that could be neurotoxic.[42] Functional neuroimaging findings will be discussed further in the next section.

Findings in Individuals at Risk for Bipolar Disorder

An approach to elucidate whether amygdala structural abnormalities are associated with risk for bipolar disorder is to assess individuals who are at elevated risk because they have a first-degree relative with bipolar disorder. Initial studies of children and adolescents at risk for bipolar disorder, including children who have already shown some signs of mood dysfunction although not full-blown manic episodes, did not detect statistically significant differences in amygdala volume.[49,50] Ladouceur and colleagues[51] found a trend toward an increase in amygdala size in at-risk adolescents. It is important to note that these adolescents were free of any Axis I disorder, and follow-up information for which adolescents developed bipolar disorder is not known, suggesting that this may be an emotionally resilient group.

Comparison to Findings in Individuals With Major Depressive Disorder

Comparing findings in adolescents with bipolar disorder to those in adolescents with major depressive disorder can suggest abnormalities that may be specific to the development of bipolar disorder. However, studies of adolescents with major depressive disorder have yielded inconsistent results. One study of unmedicated young women experiencing their first episode of major depressive disorder demonstrated amygdala volume decreases.[52] In studying children and adolescents with major depressive disorder, MacMillan and colleagues[53] instead found increases in amygdala volume; however, these results did not account for age and intracranial volume. MacMaster et al.[54] did not find significant reductions in amygdala volume in children and adolescents with major depressive disorder, but they did find reductions in hippocampus. Findings in hippocampus in bipolar disorder are variable, possibly owing to genetically separable subtypes within the disorder.[55] A study of youths with bipolar disorder did show decreases in hippocampus volume that might also depend on gender, with females displaying smaller volumes.[56] Overall, however, the literature suggests that hippocampus volume abnormalities are less consistent than amygdala abnormalities in bipolar disorder[34] and may be more consistent in major depressive disorder[57] and/or especially associated with exposure to stress.[58] Direct comparisons between individuals with bipolar disorder and with major depressive disorder are needed to better assess specificity of structural findings.

Summary

The amygdala is a main brain region of interest in bipolar disorder owing to its early and important role in emotional processing. Due to its early maturation compared to cortical regions, it may demonstrate changes early in bipolar disorder and thus be helpful for early detection. This suggestion is, to some degree, supported by the literature. Whereas studies of adults with bipolar disorder have shown inconsistent results in regard to volume increases or decreases in the amygdala, studies of adolescents with bipolar disorder have predominantly shown a decrease in amygdala volume. A study of at-risk youth who developed bipolar disorder suggests that decreased amygdala volume may be associated with risk for developing the disorder in adolescence. Longitudinal studies of youths with bipolar disorder differ in whether amygdala volume changes are detected over time. Differences in volumes in youths with bipolar disorder related to medication exposures, and the variable findings in adults, suggest that there are multiple factors that may influence amygdala volume in the disorder. In addition, there have been few direct comparisons of amygdala volume between groups with bipolar disorder and groups with other disorders, such as major depressive disorder, to assess the specificity of amygdala findings to bipolar disorder. Longitudinal studies are needed to compare adolescents with bipolar disorder and at risk for bipolar disorder to those with other disorders, which also include examination of factors that may influence amygdala volume development.

Ventral Striatum

Findings in Adults and Adolescents

The ventral striatum has not yet been as well researched in individuals with bipolar disorder as structures such as the amygdala. However, bipolar disorder researchers have interest in this brain region because the ventral striatum plays a role in motivational behaviors that are characteristically dysregulated in bipolar disorder, such as the impulsive pursuit of reward in mania and anhedonic loss of pleasure from rewarding behaviors in depression.[59] There are few studies of bipolar disorder that have focused on the ventral striatum and findings are variable. In a study of medication-naïve adults with bipolar disorder, volume differences were not detected; however, shape differences were detected,[60] suggesting morphological abnormalities. One study did demonstrate a decrease in left nucleus accumbens in children and adolescents with bipolar disorder.[41] However, in the majority of studies, differences in basal ganglia structures were not detected, and some studies reported increases in varying basal ganglia regions.[39,40,56,61–65]

The striatum may be especially sensitive to factors such as course features and exposures, including medication exposure. For example, in adults with bipolar disorder, Brambilla et al.[66] found an inverse relationship between the length of illness and the size of the left putamen. There is a body of literature supporting striatal volume increases in association with antipsychotic medications,[67,68] often used in the treatment of bipolar disorder. Neuroimaging studies specific to the ventral striatum are especially challenging to perform because the ventral striatum is a small structure with boundaries that are challenging to delineate on MRI images.

Findings in Individuals at Risk for Bipolar Disorder

The ventral striatum has also been investigated in at-risk adolescents and adults. Singh and colleagues[49] did not detect significant differences in striatum in children with subthreshold mood symptoms who had at least one parent with bipolar disorder. However, another study indicated a decrease in caudate volume in adolescents at risk for bipolar disorder.[51] Investigations of adults at risk for bipolar disorder have also shown variable results. Studies of affected and unaffected twins have shown larger left caudate volumes in both groups, compared to twin pairs without bipolar disorder,[69,70] while studies of adult siblings of individuals with bipolar disorder have shown reduced ventral striatum volume.[71] In a study of at-risk adolescents and young adults, subjects showed significantly larger caudate volumes, compared to low-risk subjects.[72] However, there was no difference in putamen volumes among these subjects, perhaps as a result of protective effects of medications.[72]

Comparison to Findings in Individuals With Major Depressive Disorder

Matsuo and colleagues[73] investigated striatal volume in medication-naïve adolescents with major depressive disorder. They found smaller right striatum volumes in the adolescents with major depressive disorder, when compared to healthy comparison adolescents. Striatal volume was also found to be inversely correlated with severity of depressive symptoms, indicating that striatal abnormalities may be present early in major depressive disorder and related to severity.[73] Adult studies have shown varied results, perhaps due to gender and medication response. Lacerda and colleagues,[74] for example, found no significant differences in striatal volumes between adults with and without major depressive disorder. On the other hand, other studies have indicated that women with major depressive disorder display decreased gray matter in the caudate, perhaps because of medication that may protect against a volume reduction.[75,76]

Summary

The ventral striatum is implicated in bipolar disorder due to the motivational abnormalities implicated in both mania and depression. However, studies in adolescents and adults with bipolar disorder and at risk for bipolar disorder have produced variable results. It is also unclear whether study findings of striatal involvement will be specific to bipolar disorder. The study of ventral striatum is an area where relatively little work has been done and more research is needed.

Prefrontal Cortex
Findings in Adults

The prefrontal cortex has long been implicated in bipolar disorder. Ventral and medial prefrontal cortex lesions have long been noted to produce symptoms that are similar to those of bipolar disorder, such as euphoric states and impulsiveness, as well as those of depressive states.[77,78] As noted above, the ventral prefrontal cortex has major connections to the amygdala, ventral striatum, and other corticolimbic regions implicated in bipolar disorder; ventral prefrontal cortex regulates their activity and, therefore, the emotional and motivational behaviors subserved by these fronto-subcortical limbic neural systems. The ventral prefrontal cortex is thus another region that has received much attention in bipolar disorder. Studies have varied widely as to how ventral prefrontal cortex regions have been delineated. For the purposes of this chapter, frontal regions that are ventral to the anterior commissure-posterior commissure plane, including orbitofrontal cortex (Brodmann areas [BAs] 11, 47), ventral anterior cingulate cortex (BAs 24, 25, 32), and ventral parts of rostral prefrontal cortex (BA 10), will be discussed together as ventral prefrontal cortex regions.

Volume decreases in ventral prefrontal cortex regions have been seen most consistently in adults with bipolar disorder. Drevets et al.[79] provided an early report of a reduction in ventral anterior cingulate cortex gray matter volume in adults with bipolar disorder. Since that time there have been multiple reports of decreases in frontal gray matter volume in adults with bipolar disorder in regions including ventral anterior cingulate cortex, orbitofrontal cortex, and inferior prefrontal cortex.[21,80–82] However, there have been several reports of either increases or no differences in frontal gray matter volume.[83,84]

Findings of prefrontal cortex volume in adults with bipolar disorder in association with mood-stabilizing medications, taken together with preclinical findings of neurotrophic and neuroprotective effects of medications,[85,86] suggest the potential for medications to reverse volume decreases. Consistent with this, Sassi and colleagues[82] studied medicated and unmedicated adults with bipolar disorder and found that only the unmedicated participants displayed a decrease in anterior cingulate cortex volume. A similar finding was demonstrated by Blumberg et al.[21] in the ventral prefrontal cortex in bipolar disorder, in which gray matter volume was significantly higher in individuals with bipolar disorder who were taking mood-stabilizing medications at the time of scanning than in those who were unmedicated. Neurotrophic and neuroprotective effects are especially implicated for lithium. Moore et al.[87] reported increases in cortical gray matter in individuals with bipolar disorder after 4 weeks of lithium treatment. Bearden and colleagues[88] conducted a study that investigated differences in a group with bipolar disorder treated with lithium for at least 2 weeks, a bipolar disorder group with no lithium treatment for a month, and a healthy comparison group. Their study revealed larger anterior cingulate cortex volumes in the group that had received lithium, compared to the two other groups. However, it remains unclear whether the effects observed on MRI scans during the short time frame of treatment with lithium represent volume changes.[89]

Findings in Adolescents

Findings in adolescents with bipolar disorder in the prefrontal cortex have been more variable, perhaps attributable, at least in part, to the dynamic developmental changes that continue in the prefrontal cortex during adolescence and early adulthood. As suggested above, during development, prefrontal cortex morphology in adolescents and young adults with and without bipolar disorder may continue to diverge and differences may be more difficult to detect until later in adolescence/young adulthood. For example, some studies of youths with bipolar disorder have found no differences in ventral prefrontal cortex volume,[41,90,91] while others have found decreases in areas such as the left anterior cingulate cortex and the orbitofrontal cortex.[63,92,93] However, mood stabilizers may increase cingulate volume in adolescents with bipolar disorder.[94] Najt and colleagues[95] found gender-related differences in children and adolescents, with males showing decreases in volume in ventral prefrontal cortex regions and females showing increases. These findings raise the possibility of interactions among the emergence of ventral prefrontal cortex differences in the disorder, age, and gender.

Blumberg et al.[21] reported ventral prefrontal cortex decreases in young adults with bipolar disorder but not in adolescents with bipolar disorder. They suggested that developmental changes in bipolar disorder might interact through adolescence so that the full extent of differences might not manifest until young adulthood. Their group reported on a small longitudinal study in which adolescents and young adults with and without bipolar disorder were scanned twice over an approximately 2-year period.[96] Individuals with bipolar disorder showed significantly more decreases in prefrontal cortex volume over the 2-year period than the individuals without bipolar disorder. The progressive differences were seen in rostral regions of ventral prefrontal cortex. The investigators suggested that the differences in the rostroventral regions might manifest relatively later in bipolar disorder than other regions such as amygdala. Volume loss over time in prefrontal cortex areas was also reported in other studies of adolescents and young adults with bipolar disorder.[97,98]

Recently, Wang et al.[99] performed a study of 41 adolescents with bipolar disorder and found gray matter volume decreases in a subset of anterior paralimbic regions termed the olfactocentric paralimbic cortices, which includes the orbitofrontal cortex, as well as the insula and temporopolar cortex. If this area of cortex was unfolded, these structures can be noted to be one continuous area of cortex. Notably, these structures are thought to develop together, sharing similar cytoarchitectural features in transitioning from agranular to granular cortex. They are strongly interconnected, as well as being highly connected with the amygdala and hypothalamus, and subserve emotional processes.[100] Thus, the olfactocentric paralimbic cortex structures are highly implicated in bipolar disorder. Little is known about the development of this cortex. Future studies will be very important in understanding the development of these regions and implications for mood disorders. Taken together with the findings noted above, the olfactocentric paralimbic cortex findings suggest that there may be a progression in the appearance of cortical abnormalities in bipolar disorder with the olfactocentric paralimbic cortex abnormalities manifesting prior to ones in more rostral, heteromodal prefrontal cortex regions.

Findings in Individuals at Risk for Bipolar Disorder

The progressive differences, especially in more rostral prefrontal cortex areas, suggest that prefrontal cortex structural abnormalities may emerge later than subcortical abnormalities. Therefore, prefrontal cortex abnormalities may be more difficult to detect early in the disorder, as well as in younger individuals with vulnerability to bipolar disorder. Some studies involving family members of those with bipolar disorder are consistent with the notion that ventral prefrontal cortex abnormalities may progress over time in the disorder. For example, Singh et al.[49] did not detect statistically significant differences in prefrontal cortex volumes in at-risk children. Similarly, Gogtay et al.[98] noted that at-risk youth did not show anterior cingulate cortex volume decreases until after the first manic episode. However, there is a study of unaffected adult siblings of adults with bipolar disorder that shows deficits in the anterior cingulate cortex,[71] indicating that differential development of anterior cingulate cortex structure into adulthood may be associated with bipolar disorder.

Comparison of Findings in Individuals With Major Depressive Disorder

Although ventral prefrontal cortex volume decreases in adults with bipolar disorder have been consistently reported, ventral prefrontal cortex volume findings in adolescents and adults with major depressive disorder are more variable. In addition to ventral anterior cingulate cortex gray matter decreases observed in bipolar disorder, Drevets et al.[79] also observed ventral anterior cingulate cortex similar decreases in major depressive disorder. Frontal volume decreases have been observed by subsequent research groups, such as in a study of treatment-naïve women with major depressive disorder.[52] Reduction in orbitofrontal cortex volumes is seen in some adult major depressive disorder samples.[101–103] However, some studies indicated no significant differences in ventral prefrontal cortex structures in major depressive disorder.[104–106] In adolescents, there does not seem to be a significant difference in ventral prefrontal cortex volume in major depressive disorder.[107] As suggested in bipolar disorder, this could be due to continued frontal development in adolescents. Therefore, it is unclear whether it will be possible to distinguish ventral prefrontal cortex volume abnormalities in adolescents with bipolar disorder and major depressive disorder; however, direct comparisons between the diagnostic groups are needed.

Summary

The ventral prefrontal cortex is highly implicated in bipolar disorder, as it is responsible for regulation of subcortical structures resulting in situationally appropriate emotional responses. Results in adults have been consistent in indicating decreases in ventral prefrontal cortex gray matter volume in bipolar disorder. However, studies with adolescents with bipolar disorder have shown varied findings. This may be due, at least in part, to continual development of the prefrontal cortex into late adolescence/early adulthood. Preliminary findings suggest that there may be a progression in the appearance of abnormalities in cortical regions from olfactocentric paralimbic cortices regions to more rostral heteromodal regions in bipolar disorder. There is also a suggestion that abnormalities in prefrontal cortex development progressing into adulthood may be related to vulnerability for bipolar disorder. However, these are early findings in a relatively young field. A great deal more work needs to be performed, particularly research studies with longitudinal designs. Findings of increased prefrontal cortex volume in association with mood-stabilizing medication suggest that volume decreases might be reversible. Moreover, as prefrontal cortex differences may be continuing to progress during adolescence and as the prefrontal cortex is quite plastic during that period, it is possible that future interventions may be able to halt the progression of prefrontal cortex abnormalities and thus improve prognosis and someday help to prevent bipolar disorder.

Functional Magnetic Resonance Imaging
Amygdala

As disturbances in emotional regulation are characteristic of bipolar disorder, and the amygdala is essential to the processing of emotional stimuli, a focus of functional neuroimaging research in bipolar disorder has been the study of amygdala responses to emotional stimuli. Different types of emotion-related tasks have been used in functional neuroimaging studies, such as ones that include the viewing of emotional scenes and/ or methods to induce differing emotional states, such as recalling personally evocative situations. Faces are evolutionarily strong automatic elicitors of emotional responses, and the amygdala is important in processing emotional faces. As abnormalities in processing emotional faces are one of the most frequent neurobehavioral findings reported in studies of youths with bipolar disorder,[108–110] scanning tasks that include presentation of faces depicting emotional expressions have been particularly fruitful in eliciting functional differences in the amygdala between individuals with and without bipolar disorder.

Findings in Adults

Studies in adults with bipolar disorder have been relatively consistent in showing increases in amygdala responses to emotional stimuli, including both emotional faces and scenes standardized to elicit particular emotional responses.[47,111–115] Increased amygdala responses have been observed in response to negative emotional stimuli.[115,116] However, there have also been reports of decreases[117] or of no differences[118] in amygdala responses.

Increased amygdala responses have been demonstrated to be especially robust for positive face stimuli in adults with bipolar disorder.[47,113,119,120] Such increases in response to positive emotional stimuli have been reported less commonly in other mood disorders than abnormalities in responses to negative emotional stimuli. Abnormalities observed in response to positive emotional stimuli in bipolar disorder have been suggested to be a potential marker for bipolar disorder, as vulnerability to extremes in positive emotional states and disinhibited responses to positive stimuli are characteristic of elevated emotional states.[47,113,119]

In some of the studies of adults with bipolar disorder, the increased responses to emotional stimuli were observed across mood states, including euthymia,[47,113,121] suggesting that the increased amygdala responses might be a trait feature of the disorder. However, there have been studies in which amygdala differences have not been detected in adults with bipolar disorder during euthymia.[122] Factors observed to influence amygdala responses might have contributed to the differences across the studies. For example, a preliminary study suggested that mood-stabilizing medication, and potentially anticonvulsant treatments in particular, may blunt excesses in amygdala responses in bipolar disorder.[47] This finding is especially of interest as it is potentially consistent with early mesial temporal sensitization models of bipolar disorder that led to anticonvulsants trials for bipolar disorder, as anticonvulsants reduce sensitization.[123]

Findings in Adolescents

Consistent with the studies of bipolar disorder in adults, fMRI studies of youths with bipolar disorder in which they perform face-processing tasks have shown excessive amygdala responses across mood states of the disorders,[42,124–126] although there also have been negative reports.[118,127] As in the adult studies, functional amygdala findings in adolescents with bipolar disorder have included increases observed during the processing of faces depicting positive and negative expressions.[42,120,128] The findings were detected when fMRI was performed during viewing tasks that required minimal cognitive effort; however, differences were less in some studies in which the fMRI activation tasks required more cognitive effort that could have inhibited amygdala responses and minimized amygdala activation. There may be particular abnormalities in youths with bipolar disorder in association with processing emotions when they are depicted on faces, as there was no difference in amygdala activation observed between adolescents with and without bipolar disorder when presented with nonfacial emotional stimuli.[129]

Increased amygdala responses to emotional faces as an early trait feature of bipolar disorder is further supported by a treatment study by Passarotti et al.[130] They scanned youths with bipolar disorder who presented in manic and hypomanic states before and after treatment with lamotrigine. Although the youths showed symptom improvement and there were changes in other brain regions, elevated amygdala responses to emotional faces persisted after the treatment.

Findings in Individuals at Risk

A study of unaffected adults with a family history of bipolar disorder, showing heightened amygdala responses to happy faces, suggests that the elevated responses to positive emotional faces may be related to vulnerability to the disorder.[131] Olsavsky and colleagues[132] reported on a study of a group of 13 at-risk children and adolescents for whom they found increased amygdala responses while the youths rated their feelings of fear when viewing fearful faces; yet differences were not observed when happy faces were viewed. It is possible that the responses to happy faces as a vulnerability factor develop later; however, the small sample size, which included preadolescents and adolescents and family members who themselves were still youths, could have influenced findings. Additionally, as above, the type of task performed might have influenced the findings.[132] In the study of adults in which amygdala differences were elicited,[131] the subjects viewed faces while performing a task orthogonal to emotional experience, that is, a gender determination. In the study of youths,[132] the task was more effortful and required the youths to assess their emotional reactions to the faces, which may have brought online other structures such as the prefrontal cortex, potentially blunting amygdala responses. The relationship of amygdala functioning to functioning of prefrontal cortex structures may be important in adolescents with the disorder. For example, one study of adolescents at risk for bipolar disorder found decreased modulation of the amygdala to emotional stimuli by the ventral prefrontal cortex.[133]

Comparison to Findings in Individuals With Major Depressive Disorder

Increases in amygdala responses are not specific to bipolar disorder; however, some features of the increases in amygdala responses may be more pronounced in the disorder.[47,113,119] For example, increases in amygdala responses to negative emotional stimuli have been shown across several disorders. They have been noted in response to negative stimuli, but not to positive stimuli, in adults and adolescents with major depressive disorder.[134–136] Lawrence et al.[113] compared 12 adults with bipolar disorder to 9 adults with major depressive disorder. They found increases in amygdala responses to negative and positive face stimuli in the bipolar disorder group, compared to responses in both the major depressive disorder group and a healthy comparison group. Notably, Grotegerd et al.[136] compared individuals with bipolar disorder directly to individuals with major depressive disorder and found that those with bipolar disorder showed amygdala increases in response to positive emotional stimuli, whereas in major depressive disorder there were increases in response to negative emotional stimuli. Although this initial study also had a modest sample size of 10 subjects in each diagnostic group, it suggests that differences in amygdala responses to emotional stimuli of particular valences may help to differentiate the disorders.

Summary

The amygdala is responsible for processing emotional stimuli and plays a key role in processing emotional faces, which is implicated as an early abnormality in bipolar disorder. Therefore, emotional stimuli are often presented in fMRI tasks in order to assess amygdala activation. Multiple studies have shown excesses in amygdala responses in adults and adolescents with bipolar disorder. Furthermore, increased amygdala response has been reported across mood states and has been seen in unaffected individuals at risk for bipolar disorder, indicating it may be a trait of the disorder. In comparison to individuals with major depressive disorder, individuals with bipolar disorder display excessive amygdala activation when presented with positive faces. Abnormal amygdala activation to positive emotional stimuli is one of the few candidate neural differences that may help to distinguish bipolar disorder from major depressive disorder. However, amygdala response is sensitive to stimulus types and other factors such as medication, and its specificity to disorders is not clear. Emerging neuroimaging methods may help to elucidate the role of the amygdala within bipolar disorder and as compared to other disorders. For example, studies are emerging in which the function of amygdala subregions can be studied,[137] and methods are used in which fMRI and other imaging modalities are paired, such as in the structure-function work of Kalmar et al.[42] These approaches may help to elucidate more specific subregions and types of pathologies involved in the amygdala in bipolar disorder.

Ventral Striatum

Findings in Adults

As with the sMRI investigations, there are fewer fMRI studies reported that have focused on functioning of the ventral striatum, as compared to the amygdala and ventral prefrontal cortex. A positron emission tomography (PET) study indicated increased caudate activity in manic subjects with bipolar disorder[138] in subjects at rest during scanning. Findings in studies of emotional face processing in bipolar disorder have been reported in striatal structures, further implicating their involvement; however, findings have primarily been of decreased activation. For example, in the study by Lawrence et al.[113] when presented with mildly happy faces, adults with bipolar disorder displayed increased striatum activation relative to major depressive disorder and healthy comparison subjects. In another study, euthymic subjects showed significant decreased putamen responses when presented with emotional faces.[122] A recent study showed decreases in ventral striatum responses to faces depicting both happy and neutral expressions in adults with bipolar disorder that were not influenced by mood state.[137] Hassel et al.[139,140] have reported increases in striatum responses, especially to happy face stimuli, in adults with bipolar disorder who were euthymic at scanning. It was noted that the findings were not influenced by medications; however, striatal findings were particularly evident in the adults who also had substance use disorders. This observation is of interest especially as the striatum is implicated in motivational states involved in substance use disorders and has shown abnormalities in individuals with substance use disorders without bipolar disorder. This finding also suggests that substance use is one possible source of heterogeneity across the studies. Further study of striatal function in adults with bipolar disorder, especially in relation to mood states, and with attention to comorbidity, is needed.

Findings in Adolescents

Studies with adolescents have tended to show increases in activation in the striatum. Dickstein and colleagues[141] investigated adolescents with bipolar disorder who were euthymic, hypomanic, and depressed at the time of scanning. Compared to healthy comparison adolescents, adolescents with bipolar disorder had increased striatal responses when encoding happy faces.[141] Chang et al.[129] also found an increase in caudate responses to positively valenced pictures. Other investigators studying adolescents with bipolar disorder have found increases in responses of the nucleus accumbens and the putamen to hostile and fearful faces,[124] as well as abnormalities in striatum responses during cognitive tasks. The latter includes increases particularly during tasks that require the inhibition of maladaptive responses and that were associated with depressive symptoms.[142–144] These findings suggest that striatal dysfunction may be an important aspect of bipolar disorder in adolescents. However, few studies included methods designed specifically to study ventral striatum function, which could be an important focus for future research.

Findings in Individuals at Risk

There has been little study of the role of the ventral striatum in individuals at risk for bipolar disorder. Studies that assessed striatal functioning during tasks that involve adaptive behavioral inhibition and cognitive flexibility found that at-risk youths showed elevated striatal responses, compared to healthy comparison youths.[145,146] The frequent observation of behavioral disinhibition in youths with bipolar disorder suggests that further study of striatal function in at-risk youths may also provide insights into the development of the disorder.

Comparison to Findings to Individuals With Major Depressive Disorder

In contrast to findings in bipolar disorder, in which striatal dysfunction tends to vary in direction, findings in major depressive disorder tend to be in the direction of decreases in responses. In particular, perhaps reflecting the more consistent tendencies for amotivational and anhedonic states, major depressive disorder is especially associated with decreased ventral striatum responses to positive emotional stimuli. Differences in responses to positive emotional stimuli between bipolar disorder and major depressive disorder were noted in the direct comparison between groups with bipolar disorder and with major depressive disorder by Lawrence and colleagues.[113] They found increased responses in bipolar disorder but decreases in responses in major depressive disorder in the striatum when individuals were presented with happy faces.[113] Individuals with major depressive disorder display a decrease in caudate responses in anticipation to positive rewards.[147,148] Additionally, striatum decreases in major depressive disorder have been noted to be "normalized" by antidepressant medication.[149,150] Taken together with the findings in bipolar disorder, these findings suggest the possibility that the direction of abnormalities in striatum responses might relate to the tendency toward both elevated and depressed mood states in bipolar disorder and toward depressed states in major depressive disorder, and that abnormalities might be influenced by treatment. However, this is speculative and more studies are very much needed in this area.

Summary

There has been limited research focusing on functioning of the ventral striatum in bipolar disorder. While results have varied in direction, ventral striatal dysfunction has been reported in numerous studies of both adults and adolescents with bipolar disorder. Reports in bipolar disorder have varied in direction, while reports in disorders such as major depressive disorder have been more consistently of decreases. Much more work is needed; ventral striatal responses to stimuli of positive or negative valence may help to identify tendencies toward particular types of episodes. However, little work has been performed to assess factors that may contribute to differing findings, and factors such as mood state and medication may be important influences.

Prefrontal Cortex

As suggested above, dysfunction in the ventral prefrontal cortex has been implicated in bipolar disorder, as ventral prefrontal cortex lesions appear to result in difficulties responding adaptively to changing emotional states and motivational situations.[151,152] This injury may lead to inappropriate disinhibited manic-like or inappropriate inhibited depressive symptoms.[153–155]

Findings in Adults

Findings across studies of adults with bipolar disorder are highly convergent in demonstrating dysfunction in ventral prefrontal cortex regions, although results differ across studies in the specific subregions and directions of findings.[122,137,156–158] Studies have reported both increases and decreases in prefrontal cortex activation during emotion face processing tasks during both manic and depressed states of bipolar disorder.[115,159,160] The emotions depicted by the face stimuli and the mood state of the subjects may have contributed to discrepancies. For example, Liu and colleagues[137] investigated state and trait characteristic in adults with bipolar disorder. Results indicated a decrease in ventral anterior cingulate cortex and orbitofrontal cortex activation to happy and neutral faces regardless of mood state, suggesting these may be trait characteristics. Additionally, subjects with an elevated mood displayed a decrease in right rostral prefrontal cortex responses to fearful and neutral faces, while those who were depressed displayed an increase in left orbitofrontal cortex to fearful faces, suggesting that these are mood-state-related bipolar disorder features. An earlier study conducted by the same research group supported a similar lateralization of prefrontal cortex activation based on mood state that was detected during a task requiring inhibition of prepotent responses.[157] Other studies have also shown that, when processing positive and negative emotional stimuli, adults with bipolar disorder displayed a decrease in ventral anterior cingulate cortex and ventral prefrontal cortex activation regardless of mood state at time of scanning.[47,79,117,161] These studies suggest that frontal dysfunction has both trait- and state-related features in bipolar disorder.

Preliminary studies suggest that medications might reverse ventral prefrontal cortex functional abnormalities of the disorder. In a preliminary report, Blumberg et al.[47] noted decreases in responses to emotional face stimuli in the ventral anterior cingulate cortex in adults with bipolar disorder who were unmedicated, but not in adults with bipolar disorder who were taking mood-stabilizing medications, suggesting that medications may "normalize" ventral anterior cingulate cortex function in bipolar disorder. Mah and colleagues[162] found an increase in anterior cingulate cortex in adults with bipolar disorder who were currently being treated with lithium. Similar results were seen in depressed adults with bipolar disorder after lamotrigine treatment.[163] Studies are needed to further investigate the effects of medications on circuitry dysfunction in bipolar disorder, including ones with larger samples and systematic study of specific medications.

Findings in Adolescents

Findings from studies of prefrontal cortex function in adolescents with bipolar disorder have differed, which may be due, at least in part, to continuing maturation of this brain region during adolescence, as discussed in the sections on structural imaging earlier. In a preliminary fMRI study in adolescents with bipolar disorder, differences were not detected in the ventral prefrontal cortex in adolescents with bipolar disorder during performance of a task requiring inhibition of prepotent responses.[142] In that study, the healthy adolescents showed increases in rostral ventral prefrontal cortex responses with age, whereas these increases were not observed in the adolescents with bipolar disorder. The authors suggested that rostral ventral prefrontal cortex functional abnormalities may progress during adolescence,[47,142] diverging over time during this epoch. However, some studies have shown abnormalities in responses of ventral prefrontal cortex in adolescents with bipolar disorder during emotional face processing.[124,125,128,129,164] As with adults, results have differed in direction and the type of stimuli that elicited functional abnormalities. For example, Ladouceur and colleagues[125] found increased ventral prefrontal cortex activation to happy faces in adolescents who had a history of manic episodes, while Rich et al.[124] found increased activation when adolescents with bipolar disorder were viewing hostile faces. It is possible that methods, such as use of emotional tasks during scanning, may provide increased sensitivity to detecting ventral prefrontal cortex dysfunction in adolescents with bipolar disorder.

Medication may also have an effect on prefrontal cortex activity in adolescents with bipolar disorder. Pavuluri and colleagues[165] investigated the effects of risperidone and divalproex on brain activation to emotional faces in manic adolescents. At baseline, the adolescents in the two medication groups did not differ. At 6-week follow-up, adolescents in the risperidone group displayed an increase in anterior cingulate cortex responses to angry faces, compared to the divalproex and healthy comparison groups. Both medication groups showed increases in ventral prefrontal cortex responses to angry faces, compared to the healthy comparison adolescents. When viewing happy faces, the only significant difference was an increase in right ventral prefrontal cortex in the risperidone group, compared to healthy comparison adolescents.[165] This suggests that medications may have differing effects on prefrontal cortex responses to different types of emotional stimuli in adolescents with bipolar disorder.

Findings in Individuals at Risk

There are few studies investigating prefrontal cortex functioning during emotional tasks in individuals at risk for bipolar disorder. Similar to findings in adults with bipolar disorder, at-risk adults showed increased responses to happy and fearful faces.[131] When presented with positive facial stimuli, adolescents who are at risk also showed ventral prefrontal cortex activation abnormalities,[133] similar to findings in adolescents with bipolar disorder. Therefore, ventral prefrontal cortex dysfunction may be an early trait feature of bipolar disorder. More studies with at-risk populations are needed in order to draw further conclusions about ventral prefrontal cortex dysfunction in risk for bipolar disorder and the timing at which ventral prefrontal cortex dysfunction emerges.

Comparison to Findings in Individuals With Major Depressive Disorder

Studies of individuals with major depressive disorder suggest that they may show differences in their patterns of ventral prefrontal cortex dysfunction, compared to individuals with bipolar disorder. Adults with major depressive disorder differ from adults with bipolar disorder in their responses to negative, and especially positive emotional face stimuli.[113] When presented with fearful face stimuli, increases in left ventral prefrontal cortex responses have been observed in depression in bipolar disorder,[137] while decreases have been noted in major depressive disorder.[166] A study that used machine learning methods suggested abnormalities in ventral prefrontal cortex responses to neutral face stimuli when individuals with bipolar disorder are presented together with happy face stimuli, but not when presented with fearful face stimuli, may distinguish between individuals with bipolar disorder or major depressive disorder.[167]

Summary

Adults with bipolar disorder have consistently shown dysfunction in ventral prefrontal cortex, although both activation increases and decreases in prefrontal cortex regions have been reported. Some ventral prefrontal cortex functional abnormalities may be related to the bipolar disorder trait, whereas others may differ depending on mood state. The types of abnormalities elicited by stimuli may depend on the valence of the stimuli, and these may help to differentiate bipolar disorder from major depressive disorder. Adolescents with bipolar disorder have displayed varying results, which may be contributed to, at least in part, by the continued maturation of the functional role of the prefrontal cortex during adolescence. Therefore, similar to morphological abnormalities, activation deficits in adolescents with bipolar disorder, relative to healthy adolescents, may still be progressing. Studies investigating at-risk individuals provide preliminary evidence that ventral prefrontal cortex dysfunction is similar to that in individuals diagnosed with bipolar disorder, supporting ventral prefrontal cortex dysfunction as a trait feature of bipolar disorder.

Studies of White Matter and Diffusion Tensor Imaging

White matter abnormalities have also long been implicated in bipolar disorder. Early in the 20th century, Starr[168] described bipolar disorder–type symptoms in association with lesions in frontal white matter and in white matter connections from the frontal lobe. Symptoms included manic-like disinhibited euphoric states, as well as tearfulness and other depressive symptoms. Abnormalities in white matter have since been a frequently reported type of abnormality in MRI research on bipolar disorder.

Early neuroimaging studies of white matter in bipolar disorder were primarily of cross-sectional areas or volumes of specific white matter structures and/or of white matter hyperintensities observed on T2-weighted MRI scans. Studies of structural abnormalities in white matter in adults with bipolar disorder have shown both decreases in volume within ventral frontal regions,[21] as well as decreases in the area or signal intensity of the corpus callosum.[169,170] Decreases in corpus callosum area, specifically in genu of the corpus callosum that provides interhemispheric connections between right and left ventral prefrontal cortices, were found in bipolar disorder in association with suicide attempts.[171]

The corpus callosum decreases were also associated with impulsivity, suggesting that abnormalities in white matter in this region might be related to the impulsiveness that can be associated with attempts. Caetano et al.[172] noted decreased signal intensity in the corpus callosum in children and adolescents with bipolar disorder, suggesting that white matter abnormalities, particularly in interhemispheric connections, might be an early feature of the disorder. Reduced left hemisphere white matter volume was also found in unaffected relative twins of subjects with bipolar disorder,[173] and decreased left frontal and temporoparietal white matter volumes were found in both subjects with bipolar disorder and their unaffected relatives,[71] suggesting that corticolimbic disconnectivity might be present in individuals at risk for bipolar disorder.

Studies of white matter hyperintensities have tended to focus on regions vulnerable to vascular insults, such as periventricular white matter regions.[174] Pompili et al.[175] noted associations between the presence of hyperintensities and history of suicide attempts in adults, suggesting that the accumulation of hyperintensities could be associated with adverse outcomes. However, Sassi et al.[176] did not find increased rates of white matter hyperintensities in a group of adults with mood disorders with a mild to moderate illness severity. In addition, a study of adolescents with bipolar disorder did not show increases in white matter hyperintensities,[90] suggesting that the increased hyperintensities seen in the disorder may be related to factors associated with age, duration of illness, and/or pathology associated with adult-onset bipolar disorder. The etiology of white matter hyperintensities is not clear. Contributing factors may include processes such as cellular loss and responses to ischemia, dilation of perivascular spaces, ependymal loss, and vascular-related demyelination. This suggests that increased white matter hyperintensities might represent interactions between pathophysiological processes of bipolar disorder and aging. However, similar white matter hyperintensities findings in youths with bipolar disorder[177,178] and in unaffected relatives of individuals with bipolar disorder have been reported,[179,180] suggesting earlier and alternate pathophysiological processes may be involved.

This section will focus on studies of white matter in bipolar disorder using DTI methods. The advent of this relatively new neuroimaging technique has made it possible to study white matter tracts providing connections between regions implicated in bipolar disorder, and measures of their microstructural integrity. A main outcome measured in DTI studies is fractional anisotropy, which is thought to be an indicator of the structural integrity and organization of fibers within a bundle, with higher fractional anisotropy reflecting more intact structure and fibers more organized along a specific direction. Next, findings will be reviewed both for intrahemispheric connections to the frontal and subcortical regions discussed earlier, as well as interhemispheric connections between frontal lobes via the corpus callosum.

Intrahemispheric Connections

Given the concentration of findings in bipolar disorder in ventral prefrontal cortex and mesial temporal structures, their strong interconnections, and the importance of their coordinated activity in regulating emotions, frontotemporal white matter bundles carrying connections between the ventral prefrontal cortex and mesial temporal structures are especially implicated in bipolar disorder. These white matter tracts include the uncinate fasciculus, which carries major connections between the ventral prefrontal cortex and amygdala, and the cingulum bundle, which carries major connections between the ventral prefrontal cortex and the hippocampus and amygdala. Additional tracts have also been implicated in bipolar disorder, including tracts that provide frontal connections to basal ganglia, thalamus, and posterior association cortices.

Frontotemporal White Matter Tracts
Findings in Adults

Altered uncinate fasciculus white matter integrity in bipolar disorder has been described by several research groups over the last decade; however, findings have varied in direction. In the left uncinate fasciculus, an increased number of fibers,[181] higher fiber density,[182] and higher fractional anisotropy values[183] have been reported in adults with bipolar disorder, compared to healthy adults. The latter study also provided evidence for decreased fractional anisotropy in the right uncinate fasciculus, in addition to greater fractional anisotropy in the left uncinate fasciculus,[183] suggesting right-left hemisphere differences in white matter abnormalities in the disorder. There have been several additional reports of findings of decreased white matter structural integrity in uncinate fasciculus and neighboring orbital frontal white matter in adults with bipolar disorder.[183–194] These more consistent findings support uncinate fasciculus decreases in bipolar disorder, although these have not lateralized consistently to the right.

Studies are emerging that link DTI findings to dysfunction in bipolar disorder. One study used an approach integrating both DTI and fMRI data acquired from the same scanning session of adults with bipolar disorder.[186] This study included a measure of functional connectivity, derived from the degree of activity coordinated in time from a seed region to different brain regions. Wang et al.[186] found that decreases in fractional anisotropy in the uncinate fasciculus were associated with decreases in functional connectivity between the perigenual anterior cingulate cortex and the amygdala during processing of emotional stimuli by adults with bipolar disorder, compared to healthy adults. This observation suggests that abnormalities in the structural integrity of uncinate fasciculus white matter connections might contribute to disruptions in the ability of the perigenual anterior cingulate cortex and amygdala to work together in the regulation of responses to emotional stimuli. In a study that integrated DTI imaging with behavioral assessment methods, Mahon et al.[195] noted decreases in fractional anisotropy in anterior components of orbital frontal white matter that were associated with both higher impulsivity and prior suicide attempts. This finding suggests that abnormalities in orbital frontal white matter might play a role in impulsivity, and specifically in impulsive suicide attempts, which are common in bipolar disorder.

Other frontotemporal white matter abnormalities have been reported, although to a lesser extent, in adults with bipolar disorder. Abnormal white matter integrity has been found in the anterior cingulum bundle.[192,196–198] This observation suggests the involvement of more extensive abnormalities in white matter providing frontotemporal connections.

Findings in Adolescents

Interestingly, children and adolescents with bipolar disorder also show findings in the ventral frontal white matter.[199,200] A recent study investigated adolescents with subthreshold bipolar disorder symptoms and found decreased fractional anisotropy values in the uncinate fasciculus,[201] suggesting that abnormalities in the uncinate fasciculus may be associated with the emergence of symptoms in the disorder. Decreased fractional anisotropy values have also been detected in more dorsal peri-cingulate regions in children and adolescents.[199,202,203] These results suggest that frontotemporal white matter abnormalities may be early abnormalities in bipolar disorder that are present by adolescence, and, as they were also reported in prepubertal children,[199,202] may be present in childhood, representing some of the earliest markers of the disorder.

Findings in Individuals at Risk

Genetic studies of bipolar disorder, which provide evidence for susceptibility in genes that can affect development of white matter connections,[204,205] implicate white matter in risk for bipolar disorder, supported by the structural imaging findings mentioned earlier. A recent study showed reduced fractional anisotropy in the right uncinate fasciculus in both adults with bipolar disorder and their unaffected first-degree relatives.[193] However, there have not yet been reports of decreased ventral frontotemporal white matter connections in at-risk youth.

Comparison of Findings to Individuals With Major Depressive Disorder

Several DTI studies of adults with major depressive disorder show abnormalities in white matter in some similar frontotemporal regions as seen in adults with bipolar disorder.[206] Fractional anisotropy reductions were observed in the uncinate fasciculus in major depressive disorder subjects compared with healthy control subjects.[207,208] Also, adolescents with major depressive disorder demonstrated lower fractional anisotropy within the frontotemporal circuitry, including in the uncinate fasciculus and anterior cingulum bundle.[209] De Kwaasteniet and colleagues[208] showed in adults with major depressive disorder, in contrast to findings in adults with bipolar disorder, an association between uncinate fasciculus abnormalities and increases in functional connectivity between the ventral anterior cingulate cortex and medial temporal lobe. This finding suggests that there may be different pathophysiologies underlying the decreases in connectivity in the two disorders that also result in the different direction of functional connectivity abnormalities paired with white matter decreases. However, due to the limited DTI studies of major depressive disorder and limited studies directly comparing bipolar disorder and major depressive disorder, a clear marker to differentiate the two disorders has not yet been identified.

Other Intrahemispheric White Matter Tracts
Findings in Adults

Abnormalities in white matter connections in adults with bipolar disorder have also been observed in connections from more dorsal frontal regions, especially to regions such as the striatum or thalamus via connections within structures, such as the anterior limb of the internal capsule.[187,210] For example, in one of the first DTI reports in bipolar disorder, Adler et al.[211] showed abnormalities in dorsal and rostral frontal white matter tracts. In addition to abnormalities in anterior white matter connections, connections from frontal and temporal structures to posterior association regions, such as through the superior longitudinal fasciculus, inferior longitudinal fasciculus, and the inferior fronto-occipital fasciculus have also been implicated in bipolar disorder.[188,189,212–214]

Findings in Adolescents

In an early DTI study of bipolar disorder adolescents experiencing their first episode of mania, fractional anisotropy values in the superior frontal region were significantly lower, compared to healthy adolescents.[215] Lower fractional anisotropy values in the corona radiata, especially in the anterior corona radiata, have been reported in several studies of youths and young adults with bipolar disorder.[216–218] Interestingly, Lu et al.[219] found a difference in pediatric and adult-onset bipolar disorder within the left anterior limb of the internal capsule; fractional anisotropy values were lower in this region in pediatric compared to adult-onset bipolar disorder, suggesting that early- and late-onset bipolar disorder might be different subtypes within the bipolar spectrum.

Findings in Individuals at Risk

In addition to decreases in frontotemporal white matter integrity, at-risk individuals have also shown reductions in fractional anisotropy in the anterior limb of the internal capsule and in frontal connections to posterior association cortices.[188,193,214,220] This includes a finding of reductions in fractional anisotropy in the superior longitudinal fasciculus in both children with bipolar disorder and those at risk for bipolar disorder.[199] Taken together with functional connectivity abnormalities to posterior association cortices found in children and adolescents with bipolar disorder,[221] this suggests that posterior white matter abnormalities may be especially early abnormalities in the disorder and could contribute to abnormalities in the development of emotional associations to environmental stimuli.

Comparison of Findings to Individuals With Major Depressive Disorder

The specificity of posterior white matter findings to bipolar disorder is not clear. One DTI study, which included a direct comparison between bipolar disorder and major depressive disorder in adults, showed more pronounced decreases in fractional anisotropy in the superior longitudinal fasciculus in bipolar disorder.[189] However, in adolescents with major depressive disorder, decreased white matter integrity was seen in the left superior longitudinal fasciculus and the inferior fronto-occipital fasciculus.[209] More studies are needed to investigate specificity for the involvement of the posterior white matter to the development of bipolar disorder.

Interhemispheric Connections

Decreases in the structural integrity of interhemispheric white matter connections have also been shown in DTI studies of adults with bipolar disorder. The relatively consistent findings in the genu of the corpus callosum are particularly of interest, as the corpus callosum genu provides right-left frontal interhemispheric connections critical for integration of emotional, cognitive, motor, and sensory information between the hemispheres, which has been hypothesized to be affected in individuals with bipolar disorder.[157,222] Abnormalities in interhemispheric connectivity have also been suggested to contribute to the hemispherically lateralized dysfunction associated with acute mood states of the disorder.[157,223]

Findings in Adults

Lower fractional anisotropy values in the anterior portions of the corpus callosum, and particularly in the genu, are some of the most consistent DTI findings in adults with bipolar disorder compared to healthy adults,[188,194,224–226] although higher corpus callosum genu fractional anisotropy values have also been reported.[227] Findings from a low-frequency resting-state fMRI study suggest that the abnormalities in interhemispheric connections might relate to abnormalities in interhemispheric functioning. That study revealed significantly increased interhemispheric correlations between the left and right ventral prefrontal cortices in an adult bipolar disorder group, relative to a healthy comparison group.[223]

Findings in Adolescents

The corpus callosum continues to show developmental changes in late adolescence and early adulthood, including continued myelination.[228] As these developmental changes also coincide with the adolescent/early adult peak in the onset of bipolar disorder, and corpus callosum abnormalities are frequently found in adolescents with bipolar disorder, this suggests that abnormalities in corpus callosum development in adolescence might contribute to bipolar disorder. Decreased fractional anisotropy values have been found in the corpus callosum in adolescents and young adults with bipolar disorder.[216,218] Decreased structural integrity of interhemispheric connections in adolescents with bipolar disorder has also been found in anterior commissure, with anterior commissure fractional anisotropy values negatively correlated with history of aggression.[229] While the structures through which decreased anterior commissure integrity may have its effects are not clear, right-left structures connected by the anterior commissure include fronto-temporal structures such as the amygdala.

Findings in Individuals at Risk

Increased genetic liability for bipolar disorder was found to be associated with a trend toward reduced fractional anisotropy in the genu of the corpus callosum, with at-risk adults showing fractional anisotropy values intermediate between healthy subjects and lower bipolar disorder values.[188] A study of at-risk youths suggested that developmental abnormalities during early adolescence might contribute to the differences, as healthy youths showed expected increases in corpus callosum fractional anisotropy values with age, while at-risk youths showed decreases in fractional anisotropy with age in the same location.[230]

Comparison of Findings to Individuals With Major Depressive Disorder

Abnormalities in the anterior interhemispheric connections provided by the corpus callosum have also been implicated in major depressive disorder. In adults with major depressive disorder, decreased fractional anisotropy has been observed in the corpus callosum, including decreases in the corpus callosum genu.[231,232] However, results in a study that directly compared individuals in late life with bipolar disorder to individuals with major depressive disorder and to healthy individuals showed significantly greater reductions in fractional anisotropy in the bipolar disorder than in the major depressive disorder group,[233] suggesting that there are more pronounced abnormalities in the structural integrity of the corpus callosum in bipolar disorder.

Summary

White matter findings in bipolar disorder are abundant in adults and recent evidence suggests intra- and interhemispheric corticolimbic white matter abnormalities are present in adolescents with bipolar disorder and in at-risk adolescents and adults. These findings together suggest that these abnormalities may be associated with genetic vulnerability to bipolar disorder. The findings in youth are indications that alterations in white matter are present early in the course of bipolar disorder and abnormalities in the maturation of white matter structures during childhood and/or adolescence may play a role in the emergence of bipolar disorder.

However, limited consistent findings from DTI studies have been reported, which may be due both to the heterogeneity of the different subject groups, as well as different methods used by different research groups. The specificity of findings to help to distinguish bipolar disorder from other disorders, such as major depressive disorder, is not clear. Future DTI research, especially investigating children and adolescent subjects with bipolar disorder and at risk for the disorder, including longitudinal studies and comparisons to other disorders, are needed.

Conclusions

Corticolimbic abnormalities have long been implicated in the development of bipolar disorder. Evidence from sMRI, fMRI, and DTI studies converges in supporting abnormalities in the structure, function, and connectivity between prefrontal cortex, amygdala, and ventral striatum in adults with bipolar disorder. Evidence from studies using these imaging modalities also supports the notion that trajectories of corticolimbic development during adolescence and young adulthood differ in bipolar disorder than in health. While some corticolimbic abnormalities appear to be established by adolescence in bipolar disorder, particularly in the subcortical amygdala and ventral striatum and in their connections to the prefrontal cortex, others appear to progress during adolescence and young adulthood.

The amygdala is a central structure in emotional processing and therefore highly implicated in bipolar disorder. Neuroimaging studies of the amygdala have yielded some of the most consistent findings in bipolar disorder. Abnormalities consistently reported in adolescents include findings of volume decreases and excessive responses to emotional stimuli. There is also some evidence supporting amygdala abnormalities in adolescents at risk for bipolar disorder, suggesting these are early abnormalities in bipolar disorder that are potential targets for early detection, treatment, and possibly prevention strategies. The ventral striatum is also highly implicated in bipolar disorder due to its role in motivational states that are altered in acute episodes of the disorder. Although there have been some reports of both structural and functional findings in the striatum in adult and adolescent bipolar disorder and at-risk individuals, there have been fewer studies of the ventral striatum, and results have varied. There have been few direct comparisons of the amygdala and ventral striatum between bipolar disorder and major depressive disorder; however, there is preliminary evidence suggesting that there may be features of abnormalities in these structures that may differ between the disorders, such as in the type of functional abnormalities that are elicited by stimuli of particular valences.

Of cortical structures, the ventral prefrontal cortex is of high interest in bipolar disorder research due to its role in regulating emotionally appropriate behavior, and in regulating the responses of the amygdala and ventral striatum. Decreases in ventral prefrontal cortex volume and dysregulated responses have been relatively consistent findings in adults with bipolar disorder. Although there are some state-related features, these have been found across mood states and in at-risk individuals, suggesting they are associated with risk for the disorder. In contrast to the subcortical abnormalities, some results suggest that, consistent with the continued maturation of the ventral prefrontal cortex during adolescence and young adulthood, ventral prefrontal cortex abnormalities progress during this epoch. This observation suggests that adolescence and young adulthood may be periods during which reduction in factors that are detrimental to ventral prefrontal cortex development, such as stress and substance abuse, may help to reduce the magnitude of abnormalities and improve course. It also suggests that if the specific risk mechanisms that contribute to the abnormalities in ventral prefrontal cortex development could be identified and targeted, it may someday be possible to halt this progression and improve prognosis in individuals who have started to show symptoms of bipolar disorder and, perhaps, to prevent it in ones who have not yet developed these symptoms.

Studies of frontotemporal connections between the brain regions described above are more recent, made possible by newer imaging methods such as DTI. DTI studies have indicated intra- and interhemispheric white matter abnormalities in adults, adolescents, and in at-risk individuals. This suggests that frontotemporal white matter alterations may be a trait of bipolar disorder, and that white matter should be considered as a candidate to target in identification, treatment, and prevention strategies.

The convergent evidence from neuroimaging findings highly implicates the brain structures described above in bipolar disorder and provides evidence to support the contribution of alterations in the development of these structures to the neural circuitry abnormalities that underlie the disorder. This work has helped to establish the location of brain abnormalities in which bipolar disorder occurs; however, the mechanisms that underlie the development of the abnormalities, such as the molecular underpinnings of these abnormalities, remain unclear. Consequently, there is a great deal of research that needs to be performed. Samples sizes have been modest and subject samples and imaging methods have varied across studies. Sources of subject heterogeneity that appear to influence findings include mood-stabilizing medication, which appears to have salutary effects on the circuitry, suggesting the potential for treatments to reverse abnormalities. However, factors that lead to discrepant findings, such as findings of both decreases and increases in volume in the amygdala in adults with bipolar disorder, are not known. There remain few longitudinal studies and studies of individuals at risk for bipolar disorder. Future such studies have the potential to reveal important insight into the pathophysiology of the disorder and to identify brain differences and mechanisms to target for early identification, intervention, and prevention strategies.

Author Disclosures

Drs. Russo and Blumberg and Ms. de Zwarte have no conflicts to disclose. Dr. Blumberg received funding from the National Institute of Mental Health, National Institute on Drug Abuse, Department of Veterans' Affairs, International Bipolar Foundation, American Foundation for Suicide Prevention, National Alliance for Research in Schizophrenia and Depression, Stanley Medical Research Institute, Attias Family Foundation, and Women's Health Research at Yale University. She has performed grant reviews for the National Institutes of Health; has given academic lectures in grand rounds, continuing medical education events, and other clinical or scientific venues; and has generated book chapters for publishers of mental health texts.

References

1. Carlson GA, Fennig S, Bromet EJ. The confusion between bipolar disorder and schizophrenia in youth: where does it stand in the 1990s? *J Am Acad Child Adolesc Psychiatry*. 1994;33(4):453–60.
2. Lish JD, Dime-Meenan S, Whybrow PC, Price RA, Hirschfeld RM. (1994). The National Depressive and Manic-Depressive Association (DMDA) survey of bipolar members. *J Affect Disord*. 1994;31(4):281–94.
3. Blumberg HP, Kaufman J, Martin A, Charney DS, Krystal JH, Peterson BS. Significance of adolescent neurodevelopment for the neural circuitry of bipolar disorder. *Ann N Y Acad Sci*. 2004;1021(1):376–83.
4. Dunner DL. Clinical consequences of under-recognized bipolar spectrum disorder. *Bipolar Disord*. 2003;5(6):456–63.
5. Thase ME. Bipolar depression: issues in diagnosis and treatment. *Harv Rev Psychiatry*. 2005;13(5):257–71.
6. Baumer FM, Howe M, Gallelli K, Simeonova DI, Hallmayer J, Chang KD. A pilot study of antidepressant-induced mania in pediatric bipolar disorder: characteristics, risk factors, and the serotonin transporter gene. *Biol Psychiatry*. 2006;60(9):1005–12.
7. Jenkins MM, Youngstrom EA, Washburn JJ, Youngstrom JK. Evidence-based strategies improve assessment of pediatric bipolar disorder by community practitioners. *Prof Psychol Res Pr*. 2011;42(2):121–9.
8. Bourgeois JP, Goldman-Rakic PS, Rakic P. Synaptogenesis in the prefrontal cortex of rhesus monkeys. *Cereb Cortex*, 1994;4(1):78–96.
9. Machado CJ, Bachevalier J. Non-human primate models of childhood psychopathology: the promise and the limitations. *J Child Psychol Psychiatry*. 2003;44(1):64–87.
10. Chugani HT. A critical period of brain development: studies of cerebral glucose utilization with PET. *Prev Med*. 1998;27(2):184–8.
11. Hare TA, Casey BJ. The neurobiology and development of cognitive and affective control. *Cogn Brain Behav*. 2005;9(3):273–86.
12. Baxter MG, Murray EA. The amygdala and reward. *Nat Rev Neurosci*. 2002;3(7):563–73.
13. Bauman MD, Lavenex P, Mason WA, Capitanio JP, Amaral DG. The development of social behavior following neonatal amygdala lesions in rhesus monkeys. *J Cogn Neurosci*. 2004;16(8):1388–411.
14. Phelps EA, LeDoux JE. Contributions of the amygdala to emotion processing: from animal models to human behavior. *Neuron*. 2005;48(2):175–87.
15. Bachevalier J, Loveland KA. The orbitofrontal-amygdala circuit and self-regulation of social-emotional behavior in autism. *Neurosci Biobehav Rev*. 2006;30(1):97–117.
16. Fried I, Cameron KA, Yashar S, Fong R, Morrow JW. Inhibitory and excitatory responses of single neurons in the human medial temporal lobe during recognition of faces and objects. *Cereb Cortex*. 2002;12(6):575–84.
17. Nauta WJ. The problem of the frontal lobe: a reinterpretation. *J Psychiatr Res*. 1971;8(3):167–87.
18. Rolls ET. *The brain and emotion*. Oxford University Press, New York, 1999
19. Passe TJ, Rajagopalan P, Tupler LA, Byrum CE, MacFall JR, Krishnan KR. Age and sex effects on brain morphology. *Prog Neuropsychopharmacol Biol Psychiatry*. 1997;21(8):1231–7.
20. Giedd JN, Blumenthal J, Jeffries NO, et al. Brain development during childhood and adolescence: a longitudinal MRI study. *Nat Neurosci*. 1999;2(10):861–3.
21. Blumberg HP, Krystal JH, Bansal R, et al. Age, rapid-cycling, and pharmacotherapy effects on ventral prefrontal cortex in bipolar disorder: a cross-sectional study. *Biol Psychiatry*. 2006;59(7):611–8.
22. Galvan A, Hare TA, Parra CE, et al. Earlier development of the accumbens relative to orbitofrontal cortex might underlie risk-taking behavior in adolescents. *J Neurosci*. 2006;26(25):6885–92.
23. Amaral DG, Price JL. Amygdalo-cortical projections in the monkey (Macaca fascicularis). *J Comp Neurol*. 1984;230(4):465–96.
24. Bachevalier J. The amygdala, social cognition, and autism. In *The amygdala: A functional analysis*, JP Aggleton (Ed.), New York, NY: Oxford University Press; 2000: 509–43.
25. Liao DL, Yeh YC, Chen HM, Chen H, Hong CJ, Tsai SJ. Association between the Ser9Gly polymorphism of the dopamine D3 receptor gene and tardive dyskinesia in Chinese schizophrenia patients. *Neuropsychobiology*. 2001;44(2):95–8.

26. Cunningham MG, Bhattacharyya S, Benes FM. Amygdalo-cortical sprouting continues into early adulthood: implications for the development of normal and abnormal function during adolescence. *J Comp Neurol*. 2002;453(2):116–30.

27. Yakovlev P, Lecours A. The mylogenetic cycles of regional maturation of the brain. In: *Regional Development of the Brain in Early Life*, Minkowski A, ed. Oxford, UK: Blackwell Scientific; 1967:3–70.

28. Courchesne E, Chisum HJ, Townsend J, et al. Normal brain development and aging: quantitative analysis at in vivo MR imaging in healthy volunteers. *Radiology*. 2000;216(3):672–82.

29. Sowell ER, Peterson BS, Thompson PM, Welcome SE, Henkenius AL, Toga AW. Mapping cortical change across the human life span. *Nat Neurosci*. 2003;6(3):309–15.

30. Bartzokis G, Lu PH, Mintz J. Quantifying age-related myelin breakdown with MRI: novel therapeutic targets for preventing cognitive decline and Alzheimer's disease. *J Alzheimers Dis*. 2004;6(6):S53–9.

31. Lenroot RK, Gogtay N, Greenstein DK, et al. Sexual dimorphism of brain developmental trajectories during childhood and adolescence. *Neuroimage*. 2007;36(4):1065–73.

32. Sowell ER, Thompson PM, Holmes CJ, Jernigan TL, Toga AW. In vivo evidence for post-adolescent brain maturation in frontal and striatal regions. *Nat Neurosci*. 1999;2(10):859–61.

33. Pearlson GD, Barta PE, Powers RE, et al. Medial and superior temporal gyral volumes and cerebral asymmetry in schizophrenia versus bipolar disorder. *Biol Psychiatry*. 1997;41(1):1–14.

34. Blumberg HP, Kaufman J, Martin A, et al. Amygdala and hippocampal volumes in adolescents and adults with bipolar disorder. *Arch Gen Psychiatry*. 2003;60(12):1201–8.

35. Strakowski SM, DelBello MP, Sax KW, et al. Brain magnetic resonance imaging of structural abnormalities in bipolar disorder. *Arch Gen Psychiatry*. 1999;56(3):254–60.

36. Altshuler LL, Bartzokis G, Grieder T, et al. An MRI study of temporal lobe structures in men with bipolar disorder or schizophrenia. *Biol Psychiatry*. 2000;48(2):147–62.

37. Brambilla P, Harenski K, Nicoletti M, et al. MRI investigation of temporal lobe structures in bipolar patients. *J Psychiatr Res*. 2003;37(4):287–95.

38. Savitz J, Nugent AC, Bogers W, et al. Amygdala volume in depressed patients with bipolar disorder assessed using high resolution 3T MR: the impact of medication. *Neuroimage*. 2010;49(4):2966–76.

39. DelBello MP, Zimmerman ME, Mills NP, Getz GE, Strakowski SM. Magnetic resonance imaging analysis of amygdala and other subcortical brain regions in adolescents with bipolar disorder. *Bipolar Disord*. 2004;6(1):43–52.

40. Chang K, Karchemskiy A, Barnea-Goraly N, Garrett A, Simeonova DI, Reiss A. Reduced amygdalar gray matter volume in familial pediatric bipolar disorder. *J Am Acad Child Adolesc Psychiatry*. 2005;44(6):565–73.

41. Dickstein DP, Milham MP, Nugent AC, et al. Frontotemporal alterations in pediatric bipolar disorder: results of a voxel-based morphometry study. *Arch Gen Psychiatry*. 2005;62(7):734–41.

42. Kalmar JH, Wang F, Chepenik LG, et al. Relation between amygdala structure and function in adolescents with bipolar disorder. *J Am Acad Child Adolesc Psychiatry*. 2009;48(6):636–42.

43. Blond BN, Fredericks CA, Blumberg HP. Functional neuroanatomy of bipolar disorder: structure, function, and connectivity in an amygdala-anterior paralimbic neural system. *Bipolar Disord*. 2012;14(4):340–55.

44. Rosso IM, Killgore WDS, Cintron CM, Gruber SA, Tohen M, Yurgelun-Todd DA. Reduced amygdala volumes in first-episode bipolar disorder and correlation with cerebral white matter. *Biol Psychiatry*. 2007;61(6):743–9.

45. Bitter SM, Mills NP, Adler CM, Strakowski SM, DelBello MP. Progression of amygdala volumetric abnormalities in adolescents after their first manic episode. *J Am Acad Child Adolesc Psychiatry*. 2011;50(10):1017–26.

46. Geller B, Harms MP, Wang L, et al. Effects of age, sex, and independent life events on amygdala and nucleus accumbens volumes in child bipolar I disorder. *Biol Psychiatry*. 2009;65(5):432–7.

47. Blumberg HP, Donegan NH, Sanislow CA, et al. Preliminary evidence for medication effects on functional abnormalities in the amygdala and anterior cingulate in bipolar disorder. *Psychopharmacology (Berl)*. 2005;183(3):308–13.

48. Chang K, Karchemskiy A, Kelley R, et al. Effect of divalproex on brain morphometry, chemistry, and function in youth at high-risk for bipolar disorder: a pilot study. *J Child Adolesc Psychopharmacol*. 2009;19(1):51–9.

49. Singh MK, Delbello MP, Adler CM, Stanford KE, Strakowski SM. Neuroanatomical characterization of child offspring of bipolar parents. *J Am Acad Child Adolesc Psychiatry*. 2008;47(5):526–31.

50. Karchemskiy A, Garrett A, Howe M, et al. Amygdalar, hippocampal, and thalamic volumes in youth at high risk for development of bipolar disorder. *Psychiatry Res*. 2011;194(3):319–25.

51. Ladouceur CD, Almeida JRC, Birmaher B, et al. Subcortical gray matter volume abnormalities in healthy bipolar offspring: potential neuroanatomical risk marker for bipolar disorder. *J Am Acad Child Adolesc Psychiatry*. 2008;47(5):532–9.

52. Tang Y, Wang F, Xie G, et al. Reduced ventral anterior cingulate and amygdala volumes in medication-naïve females with major depressive disorder: a voxel-based morphometric magnetic resonance imaging study. *Psychiatry Res*. 2007;156(1):83–6.

53. MacMillan S, Szeszko PR, Moore GJ, et al. Increased amygdala: hippocampal volume ratios associated with severity of anxiety in pediatric major depression. *J Child Adolesc Psychopharmacol*. 2003;13(1):65–73.

54. MacMaster FP, Mirza Y, Szeszko PR, et al. Amygdala and hippocampal volumes in familial early onset major depressive disorder. *Biol Psychiatry*. 2008;63(4):385–90.

55. Chepenik LG, Fredericks C, Papademetris X, et al. Effects of the brain-derived neurotrophic growth factor val66met variation on hippocampus morphology in bipolar disorder. *Neuropsychopharmacol*. 2009;34(4):944–51.

56. Frazier JA, Chiu S, Breeze JL, et al. Structural brain magnetic resonance imaging of limbic and thalamic volumes in pediatric bipolar disorder. *Am J Psych*. 2005;162(7):1256–65.

57. Sheline YI, Gado MH, Kraemer HC. Untreated depression and hippocampal volume loss. *Am J Psych*. 2003;160(8):1516–8.

58. Edmiston EE, Wang F, Mazure CM, et al. Corticostriatal-limbic gray matter morphology in adolescents with self-reported exposure to childhood maltreatment. *Arch Pediatr Adolesc Med*. 2011;165(12):1069–77.

59. Womer FY, Kalmar JH, Wang F, Blumberg HP. A ventral prefrontal-amygdala neural system in bipolar disorder: a view from neuroimaging research. *Acta Neuropsychiatr*. 2009;21(6):228–38.

60. Hwang J, Lyoo IK, Dager SR, et al. Basal ganglia shape alterations in bipolar disorder. *Am J Psychiatry*. 2006;163(2):276–85.

61. Aylward EH, Roberts-Twillie JV, Barta PE, et al. Basal ganglia volumes and white matter hyperintensities in patients with bipolar disorder. *Am J Psychiatry*. 1994;151(5):687–93.

62. Strakowski SM, DelBello MP, Zimmerman ME, et al. Ventricular and periventricular structural volumes in first- versus multiple-episode bipolar disorder. *Am J Psychiatry*. 2002;159(11):1841–7.

63. Wilke M, Kowatch RA, DelBello MP, Mills NP, Holland SK. Voxel-based morphometry in adolescents with bipolar disorder: first results. *Psychiatry Res*. 2004;131(1):57–69.

64. Sanches M, Roberts RL, Sassi RB, et al. Developmental abnormalities in striatum in young bipolar patients: a preliminary study. *Bipolar Disord*. 2005;7(2):153–8.

65. Ahn MS, Breeze JL, Makris N, et al. Anatomic brain magnetic resonance imaging of the basal ganglia in pediatric bipolar disorder. *J Affect Disord*. 2007;104(1):147–54.

66. Brambilla P, Harenski K, Nicoletti MA, et al. Anatomical MRI study of basal ganglia in bipolar disorder patients. *Psychiatry Res*. 2001;106(2):65–80.

67. Chakos MH, Lieberman JA, Bilder RM, et al. Increase in caudate nuclei volumes of first-episode schizophrenic patients taking antipsychotic drugs. *Am J Psych*. 1994;151(10):1430–6.

68. Lieberman JA, Stroup TS, McEvoy JP, et al. Effectiveness of antipsychotic drugs in patients with chronic schizophrenia. *N Engl J Med*. 2005;353(12):1209–23.

69. Noga JT, Vladar K, Torrey EF. A volumetric magnetic resonance imaging study of monozygotic twins discordant for bipolar disorder. *Psychiatry Res*. 2001;106(1):25–34.

70. van der Schot AC, Vonk R, Brans RG, et al. Influence of genes and environment on brain volumes in twin pairs concordant and discordant for bipolar disorder. *Arch Gen Psychiatry*. 2009;66(2):142–51.

71. McDonald C, Bullmore ET, Sham PC, et al. Association of genetic risks for schizophrenia and bipolar disorder with specific and generic brain structural endophenotypes. *Arch Gen Psychiatry*. 2004;61(10):974–84.

72. Hajek T, Gunde E, Slaney C, et al. Striatal volumes in affected and unaffected relatives of bipolar patients—High-risk study. *J Psychiatr Res*. 2009;43(7):724–9.

73. Matsuo K, Rosenberg DR, Easter PC, et al. Striatal volume abnormalities in treatment-naïve patients diagnosed with pediatric major depressive disorder. *J Child Adolesc Psychopharmacol.* 2008;18(2):121–31.

74. Lacerda ALT, Nicoletti MA, Brambilla P, et al. Anatomical MRI study of basal ganglia in major depressive disorder. *Psychiatry Res.* 2003;124(3):129–40.

75. Pillay SS, Renshaw PF, Bonello CM, Lafer B, Fava M, Yurgelun-Todd D. A quantitative magnetic resonance imaging study of caudate and lenticular nucleus gray matter volume in primary unipolar major depression: relationship to treatment response and clinical severity. *Psychiatry Res.* 1998;84(2):61–74.

76. Kim MJ, Hamilton JP, Gotlib IH. Reduced caudate gray matter volume in women with major depressive disorder. *Psychiatry Res.* 2008;164(2):114–22.

77. Jastrowitz M. Beiträge zur Localisation im Grosshirn und über deren praktische Verwerthung. *Dtsch Med Wochenschr.* 1888;14(05):81–3.

78. Oppenheim H. Zur Pathologie der Grosshirngeschwulste. *Arch Psychiatry.* 1889;21:560–78.

79. Drevets WC, Price JL, Simpson JR, et al. Subgenual prefrontal cortex abnormalities in mood disorders. *Nature.* 1997;386:824–7.

80. López-Larson MP, DelBello MP, Zimmerman ME, Schwiers ML, Strakowski SM. Regional prefrontal gray and white matter abnormalities in bipolar disorder. *Biol Psychiatry.* 2002;52(2):93–100.

81. Lyoo IK, Kim MJ, Stoll AL, et al. Frontal lobe gray matter density decreases in bipolar I disorder. *Biol Psychiatry.* 2004;55(6):648–51.

82. Sassi RB, Brambilla P, Hatch JP, et al. Reduced left anterior cingulate volumes in untreated bipolar patients. *Biol Psychiatry.* 2004;56(7):467–75.

83. Adler CM, Levine AD, DelBello MP, Strakowski SM. Changes in gray matter volume in patients with bipolar disorder. *Biol Psychiatry.* 2005;58(2):151–7.

84. Zimmerman ME, DelBello MP, Getz GE, Shear PK, Strakowski SM. Anterior cingulate subregion volumes and executive function in bipolar disorder. *Bipolar Disord.* 2006;8(3):281–8.

85. Manji HK, Moore GJ, Chen G. Clinical and preclinical evidence for the neurotrophic effects of mood stabilizers: implications for the pathophysiology and treatment of manic-depressive illness. *Biol Psychiatry.* 2000;48(8):740–54.

86. Moore GJ, Cortese BM, Glitz DA, et al. A longitudinal study of the effects of lithium treatment on prefrontal and subgenual prefrontal gray matter volume in treatment-responsive bipolar disorder patients. *J Clin Psychiatry.* 2009;70(5):699–705.

87. Moore GJ, Bebchuk JM, Hasanat K, et al. Lithium increases N-acetyl-aspartate in the human brain: in vivo evidence in support of bcl-2's neurotrophic effects? *Biol Psychiatry.* 2000;48(1):1–8.

88. Bearden CE, Thompson PM, Dalwani M, et al. Greater cortical gray matter density in lithium-treated patients with bipolar disorder. *Biol Psychiatry.* 2007;62(1):7–16.

89. Cousins DA, Aribisala B, Ferrier IN, Blamire AM. Lithium, gray matter, and magnetic resonance imaging signal. *Biol Psychiatry.* 2013;73(7):652–7.

90. Chang K, Barnea-Goraly N, Karchemskiy A, et al. Cortical magnetic resonance imaging findings in familial pediatric bipolar disorder. *Biol Psychiatry.* 2005;58(3):197–203.

91. Adler CM, DelBello MP, Jarvis K, Levine A, Adams J, Strakowski SM. Voxel-based study of structural changes in first-episode patients with bipolar disorder. *Biol Psychiatry.* 2007;61(6):776–81.

92. Kaur S, Sassi RB, Axelson D, et al. Cingulate cortex anatomical abnormalities in children and adolescents with bipolar disorder. *Am J Psychiatry.* 2005;162(9):1637–43.

93. Singh MK, Chang KD, Chen MC, et al. Volumetric reductions in the subgenual anterior cingulate cortex in adolescents with bipolar I disorder. *Bipolar Disord.* 2012;14(6):585–96.

94. Mitsunaga MM, Garrett A, Howe M, Karchemskiy A, Reiss A, Chang K. Increased subgenual cingulate cortex volume in pediatric bipolar disorder associated with mood stabilizer exposure. *J Child Adolesc Psychopharmacol.* 2011;21(2):149–55.

95. Najt P, Nicoletti M, Chen HH, et al. Anatomical measurements of the orbitofrontal cortex in child and adolescent patients with bipolar disorder. *Neurosci Lett.* 2007;413(3):183–6.

96. Kalmar JH, Wang F, Spencer L, et al. Preliminary evidence for progressive prefrontal abnormalities in adolescents and young adults with bipolar disorder. *J Int Neuropsychol Soc.* 2009;15(3):476–81.

97. Farrow TFD, Whitford TJ, Williams LM, Gomes L, Harris AWF. Diagnosis-related regional gray matter loss over two years in first episode schizophrenia and bipolar disorder. *Biol Psychiatry*. 2005;58(9):713–23.

98. Gogtay N, Ordonez A, Herman DH, et al. Dynamic mapping of cortical development before and after the onset of pediatric bipolar illness. *J Child Psychol Psychiatry*. 2007;48(9):852–62.

99. Wang F, Kalmar JH, Womer FY, et al. Olfactocentric paralimbic cortex morphology in adolescents with bipolar disorder. *Brain*. 2011;134(7):2005–12.

100. Mesulam MM, Mufson EJ. The insula of Reil in man and monkey: architectonics, connectivity and function. In: *Cerebral Cortex*, Peters A, Jones EG, eds. New York, NY: Plenum Press; 1985:179–226.

101. Lai TJ, Payne ME, Byrum CE, Steffens DC, Krishnan KRR. Reduction of orbital frontal cortex volume in geriatric depression. *Biol Psychiatry*. 2000;48(10):971–5.

102. Bremner JD, Vythilingam M, Vermetten E, et al. Reduced volume of orbitofrontal cortex in major depression. *Biol Psychiatry*. 2002;51(4):273–9.

103. Lacerda ALT, Keshavan MS, Hardan AY, et al. Anatomic evaluation of the orbitofrontal cortex in major depressive disorder. *Biol Psychiatry*. 2004;55(4):353–8.

104. Parashos IA, Tupler LA, Blitchington T, Krishnan KRR. Magnetic-resonance morphometry in patients with major depression. *Psychiatry Res*. 1998;84(1):7–15.

105. Hastings RS, Parsey RV, Oquendo MA, Arango V, Mann JJ. Volumetric analysis of the pre-frontal cortex, amygdala, and hippocampus in major depression. *Neuropsychopharmacology*. 2004;29(5):952–9.

106. Janssen J, Pol HEH, Lampe IK, et al. Hippocampal changes and white matter lesions in early-onset depression. *Biol Psychiatry*. 2004;56(11):825–31.

107. Chen HH, Rosenberg DR, MacMaster FP, et al. Orbitofrontal cortex volumes in medication naïve children with major depressive disorder: a magnetic resonance imaging study. *J Child Adolesc Psychopharmacol*. 2008;18(6):551–6.

108. McClure EB, Pope K, Hoberman AJ, Pine DS, Leibenluft E. Facial expression recognition in adoles-cents with mood and anxiety disorders. *Am J Psychiatry*. 2003;160(6):1172–4.

109. McClure EB, Treland JE, Snow J, et al. Deficits in social cognition and response flexibility in pediatric bipolar disorder. *Am J Psychiatry*. 2004;162(9):1644–51.

110. Brotman MA, Skup M, Rich BA, et al. Risk for bipolar disorder Is associated with face-processing deficits across emotions. *J Am Acad Child Adolesc Psychiatry*. 2008;47(12):1455–61.

111. Yurgelun-Todd DA, Gruber SA, Kanayama G, Killgore WD, Baird AA, Young AD. fMRI during affect discrimination in bipolar affective disorder. *Bipolar Disord*. 2000;2(3p2):237–48.

112. Malhi GS, Lagopoulos J, Ward PB, et al. Cognitive generation of affect in bipolar depression: an fMRI study. *Eur J Neurosci*. 2004;19(3):741–54.

113. Lawrence NS, Williams AM, Surguladze S, et al. Subcortical and ventral prefrontal cortical neural responses to facial expressions distinguish patients with bipolar disorder and major depression. *Biol Psychiatry*. 2004;55(6):578–87.

114. Altshuler L, Bookheimer S, Proenza MA, et al. Increased amygdala activation during mania: a func-tional magnetic resonance imaging study. *Am J Psych*. 2005;162(6):1211–3.

115. Chen CH, Lennox B, Jacob R, et al. Explicit and implicit facial affect recognition in manic and depressed states of bipolar disorder: a functional magnetic resonance imaging study. *Biol Psychiatry*. 2006;59(1):31–9.

116. Almeida JRC, Versace A, Hassel S, Kupfer DJ, Phillips ML. Elevated amygdala activity to sad facial expressions: a state marker of bipolar but not unipolar depression. *Biol Psychiatry*. 2010;67(5):414–21.

117. Lennox BR, Jacob R, Calder AJ, Lupson V, Bullmore ET. Behavioural and neurocognitive responses to sad facial affect are attenuated in patients with mania. *Psychol Med*. 2004;34(5):795–802.

118. Adleman NE, Kayser RR, Olsavsky AK, et al. Abnormal fusiform activation during emotional-face encoding assessed with functional magnetic resonance imaging. *Psychiatry Res*. 2013;212(2):161–3.

119. Leibenluft E, Charney DS, Pine DS. Researching the pathophysiology of pediatric bipolar disorder. *Biol Psychiatry*. 2003;53(11):1009–20.

120. Blumberg HP. Dimensions in the development of bipolar disorder. *Biol Psychiatry*. 2007;62(2):104–6.

121. Perlman SB, Almeida JRC, Kronhaus DM, et al. Amygdala activity and prefrontal cortex–amygdala effective connectivity to emerging emotional faces distinguish remitted and depressed mood states in bipolar disorder. *Bipolar Disord.* 2012;14(2):162–74.

122. Foland-Ross LC, Bookheimer SY, Lieberman MD, et al. Normal amygdala activation but deficient ventrolateral prefrontal activation in adults with bipolar disorder during euthymia. *Neuroimage.* 2012;59(1):738–44.

123. Post RM, Uhde TW, Putnam FW, Ballenger JC, Berrettini WH. Kindling and carbamazepine in affective illness. *J Nerv Ment Dis.* 1982;170(12):717–31.

124. Rich BA, Vinton DT, Roberson-Nay R, et al. Limbic hyperactivation during processing of neutral facial expressions in children with bipolar disorder. *Proc Natl Acad Sci USA.* 2006;103(23):8900–905.

125. Ladouceur CD, Farchione T, Diwadkar V, et al. Differential patterns of abnormal activity and connectivity in the amygdala–prefrontal circuitry in bipolar-I and bipolar-NOS youth. *J Am Acad Child Adolesc Psychiatry.* 2011;50(12):1275–89.

126. Garrett AS, Reiss AL, Howe ME, et al. Abnormal amygdala and prefrontal cortex activation to facial expressions in pediatric bipolar disorder. *J Am Acad Child Adolesc Psychiatry.* 2012;51(8):821–31.

127. Strakowski SM, Eliassen JC, Lamy M, et al. Functional magnetic resonance imaging brain activation in bipolar mania: evidence for disruption of the ventrolateral prefrontal-amygdala emotional pathway. *Biol Psychiatry.* 2011;69(4):381–8.

128. Pavuluri MN, O'Connor MM, Harral E, Sweeney JA. Affective neural circuitry during facial emotion processing in pediatric bipolar disorder. *Biol Psychiatry.* 2007;62(2):158–67.

129. Chang K, Adleman NE, Dienes K, Simeonova DJ, Menon V, Reiss A. Anomalous prefrontal-subcortical activation in familial pediatric bipolar disorder: a functional magnetic resonance imaging investigation. *Arch Gen Psychiatry.* 2004;61(8):781–92.

130. Passarotti AM, Sweeney JA, Pavuluri MN. Fronto-limbic dysfunction in mania pre-treatment and persistent amygdala over-activity post-treatment in pediatric bipolar disorder. *Psychopharmacology.* 2011;216(4):485–99.

131. Surguladze SA, Marshall N, Schulze K, et al. Exaggerated neural response to emotional faces in patients with bipolar disorder and their first-degree relatives. *Neuroimage.* 2010;53(1):58–64.

132. Olsavsky AK, Brotman MA, Rutenberg JG, et al. Amygdala hyperactivation during face emotion processing in unaffected youth at risk for bipolar disorder. *J Am Acad Child Adolesc Psychiatry.* 2012;51(3):294–303.

133. Ladouceur CD, Diwadkar VA, White R, et al. Fronto-limbic function in unaffected offspring at familial risk for bipolar disorder during an emotional working memory paradigm. *Dev Cogn Neurosci.* 2013;5:185–96.

134. Sheline YI, Barch DM, Donnelly JM, Ollinger JM, Snyder AZ, Mintun MA. Increased amygdala response to masked emotional faces in depressed subjects resolves with antidepressant treatment: an fMRI study. *Biol Psychiatry.* 2001;50(9):651–8.

135. Victor TA, Furey ML, Fromm SJ, Öhman A, Drevets WC. Relationship between amygdala responses to masked faces and mood state and treatment in major depressive disorder. *Arch Gen Psychiatry.* 2010;67(11):1128–38.

136. Grotegerd D, Suslow T, Bauer J, et al. Discriminating unipolar and bipolar depression by means of fMRI and pattern classification: a pilot study. *Eur Arch Psychiatry Clin Neurosci.* 2013;263(2):119–31.

137. Liu J, Blond BN, van Dyck LI, Spencer L, Wang F, Blumberg HP. Trait and state corticostriatal dysfunction in bipolar disorder during emotional face processing. *Bipolar Disord.* 2012;14(4):432–41.

138. Blumberg HP, Stern E, Martinez D, et al. Increased anterior cingulate and caudate activity in bipolar mania. *Biol Psychiatry.* 2000;48(11):1045–52.

139. Hassel S, Almeida JRC, Kerr N, et al. Elevated striatal and decreased dorsolateral prefrontal cortical activity in response to emotional stimuli in euthymic bipolar disorder: no associations with psychotropic medication load. *Bipolar Disord.* 2008;10(8):916–27.

140. Hassel S, Almeida JR, Frank E, et al. Prefrontal cortical and striatal activity to happy and fear faces in bipolar disorder is associated with comorbid substance abuse and eating disorder. *J Affect Disord.* 2009;118(1):19–27.

141. Dickstein DP, Rich BA, Roberson-Nay R, et al. Neural activation during encoding of emotional faces in pediatric bipolar disorder. *Bipolar Disord.* 2007;9(7):679–92.

142. Blumberg HP, Martin A, Kaufman J, et al. Frontostriatal abnormalities in adolescents with bipolar disorder: preliminary observations from functional MRI. *Am J Psychiatry*. 2003;160(7):1345–7.

143. Leibenluft E, Rich BA, Vinton DT, et al. Neural circuitry engaged during unsuccessful motor inhibition in pediatric bipolar disorder. *Am J Psychiatry*. 2007;164(1):52–60.

144. Adleman NE, Fromm SJ, Razdan V, et al. Cross-sectional and longitudinal abnormalities in brain structure in children with severe mood dysregulation or bipolar disorder. *J Child Psychol Psychiatry*. 2012;53(11):1149–56.

145. Deveney CM, Connolly ME, Jenkins SE, et al. Striatal dysfunction during failed motor inhibition in children at risk for bipolar disorder. *Prog Neuropsychopharmacol Biol Psychiatry*. 2012;38(2):127–33.

146. Kim P, Jenkins SE, Connolly ME, et al. Neural correlates of cognitive flexibility in children at risk for bipolar disorder. *J Psychiatr Res*. 2012;46(1):22–30.

147. Pizzagalli DA, Holmes AJ, Dillon DG, et al. Reduced caudate and nucleus accumbens response to rewards in unmedicated individuals with major depressive disorder. *Am J Psychiatry*. 2009;166(6):702–10.

148. Forbes EE, Hariri AR, Martin SL, et al. Altered striatal activation predicting real-world positive affect in adolescent major depressive disorder. *Am J Psychiatry*. 2009;166(1):64–73.

149. Fu CHY, Williams SCR, Cleare AJ, et al. Attenuation of the neural response to sad faces in major depression by antidepressant treatment: a prospective, event-related functional magnetic resonance imaging study. *Arch Gen Psychiatry*. 2004;61(9):877–89.

150. Chen CH, Ridler K, Suckling J, et al. Brain imaging correlates of depressive symptom severity and predictors of symptom improvement after antidepressant treatment. *Biol Psychiatry*. 2007;62(5):407–14.

151. Sackeim HA, Greenberg MS, Weiman AL, Gur RC, Hungerbuhler JP, Geschwind N. Hemispheric asymmetry in the expression of positive and negative emotions: neurologic evidence. *Arch Neurol*. 1982;39(4):210–8.

152. Cummings JL, Mendez MF. Secondary mania with focal cerebrovascular lesions. *Am J Psychiatry*. 1984;141(9):1084–7.

153. Damasio AR, Anderson SW. The frontal lobes. In: *Clinical Neuropsychology*, Heilman KM, Valenstein E, eds. New York, NY: Oxford University Press; 1993:409–460.

154. Schoenbaum G, Chiba AA, Gallagher M. Orbitofrontal cortex and basolateral amygdala encode expected outcomes during learning. *Nat Neurosci*. 1998;1(2):155–9.

155. Bechara A, Damasio H, Damasio AR, Lee GP. Different contributions of the human amygdala and ventromedial prefrontal cortex to decision-making. *J Neurosci*. 1999;19(13):5473–81.

156. Blumberg HP, Stern E, Ricketts S, et al. Rostral and orbital prefrontal cortex dysfunction in the manic state of bipolar disorder. *Am J Psychiatry*. 1999;156(12):1986–8.

157. Blumberg HP, Leung HC, Skudlarski P, et al. A functional magnetic resonance imaging study of bipolar disorder: state- and trait-related dysfunction in ventral prefrontal cortices. *Arch Gen Psychiatry*. 2003;60(6):601–9.

158. Jogia J, Haldane M, Cobb A, Kumari V, Frangou S. Pilot investigation of the changes in cortical activation during facial affect recognition with lamotrigine monotherapy in bipolar disorder. *Br J Psychiatry*. 2008;192(3):197–201.

159. Altshuler LL, Bookheimer SY, Townsend J, et al. Blunted activation in orbitofrontal cortex during mania: a functional magnetic resonance imaging study. *Biol Psychiatry*. 2005;58(10):763–9.

160. Foland LC, Altshuler LL, Bookheimer SY, Eisenberger N, Townsend J, Thompson PM. Evidence for deficient modulation of amygdala response by prefrontal cortex in bipolar mania. *Psychiatry Res*. 2008;162(1):27–37.

161. Malhi GS, Lagopoulos J, Sachdev PS, Ivanovski B, Shnier R, Ketter T. Is a lack of disgust something to fear? A functional magnetic resonance imaging facial emotion recognition study in euthymic bipolar disorder patients. *Bipolar Disord*. 2007;9(4):345–57.

162. Mah L, Zarater CA Jr, Singh J, et al. Regional cerebral glucose metabolic abnormalities in bipolar II depression. *Biol Psychiatry*. 2007;61(6):765–75.

163. Haldane M, Jogia J, Cobb A, Kozuch E, Kumari V, Frangou S. Changes in brain activation during working memory and facial recognition tasks in patients with bipolar disorder with Lamotrigine monotherapy. *Eur Neuropsychopharmacol*. 2008;18(1):48–54.

164. Pavuluri MN, O'Connor MM, Harral EM, Sweeney JA. An fMRI study of the interface between affective and cognitive neural circuitry in pediatric bipolar disorder. *Psychiatry Res.* 2008;162(3):244–55.

165. Pavuluri MN, Passarotti AM, Fitzgerald JM, Wegbreit E, Sweeney JA. Risperidone and divalproex differentially engage the fronto-striato-temporal circuitry in pediatric mania: a pharmacological functional magnetic resonance imaging study. *J Am Acad Child Adolesc Psychiatry.* 2012;51(2):157–70.

166. Kerestes R, Bhagwagar Z, Nathan PJ, et al. Prefrontal cortical response to emotional faces in individuals with major depressive disorder in remission. *Psychiatry Res.* 2012;202(1):30–7.

167. Mourão-Miranda J, Almeida JRC, Hassel S, et al. Pattern recognition analyses of brain activation elicited by happy and neutral faces in unipolar and bipolar depression. *Bipolar Disord.* 2012;14(4):451–60.

168. Starr MA. *Organic Nervous Diseases.* New York, NY and Philadelphia, PA: Lea Brothers; 1903.

169. Brambilla P, Nicoletti MA, Sassi RB, et al. Magnetic resonance imaging study of corpus callosum abnormalities in patients with bipolar disorder. *Biol Psychiatry.* 2003;54(11):1294–7.

170. Brambilla P, Nicoletti M, Sassi RB, et al. Corpus callosum signal intensity in patients with bipolar and unipolar disorder. *J Neurol Neurosurg Psychiatry.* 2004;75(2):221–5.

171. Matsuo K, Nielsen N, Nicoletti MA, et al. Anterior genu corpus callosum and impulsivity in suicidal patients with bipolar disorder. *Neurosci Lett.* 2010;469(1):75–80.

172. Caetano SC, Silveira CM, Kaur S, et al. Abnormal corpus callosum myelination in pediatric bipolar patients. *J Affect Disord.* 2008;108(3):297–301.

173. Kieseppä T, van Erp TG, Haukka J, et al. Reduced left hemispheric white matter volume in twins with bipolar I disorder. *Biol Psychiatry.* 2003;54(9):896–905.

174. Botteron KN, Vannier MW, Geller B, Todd RD, Lee BC. Preliminary study of magnetic resonance imaging characteristics in 8- to 16-year-olds with mania. *J Am Acad Child Adolesc Psychiatry.* 1995;34(6):742–9.

175. Pompili M, Innamorati M, Mann JJ, et al. Periventricular white matter hyperintensities as predictors of suicide attempts in bipolar disorders and unipolar depression. *Prog Neuropsychopharmacol Biol Psychiatry.* 2008;32(6):1501–7.

176. Sassi RB, Brambilla P, Nicoletti M, et al. White matter hyperintensities in bipolar and unipolar patients with relatively mild-to-moderate illness severity. *J Affect Disord.* 2003;77(3):237–45.

177. Pillai JJ, Friedman L, Stuve TA, et al. Increased presence of white matter hyperintensities in adolescent patients with bipolar disorder. *Psychiatry Res.* 2002;114(1):51–6.

178. Lyoo IK, Lee HK, Jung JH, Noam GG, Renshaw PF. White matter hyperintensities on magnetic resonance imaging of the brain in children with psychiatric disorders. *Compr Psychiatry.* 2002;43(5):361–8.

179. Ahearn EP, Steffens DC, Cassidy F, et al. Familial leukoencephalopathy in bipolar disorder. *Am J Psychiatry.* 1998;155(11):1605–7.

180. Ahearn EP, Speer MC, Chen YT, et al. Investigation of Notch3 as a candidate gene for bipolar disorder using brain hyperintensities as an endophenotype. *Am J Med Genet.* 2002;114(6):652–8.

181. Houenou J, Wessa M, Douaud G, et al. Increased white matter connectivity in euthymic bipolar patients: diffusion tensor tractography between the subgenual cingulate and the amygdalo-hippocampal complex. *Mol Psychiatry.* 2007;12(11):1001–10.

182. Torgerson CM, Irimia A, Leow AD, et al. DTI tractography and white matter fiber tract characteristics in euthymic bipolar I patients and healthy control subjects. *Brain Imaging Behav.* 2013;7(2):129–39.

183. Versace A, Almeida JR, Hassel S, et al. Elevated left and reduced right orbitomedial prefrontal fractional anisotropy in adults with bipolar disorder revealed by tract-based spatial statistics. *Arch Gen Psychiatry.* 2008;65(9):1041–52.

184. Beyer JL, Taylor WD, MacFall JR, et al. Cortical white matter microstructural abnormalities in bipolar disorder. *Neuropsychopharmacology.* 2005;30(12):2225–9.

185. McIntosh AM, Munoz Maniega S, Lymer GK, et al. White matter tractography in bipolar disorder and schizophrenia. *Biol Psychiatry.* 2008;64(12):1088–92.

186. Wang F, Kalmar JH, He Y, et al. Functional and structural connectivity between the perigenual anterior cingulate and amygdala in bipolar disorder. *Biol Psychiatry.* 2009;66(5):516–21.

187. Sussmann JE, Lymer GK, McKirdy J, et al. White matter abnormalities in bipolar disorder and schizophrenia detected using diffusion tensor magnetic resonance imaging. *Bipolar Disord.* 2009;11(1):11–8.

188. Chaddock CA, Barker GJ, Marshall N, et al. White matter microstructural impairments and genetic liability to familial bipolar I disorder. *Br J Psychiatry.* 2009;194(6):527–34.

189. Versace A, Almeida JR, Quevedo K, et al. Right orbitofrontal corticolimbic and left corticocortical white matter connectivity differentiate bipolar and unipolar depression. *Biol Psychiatry.* 2010;68(6):560–7.

190. Lin F, Weng S, Xie B, Wu G, Lei H. Abnormal frontal cortex white matter connections in bipolar disorder: a DTI tractography study. *J Affect Disord.* 2011;131(1–3):299–306.

191. Sui J, Pearlson G, Caprihan A, et al. Discriminating schizophrenia and bipolar disorder by fusing fMRI and DTI in a multimodal CCA+ joint ICA model. *Neuroimage.* 2011;57(3):839–55.

192. Benedetti F, Absinta M, Rocca MA, et al. Tract-specific white matter structural disruption in patients with bipolar disorder. *Bipolar Disord.* 2011;13(4):414–24.

193. Linke J, King AV, Poupon C, Hennerici MG, Gass A, Wessa M. Impaired anatomical connectivity and related executive functions: differentiating vulnerability and disease marker in bipolar disorder. *Biol Psychiatry.* 2013;74(12):908–16.

194. Versace A, Andreazza AC, Young LT, et al. Elevated serum measures of lipid peroxidation and abnormal prefrontal white matter in euthymic bipolar adults: toward peripheral biomarkers of bipolar disorder. *Mol Psychiatry.* 2014;19(2):200–8.

195. Mahon K, Burdick KE, Wu J, Ardekani BA, Szeszko PR. Relationship between suicidality and impulsivity in bipolar I disorder: a diffusion tensor imaging study. *Bipolar Disord.* 2012;14(1):80–9.

196. Wang F, Jackowski M, Kalmar JH, et al. Abnormal anterior cingulum integrity in bipolar disorder determined through diffusion tensor imaging. *Br J Psychiatry.* 2008;193(2):126–9.

197. Chan WY, Yang GL, Chia MY, et al. Cortical and subcortical white matter abnormalities in adults with remitted first-episode mania revealed by Tract-Based Spatial Statistics. *Bipolar Disord.* 2010;12(4):383–9.

198. Barysheva M, Jahanshad N, Foland-Ross L, Altshuler LL, Thompson PM. White matter microstructural abnormalities in bipolar disorder: a whole brain diffusion tensor imaging study. *Neuroimage.* 2013;2:558–68.

199. Frazier JA, Breeze JL, Papadimitriou G, et al. White matter abnormalities in children with and at risk for bipolar disorder. *Bipolar Disord.* 2007;9(8):799–809.

200. Kafantaris V, Kingsley P, Ardekani B, et al. Lower orbital frontal white matter integrity in adolescents with bipolar I disorder. *J Am Acad Child Adolesc Psychiatry.* 2009;48(1):79–86.

201. Paillere Martinot ML, Lemaitre H, Artiges E, et al. White-matter microstructure and gray-matter volumes in adolescents with subthreshold bipolar symptoms. *Mol Psychiatry.* 2014;19(4):462–70.

202. Gönenç A, Frazier JA, Crowley DJ, Moore CM. Combined diffusion tensor imaging and transverse relaxometry in early-onset bipolar disorder. *J Am Acad Child Adolesc Psychiatry.* 2010;49(12):1260–8.

203. Gao W, Jiao Q, Qi R, et al. Combined analyses of gray matter voxel-based morphometry and white matter tract-based spatial statistics in pediatric bipolar mania. *J Affect Disord.* 2013;150(1):70–6.

204. McIntosh AM, Moorhead TW, Job D, et al. The effects of a neuregulin 1 variant on white matter density and integrity. *Mol Psychiatry.* 2008;13(11):1054–9.

205. Cannon DM, Walshe M, Dempster E, et al. The association of white matter volume in psychotic disorders with genotypic variation in NRG1, MOG and CNP: a voxel-based analysis in affected individuals and their unaffected relatives. *Transl Psychiatry.* 2012;2(10):e167.

206. Sexton CE, Mackay CE, Ebmeier KP. A systematic review of diffusion tensor imaging studies in affective disorders. *Biol Psychiatry.* 2009;66(9):814–23.

207. Zhang A, Leow A, Ajilore O, et al. Quantitative tract-specific measures of uncinate and cingulum in major depression using diffusion tensor imaging. *Neuropsychopharmacology.* 2012;37(4):959–67.

208. de Kwaasteniet B, Ruhe E, Caan M, et al. Relation between structural and functional connectivity in major depressive disorder. *Biol Psychiatry.* 201374(1):40–7.

209. Cullen KR, Klimes-Dougan B, Muetzel R, et al. Altered white matter microstructure in adolescents with major depression: a preliminary study. *J Am Acad Child Adolesc Psychiatry*. 2010;49(2):173–83.

210. Haznedar MM, Roversi F, Pallanti S, et al. Fronto-thalamo-striatal gray and white matter volumes and anisotropy of their connections in bipolar spectrum illnesses. *Biol Psychiatry*. 2005;57(7):733–42.

211. Adler CM, Holland SK, Schmithorst V, et al. Abnormal frontal white matter tracts in bipolar disorder: a diffusion tensor imaging study. *Bipolar Disord*. 2004;6(3):197–203.

212. Bruno S, Cercignani M, Ron MA. White matter abnormalities in bipolar disorder: a voxel-based diffusion tensor imaging study. *Bipolar Disord*. 2008;10(4):460–8.

213. Vederine FE, Wessa M, Leboyer M, Houenou J. A meta-analysis of whole-brain diffusion tensor imaging studies in bipolar disorder. *Prog Neuropsychopharmacol Biol Psychiatry*. 2011;35(8):1820–6.

214. Mahon K, Burdick KE, Ikuta T, et al. Abnormal temporal lobe white matter as a biomarker for genetic risk of bipolar disorder. *Biol Psychiatry*. 2013;73(2):177–82.

215. Adler CM, Adams J, DelBello MP, et al. Evidence of white matter pathology in bipolar disorder adolescents experiencing their first episode of mania: a diffusion tensor imaging study. *Am J Psychiatry*. 2006;163(2):322–4.

216. Barnea-Goraly N, Chang KD, Karchemskiy A, Howe ME, Reiss AL. Limbic and corpus callosum aberrations in adolescents with bipolar disorder: a tract-based spatial statistics analysis. *Biol Psychiatry*. 2009;66(3):238–44.

217. Pavuluri MN, Yang S, Kamineni K, et al. Diffusion tensor imaging study of white matter fiber tracts in pediatric bipolar disorder and attention-deficit/hyperactivity disorder. *Biol Psychiatry*. 2009;65(7):586–93.

218. Lagopoulos J, Hermens DF, Hatton SN, et al. Microstructural white matter changes in the corpus callosum of young people with bipolar disorder: a diffusion tensor imaging study. *PLoS One*. 2013;8(3):e59108.

219. Lu LH, Zhou XJ, Fitzgerald J, et al. Microstructural abnormalities of white matter differentiate pediatric and adult-onset bipolar disorder. *Bipolar Disord*. 2012;14(6):597–606.

220. Sprooten E, Sussmann JE, Clugston A, et al. White matter integrity in individuals at high genetic risk of bipolar disorder. *Biol Psychiatry*. 2011;70(4):350–6.

221. Rich BA, Fromm SJ, Berghorst LH, et al. Neural connectivity in children with bipolar disorder: impairment in the face emotion processing circuit. *J Child Psychol Psychiatry*. 2008;49(1):88–96.

222. Pettigrew JD, Miller SM. A 'sticky' interhemispheric switch in bipolar disorder? *Proc Biol Sci*. 1998;265(1411):2141–8.

223. Chepenik LG, Raffo M, Hampson M, et al. Functional connectivity between ventral prefrontal cortex and amygdala at low frequency in the resting state in bipolar disorder. *Psychiatry Res*. 2010;182(3):207–10.

224. Wang F, Kalmar JH, Edmiston E, et al. Abnormal corpus callosum integrity in bipolar disorder: a diffusion tensor imaging study. *Biol Psychiatry*. 2008;64(8):730–33.

225. Haller S, Xekardaki A, Delaloye C, et al. Combined analysis of grey matter voxel-based morphometry and white matter tract-based spatial statistics in late-life bipolar disorder. *J Psychiatry Neurosci*. 2011;36(6):391–401.

226. Benedetti F, Yeh PH, Bellani M, et al. Disruption of white matter integrity in bipolar depression as a possible structural marker of illness. *Biol Psychiatry*. 2011;69(4):309–17.

227. Yurgelun-Todd DA, Silveri MM, Gruber SA, Rohan ML, Pimentel PJ. White matter abnormalities observed in bipolar disorder: a diffusion tensor imaging study. *Bipolar Disord*. 2007;9(5):504–12.

228. Keshavan MS, Diwadkar VA, DeBellis M, et al. Development of the corpus callosum in childhood, adolescence and early adulthood. *Life Sci*. 2002;70(16):1909–22.

229. Saxena K, Tamm L, Walley A, et al. A preliminary investigation of corpus callosum and anterior commissure aberrations in aggressive youth with bipolar disorders. *J Child Adolesc Psychopharmacol*. 2012;22(2):112–9.

230. Versace A, Ladouceur CD, Romero S, et al. Altered development of white matter in youth at high familial risk for bipolar disorder: a diffusion tensor imaging study. *J Am Acad Child Adolesc Psychiatry*. 2010;49(12):1249–59.

231. Kieseppä T, Eerola M, Mäntylä R, et al. Major depressive disorder and white matter abnormalities: a diffusion tensor imaging study with tract-based spatial statistics. *J Affect Disord.* 2010;120(1):240–4.

232. Xu K, Jiang W, Ren L, et al. Impaired interhemispheric connectivity in medication-naive patients with major depressive disorder. *J Psychiatry Neurosci.* 2013;38(1):43–8.

233. Sexton CE, Allan CL, Mackay CE, Ebmeier KP. White matter integrity within the corpus callosum differentiates late-life bipolar and unipolar depression. *Bipolar Disord.* 2012;14(7):790–1.

Neurobiology of Bipolar Disorder in Youth

Brain Domain Dysfunction is Translated to Decode the Pathophysiology and Understand the Nuances of the Clinical Manifestation

Mani N. Pavuluri

Introduction

Bipolar disorder in youth is a complex biological illness that impacts multiple brain functional circuits. The illness diathesis is primarily rooted in abnormally altered affective neural operations. However, neither the brain pathophysiology nor the clinical psychopathology and the neurocognitive performance described in Chapter 14 are limited to alterations in affective or emotional systems. Cognitive circuitry dysfunction is extensive, and often a rule rather than an exception, and exists alongside the affective circuitry dysfunction, especially in the early-onset variant of bipolar disorder. Modernization of medicine through multimodal imaging technology during the past decade has provided the opportunity to look into the window of how these parallel processing networks are interlinked, influence each other in amplifying the dysfunction, and show abnormal activity and connectivity patterns. This progress has charted a novel way to conceptualize pediatric psychopathology on the basis of brain circuitry dysfunction. Such complex brain pathophysiology provides explanatory power to the comorbidity that commonly occurs in early-onset bipolar disorder. Children, parents, clinicians, and scientists alike welcome the opportunity to reconceptualize the illness through understanding brain dysfunction or "wiring problems in the brain"—beyond the diagnostic nomenclature of bipolar disorder. It adds a new dimensional understanding of the intra- and interindividual variability, typical in developing brain (Chapter 11).

A Clinical Framework to Comprehend Bipolar Disorder Using Functional Magnetic Neuroimaging

Synopsis of the emerging literature unique to young people with bipolar disorder, relative to healthy peers or individuals with attention-deficit/hyperactivity disorder (ADHD), is presented under the categories of domain dysfunctions published to date. Burgeoning knowledge about fundamental domain dysfunction and the underlying neurobiological circuitry mandates a shift in thinking about targets for intervention beyond being limited by diagnosis of bipolar disorder and treating the mood instability. This approach reduces the frustration of how to conceptualize many facets of the illness. Reliable and valid clinical and multimodal imaging methods constitute the units of analysis across a range of constructs and domains in the early-onset variant of bipolar disorder, commonly referred to as pediatric bipolar disorder (PBD). The key brain regions that are functionally involved in PBD are illustrated in Figure 12.1.

Emotion Processing

Given the centrality of mood disturbance in PBD, affective circuitry function is hypothesized to be at the core of the dysfunction. Therefore, affective neuroscience systems are probed to examine automatic emotional reactivity to positive or negative stimuli, response to recognition of facial emotions, and incidental emotional response under emotional

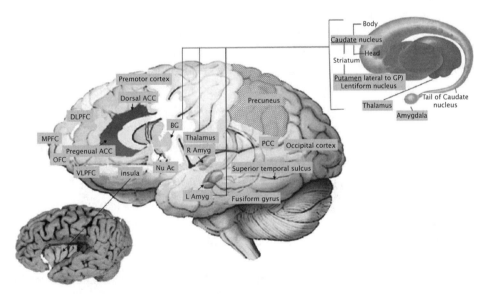

FIGURE 12.1 Orientation to key functional regions deployed in pediatric bipolar disorder. AC, nucleus accumbens; ACC, anterior cingulate cortex; BG, basal ganglia; DLPFC, dorsolateral prefrontal cortex; GP, globus pallidus; MPFC, medial prefrontal cortex; Nu OFC, orbitofrontal cortex; PBD, pediatric bipolar disorder; PCC, posterior cingulate cortex; VLPFC, ventrolateral prefrontal cortex.

challenge through words or faces during cognitive processing. Several of these proof-of-concept studies, while groundbreaking, had fewer subjects. Several of these experiments extended beyond probing the emotional systems, to delve into the intricate relationship between thinking and feeling, targeting the interface between emotional and cognitive networks. These studies helped to illustrate how negative or threatening stimuli or positive or rewarding stimuli might amplify the signal and demonstrate the abnormalities in PBD, relative to healthy controls.

Negative Valence

Across the studies, prefrontal cortex (PFC) and amygdala were found to be altered in activation, often noted as fronto-limbic dysfunction in PBD. Different tasks and type of stimuli probing the brain function, subtypes of bipolar disorder, and medication status may be primarily responsible for some variability in findings. For example, negatively valenced pictures, relative to neutral pictures, activated bilateral dorsolateral prefrontal cortex (DLPFC), ventrolateral prefrontal cortex (VLPFC), and right insula in treated patients with PBD, compared to the attentional posterior cingulate gyrus in healthy controls.[1] In another study, medication-free euthymic patients with bipolar disorder Type I, when shown threatening or angry faces relative to neutral faces, illustrated reduced activation of right VLPFC together with increased activity in right pregenual anterior cingulate (ACC), amygdala, and paralimbic cortex. Also, in this study, patients with PBD, relative to healthy controls, showed reduced activation of visual areas in occipital cortex together with greater activation in higher order visual perceptual areas, including superior temporal sulcus and fusiform gyrus with angry faces. Altered or reduced activation in VLPFC ("top") might reflect diminished top-down control, which leads to the observed exaggerated activation in amygdala and paralimbic areas ("down"). Changes in occipital areas showing reduced activation in PBD might represent an effort to gate sensory input when affective responses to the faces could not be successfully modulated. Another study reported greater VLPFC and amygdala activity in response to evaluating *hostility in neutral faces* versus nose width in medicated patients with PBD compared with non-PBD controls.[2] A point to note in this study is that the increased VLPFC activation is an incidental response during the assessment of threatening expression (i.e., fear in nonemotional faces). As in this earlier study, incidental emotions generated by actual angry and happy facial expressions during the age estimation of these faces (while evaluating age of the emotional faces, incidentally or by chance, one perceives emotion is termed *incidental emotion*), relative to labeling emotions of emotional faces (i.e., looking at the emotions and recognizing them is termed *directed emotions*), generated increased amygdala activity in euthymic unmedicated bipolar disorder Type I patients, but not in healthy controls. It is the interference of emotional challenge while performing the cognitive task that led to intrusion of the increased limbic activity in patients with PBD and may indicate more intense automatic emotional reactivity.[3] Furthermore, the right prefrontal systems that include DLPFC and VLPFC that are believed to modulate emotion are less engaged in patients with PBD regardless of whether the emotion processing is incidental or directed, which may signify reduced top-down control of emotional reactivity in PBD. Yet another study employed a completely different task that probed the functional integrity of attentional control under emotional challenge in euthymic unmedicated patients with bipolar disorder Type I and healthy controls. Matching the color of the negative disparaging or threatening words to colored dots resulted in greater activation of bilateral pregenual ACC and left amygdala, and it decreased activation in the right VLPFC and DLPFC junction.[4]

A cohort of these earlier studies used block design to preserve power (where several trials are presented in one block without any gap to ramp up brain activity) except in the study by Rich and colleagues[2] that implemented event-related (ER) design where each event (i.e., presenting the stimuli) is separated from one another. In another study that grouped adult and child bipolar subjects together, right amygdala showed hyperactivity in response to fear faces, relative to healthy controls. But pediatric patients differed from healthy controls with right amygdala hyperactivity only when fear faces were combined with angry and neutral faces in the analyses.[5] These findings leave the question open of whether response to fear faces is driven by adult patients, as not until angry faces (and neutral faces) were added to the pool instead of just fear stimuli did the pediatric patients differ from healthy controls or adult patients. It could be that children perceive threat more strongly from angry faces and/or misinterpret neutral faces. Therefore, another study with ER design was designed to see whether fear poses threat (similar to anger in block and ER design studies) in a larger sample of psychotropic naïve patients with PBD versus healthy controls.[6] Adolescents with bipolar disorder (ABD) and matched healthy controls completed a slow event-related affective hemodynamic probe task that required indicating the gender of fearful and neutral faces. Patients with ABD showed higher activity for fearful relative to neutral faces in the amygdala and prefrontal cortex and a delayed hemodynamic response to fearful faces in DLPFC and VLPFC, as well as bilateral amygdala and caudate. Furthermore, the ABD group, relative to healthy controls, showed a prolonged response to fearful faces in the right DLPFC. Clinical measures of mania and depression severity correlated with increased processing delays in the amygdala and striatum. By design, the task contained fewer, more widely spaced stimuli, possibly reducing its power to detect group differences. The use of fearful faces may not equate the negative effect elicited by angry faces in ABD.

Neuroscience Insights of Probing Emotion Processing Circuitry

Despite variable stimuli such as faces, scenes, or words, negative emotional stimuli consistently elicited fronto-limbic abnormalities in PBD. Anger is highly provocative in eliciting emotional circuitry activity. Emotional impact of anger and fear has not been directly tested. VLPFC, the emotional control region, appears to exert top-down control over overactive amygdala. It is not definitive if greater amygdala activity to negative stimuli (bottom-up) is equally challenging VLPFC's ability to regulate sub-cortical activity in PBD. Severely ill bipolar disorder Type I or threatening angry face stimuli repeatedly elicited decreased VLPFC and DLPFC activity,[3,4] while the same PFC regions showed increased activity in case of mixed samples (manic and hypo-manic), medicated subjects, or fear stimuli.[1,6] This is akin to the analogy of stretching an elastic band with increased VLPFC-DLPFC activity—with mild to moderate nega-tive stimuli or mixed samples that included subjects with hypomania that stimulate to increase activity—that can reach a breaking point with decreased VLPFC-DLPFC activity, when facing stronger negative stimuli or severe illness. Automatic emotion processing (vs. voluntary regulation or cognitive reappraisal tasks) involves the inter-face of VLPFC and DLPFC. Animal studies showed strong connectivity between VLPFC, amygdala, ACC, and insula[7] with the pregenual ACC acting as intermediary compensatory emotional control region.[8] The insula is posteriorly contiguous with VLPFC and engages in processing negative emotions.

Translational Clinical Significance of Neural Deficits Underlying Emotion Processing

1. Prefrontal cortex, specifically the right VLPFC in conjunction with the DLPFC, mod-ulates the amygdala response to threat. Although not directly compared, robust find-ings of amygdala overactivation and PFC underactivation are published in response to anger in PBD, suggesting that these individuals are more sensitive and reactive to anger. This finding is applicable to a child's responses in classroom setting when working with strict and real or perceived angry reactions from the teacher. While not directly tested, this finding led me often to suggest parents to choose compassionate teacher versus the strict and organized teacher.

2. It is also possible that PFC regions may be inherently underfunctioning and cannot efficiently modulate amygdala activity particularly when the illness is severe. Indeed, if clinical symptoms are severe, when exposed to negative emotion such as fear, the deeply seated evolutionarily old brain regions that process emotion (e.g., amygdala or striatum) show impaired rise and fall in blood flow consistent with poor processing.[6] Therefore, medications that reduce amygdala activity and increase PFC activity are important, regardless of the diagnosis if there is affective circuitry dysfunction, no matter how specific the diagnosis is, within the spectrum of bipolar disorder 1, 2, or perhaps the not otherwise specified (NOS) category.

3. Even though initial studies were designed to elicit automatic emotional responses to emotional stimuli[1-5] (though not necessarily conscious regulation), this phenomenon engaged DLPFC-striatum in the dorsal part of the brain, VLPFC-amygdala in the ventral part of the brain, occipital cortex-posterior cingulate in the posterior region, and temporal cortex in recognizing the salient stimuli. These are critical connections in appraising facial emotions, appraising and modulating one's own emotions.

4. Another critical finding was that amygdala activity was lower when labeling an emotion (be it happy or angry face) compared to attending to nonemotional problem solving (e.g., estimating age of the face) under emotional challenge[3] in PBD, relative to healthy subjects. So consciously focusing on labeling a facial emotion may help PFC better regulate amygdala in PBD. Conversely, the undivided attention toward visually looking at the emotional face and labeling that same emotion may be less taxing to the PFC in regulating amygdala activity in PBD. This finding could be applied in real-life treatment in which individuals with PBD could be taught to focus on identifying other people's facial emotions and consciously process them to avoid automatic excessive reactivity.

Positive Valence

Understanding response to positive stimuli—that is, emotion processing of positive stimuli—offers insight into the state and trait abnormalities of probing affective circuitry and eliciting the level of excitability in youth with mania, euthymia, and depression. In medicated subjects with bipolar disorder, positive emotional pictures led to increased activity in bilateral caudate and thalamus, and left DLPFC and pregenual ACC.[1] Trait deficits in euthymic unmedicated bipolar youth, in response to passive viewing of happy faces relative to neutral faces, elicited reduced right VLPFC and bilateral occipital cortex activation, and increased right pregenual ACC, amygdala, paralimbic cortex, and higher order perceptual region of posterior parietal cortex.[9] However, in response to matching colors to positive words, healthy and bipolar groups did not differ as words may not have been as strong as stimuli as faces.[10] Region of interest analyses of event-related designs (vs. whole-brain analyses in block designs in the aforementioned studies) illustrated greater amygdala, medial PFC, and DLPFC activity in response to happy faces relative to neutral faces in bipolar disorder Type I versus healthy subjects.[11]

A related crucial construct in the domain of positive valence that has particular relevance to treatment rather than diagnosis is *Reward Learning* that includes reinforcement learning. *Expectancy or Anticipation of Reward* is closely linked to *Motivation* (Italicized names of the cognitive domains in this chapter indicate the terms from the workshops conducted on research domain criteria [RDoC] at the National Institute for Mental Health). Patients with bipolar disorder are hyperresponsive to reward and are sensitized to rejection or negative consequences. Clinically, this complex process manifests as emotional reactivity to stimuli (affective), hyperarousal (neurophysiological), and mistimed response inhibition (behavioral), thereby rendering reinforcement learning a treatment challenge. A task that informed such neurophysiological alterations is the Affective Posner Task,[3,12] which is a spatial orienting attention paradigm modified to include reward-punishment contingencies and rigged negative feedback to measure induced frustration. Subjects with bipolar disorder reported significantly higher negative affect and displayed attenuated P3 event-related potential (ERP) amplitude when frustrated by punishment and rigged feedback and delayed or ill-timed response. Specifically, proportional to the increase in emotional demands, attentional allocation was lowered as shown by reduced P3 amplitude.

Using magnetoencephalography (MEG) that offers higher temporal resolution (at a millisecond level) than functional magnetic resonance imaging (fMRI) and spatial resolution than electroencephalography (EEG), during the Affective Posner Task,[12] PBD showed lower theta power in the same regions, relative to healthy subjects, in response to positive feedback. Conversely, greater theta oscillations were observed in PBD in the right ACC and the bilateral parietal lobes in response to negative feedback. These findings may mean that PBD may be more affected in response to positive or negative consequences by recruiting these regions of emotional and attentional interface. These findings are highly relevant in crafting school-based interventions, rethinking the use of contingency-based behavioral management strategies. These findings indicate why individuals with PBD react excessively to negative feedback and lash out or why they are caught up in reaping the positive rewards even before they are earned. Altered brain activity at the ACC-parietal regions explains the compensatory intermediary level of emotional and cognitive control exercised in PBD when higher cortical VLPFC and DLPFC are underfunctioning.

Reward processing was also examined in PBD using an event-related Affective Priming Task.[13] This task involved increasing expectation to gain reward prior to the anticipation, followed by a phase of anticipation, and then the actual reward or loss. The findings from this study illustrated decreased activation while anticipating gains and increased activation while anticipating losses in PBD relative to healthy subjects, a pattern that is in a similar direction as the prior study using MEG.[12] Decreased activation was seen in inferior temporal and thalamic regions, with anticipated gains and increased activation with anticipated losses in DLPFC and parietal cortex in PBD relative to healthy subjects.[13] The fronto-parietal increase in activation in response to anticipated loss and decreased orbito-frontal cortex and subgenual cingulate activation in response to anticipated gain was similar to that noted with negative and positive consequences, respectively, in the MEG study.[12] However, actual losses led to decreased activation in superior frontal-thalamic-inferior parietal regions in PBD[13] and must be better understood through replication in the future studies.

Neuroscience Insights of Probing Reward Processing and Positive Valence Circuitry

Reward circuitry involves several components such as emotional evaluation, motivation, decision making, and response to reward with parallel processing circuits in operation. In case of PBD, dysfunction could be at the interface of the reward-centric OFC-ventral striatal circuitry and the emotion-centric DLPFC-VLPFC-ACC-limbic circuitry. In addition to the studies in PBD, normative studies illustrated greater activation in orbitofrontal cortex and the subcortical regions of amygdala and nucleus accumbens during winning than losing; and with greater versus smaller rewards across adolescents and adults.[14–16] This finding held true with greater striatal activation in response to reward,[14] and reduced activation during reward anticipation[16] in adolescents relative to adults. Generated from concepts independently published in the PBD literature on emotion processing and reward, and normative studies on reward in adolescents, it is reasonable to hypothesize that the reward system is altered in PBD. These patients may show altered evaluation and appraisal of reward contingencies with *impaired consummation* resulting in excessive excitability or frustration, and *impaired motivation* illustrated in response to anticipation, possibly due to poor executive function (see Chapter 14).

Translational Clinical Significance of Neural Deficits Underlying Reward Processing and Positive Valence Circuitry

Understanding the underlying motivational and consequence-based physiological regulatory forces is critical to understand how behavior is shaped in response to any given environment. Emotional reactivity with extreme highs and lows, associated hyperarousal, and ill-timed responses to altered mental appraisal are potentially relevant and can be explained by deficits in fronto-temporo-parieto-subcortical circuits. The ventral circuits, that is, fronto-limbic and fronto-striatal circuits, may be predominantly involved in PBD.[17] Increased incidence of substance abuse in PBD, or intensity often described by parents as "mission mode" or "obsession" in seeking reward, or explosive behavior if denied, can be explained by the complex brain pathophysiology underlying the extremes of anticipation and reward or loss. Science is still unrefined in linking precise behavioral data with the brain circuitry abnormalities that underlie reward mechanisms, but current evidence paired with clinical understanding of these patients generates novel hypotheses. To give an example, a child with PBD may repeatedly insist that parents purchase a video game, and such an incessant request is often termed "obsession" by parents. Instead, it could be an intense desire to possess the reward, characterized by inability to postpone gratification paired with poor inhibition control (VLPFC-straital impairment). If parents say "no" to such demands in which reward is yet to be earned by the child or when a negative consequence is due, it would lead to excessive reactivity explained by presumably the impaired affective circuitry (VLPFC-amygdala impairment).

Attention–Impulse Control–Response Inhibition

Attention refers to a range of processes that regulate access to capacity-limited systems, such as awareness, higher perceptual processes, and motor action. The concepts of capacity limitation and competition are inherent to the concepts of selective and divided attention.[18] Response inhibition, closely linked to attention, engages the system that modulates the operation of cognitive and emotional systems, in the service of goal-directed behavior, when a prepotent response needs to be inhibited to meet the demands of the current context. There are several studies that examined the closely interrelated components of attention control and ability to stop and control impulsivity in responding in bipolar disorder with or without ADHD or contrasting bipolar disorder with ADHD. Adolescents with bipolar disorder and comorbid ADHD showed reduced VLPFC activity and greater posterior parieto-temporal activity while performing a block design single digit-continuous performance test.[19] This simple attention task illustrated how attentional resources were limited in adolescent bipolar disorder with comorbid ADHD, so that subjects recruited posterior attentional brain regions versus anterior VLPFC and ACC. In another study, Continuous Performance Test (CPT) with a response inhibition component elicited increased left parahippocampal activation in association with mania[20] versus increased superior temporal lobe activity during successful inhibition in ADHD. In another study, the Stop Signal Task, designed to examine the ability to stop a motor response to act that is already initiated, was used to compare PBD, ADHD, and healthy subjects. Subjects with PBD showed underactivity at the interface of left VLPFC and DLPFC as well as right ACC relative to healthy subjects, while the ADHD group showed increased bilateral caudate activity in addition to extensive bilateral VLPFC and DLPFC underactivity during the inhibitory process. Impulse control, therefore, was more closely tied to dysfunction in emotional control regions in PBD while they also engaged cortico-subcortical motor control regions in ADHD relative to PBD or healthy subjects. In an event-related study that examined just the PBD group, in failed trials, that is, when response inhibition was compromised, subjects showed reduced VLPFC-striatal activation.[21] This finding illustrated how the motoric response inhibition circuit is impaired in PBD, relative to healthy subjects. The impact of ADHD was not clear, and medication status did not make a difference. Another related study with an overlapping sample showed that the PBD group, relative to subjects with severe mood dysregulation (SMD) and healthy individuals, showed decreased activity in right ACC and nucleus accumbens.[22] Again, the overlapping sample of PBD from the aforementioned studies was compared with adult bipolar disorder using the same task and examining correlates of failed inhibition.[23] This study illustrated underactivity of ACC in PBD relative to adult bipolar disorder and healthy teens, as well as overactivity in adult bipolar disorder relative to healthy adults. The VLPFC-nucleus accumbens underactivity was noted with all bipolar subjects across age underscoring fronto-striatal dysfunction during motoric inhibition in bipolar disorder. In bipolar depression in youth, in a Go-NoGo Task, there was single study showing increased bilateral VLPFC and superior temporal cortex activation during failed response inhibition and just bilateral VLPFC activity during the go condition.[24] In a PBD manic and hypomanic sample, successful NoGo trials show increased neural activation in DLPFC underscoring the executive functional capability of this PFC region.[25]

Neuroscience Insights of Probing Attention–Impulse Control–Response Inhibition

Regardless of the task or sample within bipolar spectrum disorders in youth, there is consistency in the results, apparent from the summarized studies and relative to healthy individuals, illustrating VLPFC and ACC underactivity. The dual role of emotional and motor control (motor inhibition) of VLPFC region and the dual role of emotional processing and cognitive error correction by ACC may explain the involvement of these two regions in modulating both emotions and response inhibition. Two contiguous pathophysiological processes that are engaged in this process are (1) the role of DLPFC along with VLPFC in executive function, and (2) the role of temporal-parietal regions while paying attention, challenged by additional cognitive deficits with or without comorbid ADHD. Relative to those with ADHD who demonstrate cognitively driven impulsivity, people with PBD suffer from both cognitive and emotional impulsivity, thereby engaging fronto-striatal[21-23] and fronto-limbic[17,20] circuitry regions in apparent attempts to compensate for deficits.

Translational Clinical Significance of Neural Deficits Underlying Attention–Impulse Control–Response Inhibition

Inattention and failure to inhibit impulsive responses are common deficits either due to comorbid ADHD or specific cognitive deficits that are prominent in early-onset bipolar disorder.[26-29] Given that bipolar disorder is an emotional and cognitive illness, regions that have dual roles in both the emotional and cognitive processes such as (1) higher cortical centers like VLPFC, (2) intermediary cortical centers such as ACC, and (3) subcortical regions such as striatum are all involved in the illness and may show increased activity with effort or show decreased activity as the patients fail to inhibit. When attention is deployed, higher frontal cortical regions such as VLPFC and DLPFC appear to be underfunctioning and posterior cortical regions such as temporal and parietal regions and or subcortical region such as basal ganglia may be deployed to compensate. An especially consistent finding in PBD is the underfunctioning of interface (of emotional and cognitive processing) area plus error detection and correction area, that is, the ACC. Treatment interventions may serve well to target mood regulation as well as improve cognitive control and error detection to improve brain function.

Working Memory

Working memory is holding and updating information online, conducive to accomplishing the task at hand that requires maintaining information while withstanding interference. Given the intricate nature of the physiological disturbance with multiple interconnected cognitive circuits being affected in this early-onset illness, working memory impairment is often found in PBD. This domain is probed either with pure working memory tasks, or shapes and faces with or without emotions probing the interface of working memory and emotion processing. One of the earlier pioneering studies that examined visuospatial working memory in males with familial bipolar disorder and healthy males using a block design two-back memory task revealed greater activity in left DLPFC, putamen, and thalamus as well as bilateral ACC in the former.[1] Another block design working memory task that directly probed the interfacing function of emotion processing while engaged in working memory was able to parse differences between PBD, ADHD, and healthy subjects.[30] In response to remembering angry faces relative to neutral faces, PBD patients showed greater activity in orbitofrontal cortex and subgenual cingulate, while the ADHD individuals showed greater activity in DLPFC and premotor cortex. Also, PBD subjects showed decreased activity in VLPFC and DLPFC relative to healthy individuals; in contrast, ADHD relative to healthy subjects showed more widespread fronto-striatal and fronto-parietal dysfunction (i.e., reduced activation). In contrast to angry faces, happy face contrasts led to increased caudate activation in PBD and increased fronto-striatal and -parietal activation in ADHD relative to the other groups. In another study using independent component analyses (ICA) examining networks engaged during a working memory task with angry faces in PBD relative to healthy subjects, two circuits were engaged: (1) an affect evaluation and regulation network and (2) an affective working memory network.[31] Affect evaluation and regulation networks showed decreased connectivity of amygdala and VLPFC in PBD. Also, the emotional evaluative region (i.e., medial PFC) was more connected in PBD. Furthermore, in the affective working memory circuit, the affective regions were poorly functionally connected in right amygdala and bilateral temporal regions responsible for facial emotion decoding as well as higher cortical VLPFC-DLPFC emotion control regions; these abnormalities were accompanied by increased connectivity of the cognitive regions: left DLPFC, right VLPFC, and left caudate.

An emotional faces followed by a surprise postscan memory task (after 30 min of scanning) revealed reduced memory for emotional faces, specifically fearful faces, in PBD relative to healthy subjects.[32] PBD showed increased activation in frontostriatal regions, specifically in ACC and striatum, while successfully encoding happy faces, and in orbitofrontal cortex while encoding angry faces. This task was a default short-term memory task and not a working memory task where subjects were trained ahead to remember the things shown in the scanner "to keep them on line" to recall later.

Neuroscience Insights of Probing Working Memory

Emerging evidence in PBD (1) coupled with what is implicated in working memory domain dysfunction[33] points to impairment in DLPFC-ACC-thalamic-basal ganglia circuitry. In PBD, relative to ADHD, a task involving working memory under emotional challenge led to deployment of the emotional circuitry regions: orbitofrontal cortex and subgenual cingulate.[30] On the same task, ADHD, when directly compared to PBD, engaged only the dorsal cognitive fronto-striatal and frontoparietal circuits. However, when PBD or ADHD is compared to healthy individuals, both the cognitive and emotional regions are underactive. Another critical finding from these results is that the very regions of cognitive and affective circuitry that are underactive with angry/negative emotions are overactive with happy emotions in PBD. It is possible that the emotional impact imposed by negative stimuli may take a greater toll on the PBD brain's ability to function and may "switch off" or fail to meet the challenge while managing negative stimuli. While positive stimuli impose burden in requiring greater effort manifested as increased activity in PBD relative to their healthy counterparts, the impact may be potentially greater with negative stimuli. This pattern has been replicated across several studies in PBD.[10] A study unraveling the brain network connectivity showed that the affective network circuitry (VLPFC-amygdala) and the facial emotion processing circuitry (fronto-temporo-amygdala) regions are not "firing" in synchrony with the rest of the corresponding brain network regions in PBD versus healthy youth, or conversely, not well connected into the network serving the affective and face processing function.[30] Furthermore, the key operators of working memory (i.e., fronto-striatal regions) are overengaged or hyperconnected into the network serving this domain function in PBD relative to healthy youth.[31] This pattern of abnormalities illustrates interlinked compensatory processes at the interface of emotional and cognitive networks in PBD.

Another interesting observation is that the brain regions deployed while performing working memory, such as keeping a short list of things online while performing a task,[30] and short-term memory functions, such as recall from recent memory for events that occurred,[32] in PBD, reportedly overlap. Despite the difference in the physiological processing, when it pertains to immediate memory, the subcortical region caudate is engaged with positive stimuli and OFC is engaged with negative stimuli. These findings inform us that memory domain may be served by similar regions during simultaneous emotion processing or we need more sophisticated tasks to tease out the effects of working memory from short-term memory. Also these findings inform that PFC region is involved in having to evaluate or negotiate greater emotional challenges (negative stimuli) and subcortical regions may deploy less challenging emotional stimuli. Conversely, these regions may be specific biomarkers of response to emotional impact while performing cognitive tasks.

Translational Clinical Significance of Neural Deficits Underlying Working Memory

In paraphrasing the meaning and relevance from the findings described previously, it is accurate to note that working memory circuitry is impaired in PBD along with affective circuitry. This pattern may explain why children with PBD present with ADHD-like symptoms described in up to 98% of cases.[34,35] Working memory is one of the common domains affected in ADHD. The symptoms of ADHD often precede the emergence or diagnosis of ADHD. Subsequent to the onset of PBD and recognition of the diagnosis, inattention and working memory problems that often present in PBD are reconciled as either due to coexisting ADHD that precedes the onset of PBD or emerge as a result of PBD. Unless the domain dysfunction such as working memory and attention are tracked prospectively, clinical onset of ADHD may often be based on information provided by parents. In PBD, cognitive working memory circuitry is often impaired in addition to abnormalities in emotion circuitry. This pattern may explain why negative stimuli or positive stimuli add additional burden while performing a working memory function, and why reactivity to negative stimuli appears to be more severe. While working memory circuits are impaired in PBD and ADHD categories, it is apparent that emotionally driven ventral brain circuitry dysfunction is greater or more inclusive in explaining the deficits in PBD, while the dorsal circuitry function is predominant in ADHD. Additionally, it is apparent from the brain network connectivity studies that underconnectivity of regions implicated in emotion processing and overconnectivity of regions involved in working memory speak to the dysfunction or compensation at the interface of cognitive function under emotional challenge. The clinical consequences of these considerations suggest that reducing exposure, especially to negative stimuli, may preserve or foster cognitive function and learning processes in people with PBD.

Mental Flexibility and Feedback

Mental flexibility is a specific subdomain of executive function that represents the ability to shift from one task to another on demand, without being rigid and inflexible, or to yield to frustration due to feedback or any other emotional interference. This domain was explored with a reversal learning neurocognitive task described in Chapter 14.[36] In this type of task, subjects acquire stimulus–response relationships through trial-and-error learning of the rules to identify response-outcome associations. When participants receive an unexpected incorrect feedback, it should lead to exploring other options demonstrating mental flexibility. Cognitive switching under emotional challenge such as receiving negative feedback to incorrect response makes this an ideally suited task to evaluate how PBD differs from healthy subjects in their neural response to feedback and switching. Using an event-related design of a probabilistic reversal learning task, euthymic subjects with PBD, relative to healthy youth, showed increased DLPFC-ACC-parietal activity, recruiting regions responsible for cognitive control/conflict and visuo-spatial strategies.[37] This maladaptive activity is greater in response to failed reversal trials paired with punishment, that is, losing points, illustrated in precuneus and posterior cingulate cortex. Using the same task and in an expanded sample, severe mood dysregulation (SMD) was compared with PBD.[38] This region of interest (ROI) study examined activation during incorrect and correct responses in specific selected regions of the brain implicated in mental flexibility and found no significant differences between PBD and SMD in subcortical caudate that showed decreased activity in both groups relative to healthy subjects. But VLPFC activity was decreased in SMD, but not in PBD or healthy controls.

Neuroscience Insights of Probing Mental Flexibility and Feedback

Essentially, any failure to learn new rules and switch, especially if subjects receive punishment, would imply impaired circuitry activity in DLPFC-ACC-parietal regions. There may be less difference in subcortical level responsible for switching and learning new rules in PBD and SMD, with additional prefrontal abnormalities in SMD alone.

Translational Clinical Significance of Neural Deficits Underlying Mental Flexibility and Feedback

It is a common clinical problem for individuals with PBD to become frustrated and unable to switch from one activity to the other. The difficulty in switching is especially difficult when challenged with negative consequences to shape the behavior. When decisions are to be made and alternative choices have to be figured by exercising flexibility, patients with PBD, relative to healthy individuals and SMD, showed greater activity in fronto-parietal regions. These results, while they attest to some differences between SMD and PBD, may point to shared abnormalities within a mood-disorder spectrum.

Executive Function and Emotion Interface

Executive function is a higher cortical process that encompasses organization, planning, flexibility, and problem solving. Often emotion regulation is closely linked with cognitive functions, especially at the prefrontal level, and is construed as an intrinsic part of the executive function. Mental flexibility under emotional feedback, working memory under emotional challenge, reward processing paired with feedback, and incidental emotion processing are several of the tasks that utilize the interlinked cognitive and emotional functions that can be considered as executive function. In this section, executive function as a broader higher cortical domain includes attentional control, problem solving, and emotion processing and regulation to accomplish the tasks that combine automatic and conscious acts—closer to the real-life daily operations in case of PBD or healthy subjects.

In one study, individuals with PBD and health subjects performed a color matching block design task matching the color of an emotional word with the color of a dot presented below it.[10] PBD subjects, relative to healthy youth, during the matching of hurtful negative words like "jerk" or "stupid," showed underactivity of the higher cortical emotion and cognitive control regions of the right VLPFC and DLPFC, respectively, and overactivity of bilateral pregenual cingulate and left amygdala. Such a pattern of dysfunction was not seen while matching the color of positive words. This finding suggests disinhibition of emotional control systems and the dysfunction of cognitive higher cortical regions of DLPFC due to adverse impact of exaggerated responsivity to negative emotions. When the same task was administered to youth with ADHD, and three-way group comparisons were made, a clear pattern emerged in which DLPFC and VLPFC were both underactive in ADHD relative to healthy subjects and VLPFC was overactive, especially in PBD, potentially to modulate emotions, both negative and positive, that interfered during attentional control in matching colors.[30] This difference in VLPFC overactivity in PBD was also found on direct comparison between PBD and ADHD on post-hoc comparisons.

Neuroscience Insights of Probing Executive Function and Emotion Interface

The experiments described previously involving attentional control and problem solving under negative emotional challenge illustrate the joint dysfunction of cognitive and emotional higher cortical regions in PBD. It appears that the intermediary cortex consisting of cognitive and emotional interface regions—pregenual ACC—is compensatory and is also overactive. Furthermore, limbic overactivity is significant with mainly negative emotions, and not with positive emotions, when PBD and healthy subjects are compared directly. These results suggest that negative emotions may impact cognitive systems more than positive emotions in PBD. Especially, VLPFC dysfunction distinguishes PBD from ADHD with over and underactivity, very similar to that seen when probing working memory.[30,39]

Translational Clinical Significance of Neural Deficits Underlying Executive Function and Emotion Interface

These results are informative for illustrating how negative emotional stimuli can destabilize cognitive ability in youth with PBD. In fact, both PBD and ADHD groups show higher cortical dysfunction with either positive or negative emotions, with abnormal VLPFC activation being specifically implicated in PBD. These results suggest, indirectly, several things that can be potentially transferred to real-life settings: (1) Negative consequences may result in poor functioning of cortical cognitive control regions along with emotion control regions of the brain. This dysfunction could be originating from poor amygdala control or poor cortical control. (2) Psychotherapy must be crafted with principles of working on strengths, using the right timing, tone of voice, and measured language in any corrective feedback. (3) Choosing classes with teachers who are compassionate may be more conducive to learning than those who impose strict structure that engenders conflict, complicated by negative emotional exchanges. These speculations are meant to only generate hypotheses, as research must serve a purpose toward solving real-life problems.

Resting-States Functional Networks

Resting-state functional activity in brain involves low-frequency (0.01–0.1 Hz) BOLD signals that reveal the brain's intrinsic neural activity that is also thought to be abnormal in mania. Synchronized brain circuits at rest have been consistently identified that are often influenced by the prior history of coactivation during active behavior.[40] There are two resting-state network studies in PBD. One of the earlier studies of treated PBD, relative to healthy subjects, demonstrated negative resting-state connectivity between left DLPFC and right superior temporal gyrus.[37] A more recent study mapped the resting-state connectivity using a model-free ICA in untreated early-onset youth with PBD, relative to healthy subjects.[41] This study revealed three distinct resting-state networks corresponding to affective, executive, and sensorimotor functions that emerged as being significantly different between PBD and healthy subjects. Certain regions in all three networks were hyperconnected in the PBD; specifically, connectivity of the dorsal ACC differentiated bipolar from healthy subjects in both the affective and the executive networks. Greater connectivity of the right amygdala within the affective network was associated with better executive function in PBD, but not in healthy subjects. Abnormally engaged resting-state affective, executive, and sensorimotor networks in untreated PBD may be responsible for abnormal task-based brain activity and vice versa. Dual engagement of dorsal ACC in affective and executive networks supports dysfunction of these networks in PBD. Furthermore, the amygdala's engagement in moderating executive function further illustrates an altered intricate interplay of affective and cognitive operations.

Magnetic Resonance Spectroscopic Studies in Pediatric Bipolar Disorder

Unlike fMRI, which measures changes in cerebral blood flow in response to relatively transient cognitive demands, MRS investigates localized alterations in neurometabolites, which are indicators of functional integrity of neural circuits. The most commonly studied chemical, N-acetyl aspartate (NAA), plays a pivotal role in synaptic maintenance, myelination, and neuronal metabolism and is an indicator of neuronal integrity.[42] Many studies have attempted to highlight MRS profiles of PBD participants in different phases of their illness and characterize trait versus state neurometabolite profiles. This undertaking provides important supportive evidence toward understanding the functional pathophysiology of PBD.

MRS studies demonstrated biochemical abnormalities such as low NAA in regions of frontal lobe, including ACC and DLPFC in PBD.[43–45] Abnormalities such as decreased NAA and creatine (Cr) in the cerebellar vermis and increased myo-inositol in the frontal lobe were also found in children at risk for bipolar disorder and may represent putative biomarkers of PBD.[46] Lower NAA in the left DLPFC of children and adolescents with bipolar disorder may indicate abnormal dendritic arborization in the prefrontal cortex of these patients.[47] Measuring NAA levels, a marker of viable neuroaxonal tissue, provides invaluable supportive evidence to help localize areas of dysfunctional neural circuits to predominantly the PFC. Thus, MRS studies provide an important method for measuring deficits found in PBD at the neurocellular level in vivo. In addition, MRS research in PBD patients may help spur research into drug development by providing metabolic information about the effects of drugs over time.

Longitudinal Studies and Medication Effects: Precision Medicine

While the placebo-controlled trials of monotherapy determine the efficacy of the medications tested, it is studies of medication effects on brain that will unlock how each medication moderates the plasticity of the affective and cognitive circuits. Key observations are summarized here, as medication effects are extensively addressed in Chapter 12.

- PFC regions are immediately modified and/or normalized by medications, while the subcortical regions take longer to reach normality.[48] While there is decreased activity in amygdala with treatment for mania or depression among youth with PBD (a sign of improvement), there appears to be residual increased amygdala activity regardless of recovery, possibly a trait marker in PBD.[49]
- Functional studies are beginning to unravel the improved function in the fronto-limbic and fronto-temporal affective circuitry.[1,50] Contingent on the paradigm administered, especially when the interfacing cognitive and affective circuits are probed, dysfunction appears wider across fronto-striato-temporo-parietal regions that alter with treatment.[31,50]
- Medications increased amygdala connectivity in fronto-limbic circuitry in PBD versus healthy controls.[7]
- Increased baseline activation of VLPFC when performing an affective task may predict greater response to medications in PBD, mania, or depression,[24] while increased baseline amygdala activity indicated poor outcome in mania, observed in response to mood stabilizers and antipsychotics alike.[51] It may be that better PFC function at baseline yields better outcomes, while baseline hyperactive amygdala poses a challenge to modulate in nonresponders.
- MRS studies illustrated that remitters exhibited a greater increase in VMPFC NAA compared with nonremitters. The authors proposed that remission indicated increased ventral prefrontal neuronal viability and function.[52] These results are similar to those using fMRI activation as an outcome measure, illustrating a distinct state response in VLPFC in PBD.

Structural Findings: A Topography Underlying Functional Disturbance

Abnormal *gray matter structural findings* in PBD include decreased volume in the anterior cingulate cortex (ACC),[53] dorsolateral prefrontal cortex (DLPFC), and amygdala[54] and increased volume in the basal ganglia.[55–57] *Altered white matter integrity* with lower fractional anisotropy has also been reported, using diffusion tensor imaging studies, in the U fibers of fronto-limbic system, anterior and posterior corona radiata, and the corpus callosum.[58–62]

Genetic Studies

Genetic studies are sparse in PBD and are summarized by Mick and Faraone.[63] Elevated risk for bipolar disorder and unipolar depression was noted in relatives of early-onset probands greater than late-onset probands.[64] Also, increased lifetime rates of bipolar disorder are seen among those who experienced first onset of affective symptoms prior to age 12, relative to those older than 12.[65] Therefore, evidence points to increased familial risk for PBD among those with early-onset bipolar disorder.[63,66] Secondary analyses of linkage studies in adults stratified by age indicated region of linkage to loci on chromosomes that ranged from 12p, 14q, 15q,[67] 6q25, 9q34, 20q11,[68] 21q22.13, 18p11.2,[69] 3p14,[70] and 3q28.[71] None of these findings were replicated despite significant association in early-onset illness across these studies. Genetic studies of candidate genes were conducted in trios that published odds ratio of more than 1 in COMT Val158Met,[63] BDNF Val66Met,[72] SLC6A4 HTTLPR,[73] SLC6A3 rs41084,[74] and GAD1 rs2241165.[75] Furthermore, BDNF variant predicted rapid cycling variant in PBD.[76] Treatment with mood stabilizers over 8 weeks has normalized BDNF mRNA levels in PBD.[77]

Secondary analyses of adult bipolar data indicate genome-wide significant associations with ANK3 and CACNA1C suggesting calcium channel abnormalities.[78] Notwithstanding the phenotypic or etiologic restrictions, these genes may also explain etiology behind affect regulation or cognitive difficulties and need to be understood in larger samples. Most recent findings alert to the possibility that clinicians must be alert to the potential that relatives of patients with ADHD may have bipolar disorder.[79,80]

Conclusion: Laying Inroads for Future Breakthroughs

Overall, there is remarkable uniformity in findings from whole-brain conventional fMRI studies and the connectivity studies showing impairment in the implicated regions regardless of design or sample size differences. While earlier block design studies garnered greater statistical power to the data illustrating functional disturbance in PBD that laid groundwork and the latter ER designs continue to drive better temporal specificity with task events, there is basic consistency in findings across outcomes with either design. Furthermore, structural abnormalities in the higher cortical PFC regions and the subcortical amygdala and basal ganglia regions align with functional disturbance and may be serving as hubs of functional communication. Genetic and structural abnormalities may influence brain function, but exact relationships across these modalities are yet to be explored. Also, the intricate whole-brain functional connectivity, the relationship between resting- and task-based activity, and how the neuronal messages are conveyed between the white matter fiber tracts that end and begin around the areas of functional gray matter are all open for future investigation.

On in-depth review of functional studies, qualitatively, four major things appear to influence findings: whether the samples include bipolar disorder Type I or II or spectrum of bipolar disorders, the domain probed by the task, comorbidity, and type of intervention such as specific medications. However, it is hard to attribute specific effects if all confounds appear in irregular combinations across studies. The findings contingent on the domain that is probed, by far, has the strongest impact in dictating the brain activity pattern with consistency. However, affective circuitry regions are always engaged and impaired in bipolar illness regardless of any cognitive domain that is probed. The issue of multiple-domain dysfunction versus categorical comorbidity will continue to challenge decoding this complex disorder. The domain-specific circuits that are affected can serve as new targets for treatment selection and development. They provide pathways by which research findings can be translated into changes in clinical decision making. Some of the consistent findings are as follows:

1. Emotions impact cognition and emotion regulation, but negative emotions, especially angry emotions, have greater impact than positive emotions.
2. Reward studies, informed by experiments probing emotion, point to caution against imposing negative behavioral consequences in children with PBD.
3. Working memory, attention, response inhibition, and problem solving are inherently impaired in PBD (Chapter 14); functional studies complement the findings in illustrating how negative emotional stimuli amplify dysfunctional interlinked cognitive and affective circuitry brain function in PBD.

Dorsal cognitive circuits and ventral emotional circuits are engaged in combination while performing interface tasks. It is the cognitive (DLPFC) and emotional (VLPFC, MPFC) prefrontal regions that work in concert and tend to be more immediately plastic with treatment than subcortical regions such as amygdala that take time to normalize.

Specific medication choices may have added advantages in improving either or both emotional and cognitive function, and the future holds promise for brain-based pharmacotherapy algorithm. The critical mass of powerful findings accrued from the first decade of imaging studies in PBD pave the path to a future wave of fine-grained domain-based explorations as well as dictate the need to shape our interventions in cognitive-behavioral psychotherapy techniques and better refined classroom interventions in addressing combined affective and cognitive dysfunction.

Author Disclosures

Dr. Pavuluri receives or has received grant support from the following sources: National Institutes of Health (NIH), the National Institute of Mental Health, the National Alliance for Research on Schizophrenia and Depression (NARSAD), the American Foundation for Suicide Prevention, and the Marshall Reynolds Foundation. She is the recipient of the Berger-Colbeth Term Chair in Child Psychiatry and participated in the Otsuka Pharmaceuticals National Advisory Board meeting in 2013.

References

1. Chang K, Adleman NE, Dienes K, Simeonova DI, Menon V, Reiss A. Anomalous prefrontal-subcortical activation in familial pediatric bipolar disorder: a functional magnetic resonance imaging investigation. *Arch Gen Psychiatry.* 2004;61(8):781–92.

2. Pavuluri MN, O'Connor MM, Harral E, Sweeney JA. Affective neural circuitry during facial emotion processing in pediatric bipolar disorder. *Biol Psychiatry*. 2007;62(2):158–67.

3. Rich BA, Schmajuk M, Perez-Edgar KE, Pine DS, Fox NA, Leibenluft E. The impact of reward, punishment, and frustration on attention in pediatric bipolar disorder. *Biol Psychiatry*. 2005;58(7):532–9.

4. Pavuluri MN, Passarotti AM, Harral EM, Sweeney JA. An fMRI study of the neural correlates of incidental versus directed emotion processing in pediatric bipolar disorder. *J Am Acad Child Adolesc Psychiatry*. 2009;48(3):308–19.

5. Pavuluri MN, O'Connor MM, Harral EM, Sweeney JA. An fMRI study of the interface between affective and cognitive neural circuitry in pediatric bipolar disorder. *Psychiatry Res*. 2008;162(3):244–55.

6. Kim P, Thomas LA, Rosen BH, et al. Differing amygdala responses to facial expressions in children and adults with bipolar disorder. *Am J Psychiatry*. 2012;169(6):642–9.

7. Wegbreit E, Passarotti AM, Ellis JA, et al. Where, when, how high, and how long? The hemodynamics of emotional response in psychotropic-naive patients with adolescent bipolar disorder. *J Affect Disord*. 2013;147(1–3):304–11.

8. Goldman-Rakic PS. Topography of cognition: parallel distributed networks in primate association cortex. Annual review of neuroscience*Annu Rev Neurosci*. 1988;11:137–56.

9. Pavuluri MN, Schenkel LS, Aryal S, et al. Neurocognitive function in unmedicated manic and medicated euthymic pediatric bipolar patients. *Am J Psychiatry*. 2006;163(2):286–93.

10. Pavuluri MN, Passarotti A. Neural bases of emotional processing in pediatric bipolar disorder. *Expert Rev Neurotherap*. 2008;8(9):1381–7.

11. Ladouceur CD, Farchione T, Diwadkar V, et al. Differential patterns of abnormal activity and connectivity in the amygdala-prefrontal circuitry in bipolar-I and bipolar-NOS youth. *J Am Acad Child Adolesc Psychiatry*. 2011;50(12):1275–89.

12. Rich BA, Brotman MA, Dickstein DP, Mitchell DG, Blair RJ, Leibenluft E. Deficits in attention to emotional stimuli distinguish youth with severe mood dysregulation from youth with bipolar disorder. *J Abnorm Child Psychology*. 2010;38(5):695–706.

13. Singh MK, Chang KD, Kelley RG, et al. Reward processing in adolescents with bipolar I disorder. *J Am Acad Child Adolesc Psychiatry*. 2013;52(1):68–83.

14. Ernst M, Nelson EE, Jazbec S, et al. Amygdala and nucleus accumbens in responses to receipt and omission of gains in adults and adolescents. *NeuroImage*. 2005;25(4):1279–91.

15. May JC, Delgado MR, Dahl RE, et al. Event-related functional magnetic resonance imaging of reward-related brain circuitry in children and adolescents. *Biol Psychiatry*. 2004;55(4):359–66.

16. Bjork JM, Hommer DW. Anticipating instrumentally obtained and passively-received rewards: a factorial fMRI investigation. *Behav Brain Res*. 2007;177(1):165–70.

17. Passarotti AM, Sweeney JA, Pavuluri MN. Fronto-limbic dysfunction in mania pre-treatment and persistent amygdala over-activity post-treatment in pediatric bipolar disorder. *Psychopharmacology*. 2011;216(4):485–99.

18. Workshop on the Cognitive Systems Domain2011 October 23–25, 2011; Rockville, MD: Research domain criteria (RDoC) project. http://www.nimh.nih.gov/research-priorities/rdoc/cognitive-systems-workshop-proceedings.shtml

19. Adler CM, Delbello MP, Mills NP, Schmithorst V, Holland S, Strakowski SM. Comorbid ADHD is associated with altered patterns of neuronal activation in adolescents with bipolar disorder performing a simple attention task. *Bipolar Disord*. 2005;7(6):577–88.

20. Cerullo MA, Adler CM, Lamy M, et al. Differential brain activation during response inhibition in bipolar and attention-deficit hyperactivity disorders. *Early Intervent Psychiatry*. 2009;3(3):189–97.

21. Leibenluft E, Rich BA, Vinton DT, et al. Neural circuitry engaged during unsuccessful motor inhibition in pediatric bipolar disorder. *Am J Psychiatry*. 2007;164(1):52–60.

22. Deveney CM, Connolly ME, Jenkins SE, et al. Neural recruitment during failed motor inhibition differentiates youths with bipolar disorder and severe mood dysregulation. *Biol Psychol*. 2012;89(1):148–55.

23. Weathers JD, Stringaris A, Deveney CM, et al. A developmental study of the neural circuitry mediating motor inhibition in bipolar disorder. *Am J Psychiatry*. 2012;169(6):633–41.

24. Diler RS, Segreti AM, Ladouceur CD, et al. Neural correlates of treatment in adolescents with bipolar depression during response inhibition. *J Child Adolesc Psychopharmacol*. 2013;23(3):214–21.

25. Singh MK, DelBello MP, Fleck DE, Shear PK, Strakowski SM. Inhibition and attention in adolescents with nonmanic mood disorders and a high risk for developing mania. *J Clin Exp Neuropsychol.* 2009;31(1):1–7.

26. Birmaher B, Axelson D, Goldstein B, et al. Psychiatric disorders in preschool offspring of parents with bipolar disorder: the Pittsburgh Bipolar Offspring Study (BIOS). *Am J Psychiatry.* 2010;167(3):321–30.

27. Geller B, Tillman R, Craney JL, Bolhofner K. Four-year prospective outcome and natural history of mania in children with a prepubertal and early adolescent bipolar disorder phenotype. *Arch Gen Psychiatry.* 2004;61(5):459–67.

28. Pavuluri MN, Birmaher B, Naylor MW. Pediatric bipolar disorder: a review of the past 10 years. *J Am Acad Child Adolesc Psychiatry.* 2005;44(9):846–71.

29. Pavuluri MN, West A, Hill SK, Jindal K, Sweeney JA. Neurocognitive function in pediatric bipolar disorder: 3-year follow-up shows cognitive development lagging behind healthy youths. *J Am Acad Child Adolesc Psychiatry.* 2009;48(3):299–307.

30. Passarotti AM, Sweeney JA, Pavuluri MN. Emotion processing influences working memory circuits in pediatric bipolar disorder and attention-deficit/hyperactivity disorder. *J Am Acad Child Adolesc Psychiatry.* 2010;49(10):1064–80.

31. Passarotti AM, Ellis J, Wegbreit E, Stevens MC, Pavuluri MN. Reduced functional connectivity of prefrontal regions and amygdala within affect and working memory networks in pediatric bipolar disorder. *Brain Connect.* 2012;2(6):320–34.

32. Dickstein DP, Rich BA, Roberson-Nay R, et al. Neural activation during encoding of emotional faces in pediatric bipolar disorder. *Bipolar Disord.* 2007;9(7):679–92.

33. Adler CM, DelBello MP, Strakowski SM. Brain network dysfunction in bipolar disorder. *CNS Spectrums.* 2006;11(4):312–20; quiz 23–4.

34. Geller B, Zimerman B, Williams M, et al. Diagnostic characteristics of 93 cases of a prepubertal and early adolescent bipolar disorder phenotype by gender, puberty and comorbid attention deficit hyperactivity disorder. *J Child Adolesc Psychopharmacol.* 2000;10(3):157–64.

35. Geller D, Biederman J, Jones J, et al. Is juvenile obsessive-compulsive disorder a developmental subtype of the disorder? A review of the pediatric literature. *J Am Acad Child Adolesc Psychiatry.* 1998;37(4):420–7.

36. Ghahremani DG, Monterosso J, Jentsch JD, Bilder RM, Poldrack RA. Neural components underlying behavioral flexibility in human reversal learning. *Cerebral Cortex.* 2010;20(8):1843–52.

37. Dickstein DP, Gorrostieta C, Ombao H, et al. Fronto-temporal spontaneous resting state functional connectivity in pediatric bipolar disorder. *Biol Psychiatry.* 2010;68(9):839–46.

38. Adleman NE, Fromm SJ, Razdan V, et al. Cross-sectional and longitudinal abnormalities in brain structure in children with severe mood dysregulation or bipolar disorder. *J Child Psychol Psychiatry Allied Discip.* 2012;53(11):1149–56.

39. Passarotti AM, Sweeney JA, Pavuluri MN. Neural correlates of response inhibition in pediatric bipolar disorder and attention deficit hyperactivity disorder. *Psychiatry Res.* 2010;181(1):36–43.

40. Deco G, Rolls ET, Romo R. Synaptic dynamics and decision making. *Proc Natl Acad Sci USA.* 2010;107(16):7545–9.

41. Wu M, Lu LH, Passarotti AM, Wegbreit E, Fitzgerald J, Pavuluri MN. Altered affective, executive and sensorimotor resting state networks in patients with pediatric mania. *J Psychiatry Neurosci (JPN).* 2013;38(4):232–40.

42. Friedman SD, Shaw DW, Artru AA, et al. Regional brain chemical alterations in young children with autism spectrum disorder. *Neurology.* 2003;60(1):100–7.

43. Olvera RL, Caetano SC, Fonseca M, et al. Low levels of N-acetyl aspartate in the left dorsolateral prefrontal cortex of pediatric bipolar patients. *J Child Adolesc Psychopharmacol.* 2007;17(4):461–73.

44. Caetano SC, Olvera RL, Hatch JP, et al. Lower N-acetyl-aspartate levels in prefrontal cortices in pediatric bipolar disorder: a (1)H magnetic resonance spectroscopy study. *J Am Acad Child Adolesc Psychiatry.* 2011;50(1):85–94.

45. Patel NC, Cecil KM, Strakowski SM, Adler CM, DelBello MP. Neurochemical alterations in adolescent bipolar depression: a proton magnetic resonance spectroscopy pilot study of the prefrontal cortex. *J Child Adolesc Psychopharmacol.* 2008;18(6):623–7.

46. Cecil KM, DelBello MP, Sellars MC, Strakowski SM. Proton magnetic resonance spectroscopy of the frontal lobe and cerebellar vermis in children with a mood disorder and a familial risk for bipolar disorders. *J Child Adolesc Psychopharmacol.* 2003;13(4):545–55.

47. Sassi RB, Stanley JA, Axelson D, et al. Reduced NAA levels in the dorsolateral prefrontal cortex of young bipolar patients. *Am J Psychiatry.* 2005;162(11):2109–15.

48. Yang H, Lu LH, Wu M, et al. Time course of recovery showing initial prefrontal cortex changes at 16 weeks, extending to subcortical changes by 3 years in pediatric bipolar disorder. *J Affect Disord.* 2013;150(2):571–7.

49. Mayanil T, Wegbreit E, Fitzgerald J, Pavuluri M. Emerging biosignature of brain function and intervention in pediatric bipolar disorder. *Minerva Pediatrica.* 2011;63(3):183–200.

50. Pavuluri MN, Passarotti AM, Fitzgerald JM, Wegbreit E, Sweeney JA. Risperidone and divalproex differentially engage the fronto-striato-temporal circuitry in pediatric mania: a pharmacological functional magnetic resonance imaging study. *J Am Acad Child Adolesc Psychiatry.* 2012;51(2):157–70 e5.

51. Pavuluri MN, Passarotti AM, Lu LH, Carbray JA, Sweeney JA. Double-blind randomized trial of risperidone versus divalproex in pediatric bipolar disorder: fMRI outcomes. *Psychiatry Res.* 2011;193(1):28–37.

52. DelBello MP, Cecil KM, Adler CM, Daniels JP, Strakowski SM. Neurochemical effects of olanzapine in first-hospitalization manic adolescents: a proton magnetic resonance spectroscopy study. *Neuropsychopharmacology.* 2006;31(6):1264–73.

53. Chiu S, Widjaja F, Bates ME, et al. Anterior cingulate volume in pediatric bipolar disorder and autism. *J Affect Disord.* 2008;105(1–3):93–9.0

54. Dickstein DP, Milham MP, Nugent AC, et al. Frontotemporal alterations in pediatric bipolar disorder: results of a voxel-based morphometry study. *Arch Gen Psychiatry.* 2005;62(7):734–41.

55. DelBello MP, Zimmerman ME, Mills NP, Getz GE, Strakowski SM. Magnetic resonance imaging analysis of amygdala and other subcortical brain regions in adolescents with bipolar disorder. *Bipolar Disord.* 2004;6(1):43–52.

56. Frazier JA, Chiu S, Breeze JL, et al. Structural brain magnetic resonance imaging of limbic and thalamic volumes in pediatric bipolar disorder. *Am J Psychiatry.* 2005;162(7):1256–65.

57. Wilke M, Kowatch RA, DelBello MP, Mills NP, Holland SK. Voxel-based morphometry in adolescents with bipolar disorder: first results. *Psychiatry Res.* 2004;131(1):57–69.

58. Adler CM, Adams J, DelBello MP, et al. Evidence of white matter pathology in bipolar disorder adolescents experiencing their first episode of mania: a diffusion tensor imaging study. *Am J Psychiatry.* 2006;163(2):322–4.

59. Barnea-Goraly N, Chang KD, Karchemskiy A, Howe ME, Reiss AL. Limbic and corpus callosum aberrations in adolescents with bipolar disorder: a tract-based spatial statistics analysis. *Biol Psychiatry.* 2009;66(3):238–44.

60. Frazier JA, Breeze JL, Papadimitriou G, et al. White matter abnormalities in children with and at risk for bipolar disorder. *Bipolar Disord.* 2007;9(8):799–809.

61. Kafantaris V, Kingsley P, Ardekani B, et al. Lower orbital frontal white matter integrity in adolescents with bipolar I disorder. *J Am Acad Child Adolesc Psychiatry.* 2009;48(1):79–86.

62. Pavuluri MN, Yang S, Kamineni K, et al. Diffusion tensor imaging study of white matter fiber tracts in pediatric bipolar disorder and attention-deficit/hyperactivity disorder. *Biol Psychiatry.* 2009;65(7):586–93.

63. Mick E, Faraone SV. Family and genetic association studies of bipolar disorder in children. *Child Adolesc Psychiatric Clin North Am.* 2009;18(2):441–53, x.

64. M T, Faraone SV. *The Genetics of Mood Disorders.* Baltimore, MD: The John Hopkins University Press; 1990.

65. Pauls DL, Morton LA, Egeland JA. Risks of affective illness among first-degree relatives of bipolar I old-order Amish probands. *Arch Gen Psychiatry.* 1992;49(9):703–8.

66. Bellivier F, Golmard JL, Rietschel M, et al. Age at onset in bipolar I affective disorder: further evidence for three subgroups. *Am J Psychiatry.* 2003;160(5):999–1001.

67. Faraone SV, Glatt SJ, Su J, Tsuang MT. Three potential susceptibility loci shown by a genome-wide scan for regions influencing the age at onset of mania. *Am J Psychiatry.* 2004;161(4):625–30.

68. Faraone SV, Lasky-Su J, Glatt SJ, Van Eerdewegh P, Tsuang MT. Early onset bipolar disorder: possible linkage to chromosome 9q34. *Bipolar Disord.* 2006;8(2):144–51.

69. Lin PI, McInnis MG, Potash JB, et al. Assessment of the effect of age at onset on linkage to bipolar disorder: evidence on chromosomes 18p and 21q. *Am J Hum Genetics.* 2005;77(4):545–55.

70. Etain B, Mathieu F, Rietschel M, et al. Genome-wide scan for genes involved in bipolar affective disorder in 70 European families ascertained through a bipolar type I early-onset proband: supportive evidence for linkage at 3p14. *Mol Psychiatry.* 2006;11(7):685–94.

71. Zandi PP, Badner JA, Steele J, et al. Genome-wide linkage scan of 98 bipolar pedigrees and analysis of clinical covariates. *Mol Psychiatry.* 2007;12(7):630–9.

72. Geller B, Badner JA, Tillman R, Christian SL, Bolhofner K, Cook EH, Jr. Linkage disequilibrium of the brain-derived neurotrophic factor Val66Met polymorphism in children with a prepubertal and early adolescent bipolar disorder phenotype. *Am J Psychiatry.* 2004;161(9):1698–700.

73. Geller B, Cook EH Jr. Serotonin transporter gene (HTTLPR) is not in linkage disequilibrium with prepubertal and early adolescent bipolarity. *Biol Psychiatry.* 1999;45(9):1230–3.

74. Mick E, Kim JW, Biederman J, et al. Family based association study of pediatric bipolar disorder and the dopamine transporter gene (SLC6A3). *Am J Med Genet B Neuropsychiatric Genet.* 2008;147B(7):1182–5.

75. Geller B, Tillman R, Bolhofner K, Hennessy K, Cook EH Jr. GAD1 single nucleotide polymorphism is in linkage disequilibrium with a child bipolar I disorder phenotype. *J Child Adolesc Psychopharmacol.* 2008;18(1):25–9.

76. Muller DJ, de Luca V, Sicard T, King N, Strauss J, Kennedy JL. Brain-derived neurotrophic factor (BDNF) gene and rapid-cycling bipolar disorder: family-based association study. *Br J Psychiatry.* 2006;189:317–23.

77. Pandey GN, Rizavi HS, Dwivedi Y, Pavuluri MN. Brain-derived neurotrophic factor gene expression in pediatric bipolar disorder: effects of treatment and clinical response. *J Am Acad Child Adolesc Psychiatry.* 2008;47(9):1077–85.

78. Ferreira MA, O'Donovan MC, Meng YA, et al. Collaborative genome-wide association analysis supports a role for ANK3 and CACNA1C in bipolar disorder. *Nature Genet.* 2008;40(9):1056–8.

79. Larsson H, Ryden E, Boman M, Langstrom N, Lichtenstein P, Landen M. Risk of bipolar disorder and schizophrenia in relatives of people with attention-deficit hyperactivity disorder. *Br J Psychiatry.* 2013;203(2):103–6.

80. Biederman J, Faraone SV, Petty C, Martelon M, Woodworth KY, Wozniak J. Further evidence that pediatric-onset bipolar disorder comorbid with ADHD represents a distinct subtype: results from a large controlled family study. *J Psychiatr Res.* 2013;47(1):15–22.

Neurocognitive Models of Evolving Bipolar Disorder in Youth

Alessandra M. Passarotti

Toward Understanding the Neurocognitive Endophenotype of Bipolar Disorder in Youth

Bipolar disorder in youth is primarily characterized as an illness of chronic mood dysregulation. In fact, until recently, cognitive problems were overlooked or seen as caused by the chronic affective dysfunction. However, more attention has recently been devoted to the presence of *cognitive and information processing deficits* in youth with bipolar disorder—particularly in the domains of emotion processing, working memory, attention, cognitive flexibility, and executive functions.[1-3] Of further significance, these deficits persist during interepisodic, euthymic periods[2]; they tend to worsen with development[3] and with progression of the illness[4]; and they lead to poor psychosocial functioning.[5] Therefore, cognitive deficits could potentially be markers of neuropathology and disease vulnerability in youth with bipolar disorder. In the field of child and adolescent psychiatry there is also growing awareness of the intricate interconnection between affective dysfunction and cognitive deficits in bipolar disorder.

In an effort to better identify the cognitive operations that are deficient in bipolar disorder, a useful approach has been that of using neuroscience-based tasks to test different domains, based on the Research Domain Criteria (RDoC) approach recently proposed by The National Institute of Health.[6] Brain imaging and functional magnetic resonance imaging (fMRI) studies on bipolar disorder have thrived in the past 15–20 years, revealing specific neural dysfunction in the connectivity between prefrontal cortex and limbic systems.[7] On the other hand, the investigation of cognitive deficits in bipolar disorder

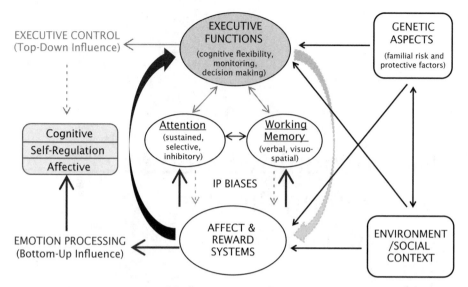

FIGURE 13.1 A neurocognitive model of cognitive and affective systems, and their interactions, in bipolar disorder. Thicker lines indicate greater influence; dotted lines indicate weaker influence. Genetic and environmental aspects are represented as well. Note that self-regulation involves both cognitive and affective components. IP, information processing.

has lagged behind, possibly because of the lack of strong neurocognitive models to guide clinical research toward explaining the mental constructs underlying bipolar disorder symptoms, and the scarcity of standardized behavioral tasks that are sensitive enough to differentiate performance in bipolar disorder youth relative to healthy youth. However, as we progress in defining the dysfunctional emotional and cognitive circuits in bipolar disorder, it is even more important to better examine and explain the relationship between neurocognitive deficits and brain imaging findings.[8]

In this chapter we will discuss the existing evidence on neurocognitive deficits in bipolar disorder youth and their clinical relevance within the context of a proposed model of cognitive (i.e., prefrontal cortex circuits) and affective (i.e., limbic circuits) systems. The central focus will be the unbalanced interactions between the two systems, due to the overreactivity of the affective system that can hinder or bias cognitive operations in challenging situations. Genetic aspects interacting with the cognitive and affective systems are also touched upon toward the end of the chapter (Fig. 13.1).

Emotion Processing Deficits in Bipolar Disorder Youth

While we know that emotion processing differs in children with bipolar disorder relative to healthy children, we are just starting to understand the mental constructs and the neural underpinnings of the developmental deviation that lead to the bipolar disorder profile of chronic affective dysregulation.[9] Studies on younger children with bipolar disorder are still scant[10–12]; however, there is an increasing body of research with older children and adolescents with bipolar disorder. Typically, bipolar disorder youth exhibit significant deficits both in terms of experiencing and understanding their own emotions, and in perceiving and understanding those of others. Because these skills are so important for psychosocial functioning, an extensive area of investigation in bipolar disorder studies is that of facial emotion processing, using basic and universally recognized emotions. With regard to the ability to discriminate between different facial emotions, Brotman et al.[13] found deficits in facial emotion labeling across a variety of emotions (i.e., happiness, surprise, fear, sadness, anger, disgust) in euthymic bipolar disorder youth, relative to comparison subjects, during an "Emotional Expression Multimorph Task" with gradations of facial emotions from 100% neutrality to 100% emotional expression. The fact that the individuals were euthymic suggests that these may be "trait deficits." Further confirming this point, in this study no significant differences were found between youth with bipolar disorder and youth at familial risk for bipolar disorder, suggesting that these emotion processing difficulties may be an endophenotype of bipolar disorder. Youth with bipolar disorder may also have a higher threshold for discriminating between different facial emotions. Indeed, McClure and colleagues[14] found that during a task requiring one to discriminate between facial emotions of different intensity, individuals with bipolar disorder were comparable in performance to healthy youth for high-intensity emotional faces but exhibited deficits specifically when identifying low-intensity facial expressions.

Emotion processing deficits seem to be present also when children with bipolar disorder process child faces instead of adult faces. In fact, Seymour et al.[15] found deficits in emotional face identification in 7- to 17-year-old youth with bipolar disorder (narrow phenotype) using emotional faces with either low or high emotional intensity (i.e., happy, sad, angry, fearful) from the Diagnostic Analysis of Nonverbal Accuracy (DANVA)[16]. Bipolar youth made significantly more identification errors on child happy faces than either healthy youth or individuals with attention-deficit/hyperactivity disorder (ADHD). Furthermore, indicating an illness-specific deficit, youth with bipolar disorder were more likely than youth with ADHD to make errors on low-intensity happy faces, but not high-intensity happy faces, suggesting increased difficulties with ambiguous face emotional information.

It is possible that the deficits in face emotion processing in bipolar disorder are due to less efficient allocation of attention to certain aspects of faces rather than others. In fact, Kim et al.[17] found that during a facial emotion labeling task involving varying emotions (i.e., anger, fear, sadness, happiness, neutral) and emotional intensity levels (60%, 80%, 100%) children with bipolar disorder, compared with healthy youth, revealed decreased fixations to eyes that were also correlated with lower labeling accuracy across emotions.

Moreover, it is remarkable that there are not only difficulties in emotion processing and discrimination but also intrinsic biases toward negative emotions (see also

Chapter 12, for brain imaging findings on this issue). For instance, during a face recognition task, Rich et al.[18] found increased perception of hostility in bipolar disorder youth relative to healthy youth while looking at faces with neutral emotions, suggesting a bias to interpret neutral emotions as negative. In addition, Shankman and colleagues[19] found that during the Emotion Recognition Test (ER-40), from the Penn Computerized Neuropsychological Battery,[20] 8- to 17-year-old youth with bipolar disorder showed specific impairment in performance for faces with negative emotions such as "sad" and "fearful," relative to healthy youth. Moreover, in an additional task called the Chicago Pediatric Emotional Acuity Task (Chicago-PEAT), which is a modified version of the Penn Emotional Acuity Task (PEAT), gender effects were found, such that girls with bipolar disorder mislabeled "very angry" faces more frequently than boys with bipolar disorder relative to healthy youth while differentiating intensity levels for angry and happy expressions. Interestingly, analyses revealed that this gender effect was mediated specifically by irritability, as assessed through self-report. Irritability, defined as an emotional reaction of anger or frustration to internal or external stimulation, is very common in bipolar disorder youth.[21,22] Moreover, there is evidence that bipolar disorder girls show greater emotional intensity than boys.[23] It is possible that irritability may mediate deficits in emotion recognition by impairing attention and overfocusing on one's own feelings rather than others' feelings.[24] Hence, psychosocial interventions to improve interpersonal skills should address these deficits while also targeting irritability problems in bipolar disorder.

There is also growing evidence that the emotion processing deficits in bipolar disorder youth are both state and trait dependent. Schenkel et al.[25] examined facial affect processing in 8- to 18-year-old bipolar disorder youth who were either acutely ill/unmedicated or clinically stable/medicated, relative to healthy youth. Two tasks were administered: a Penn Emotional Acuity Test[20] tested the ability to identify facial expressions such as "happy" and "sad," ranging from neutral to extreme in emotional intensity; an Emotion Differentiation Task measured the ability to differentiate between two emotional faces, presented simultaneously, which exhibited slight variations in intensity of the same emotion, which was either "happy" or "sad" (e.g., "are both faces equally happy?"). For the Emotional Acuity Test, while there were no group differences for neutral faces, bipolar disorder youth, relative to healthy youth, exhibited a bias to misjudge the intense emotions as mild. This pattern was found regardless of medication and clinical status, suggesting the presence of both state and trait deficits.

A possible explanation for these results is that pediatric bipolar individuals exhibit very intense emotions, and this may alter their perception of what intense emotions, as perceived by healthy youth, may be. Importantly, in the bipolar disorder group a younger age of onset was associated with more severe deficits in emotion processing, suggesting that with early illness onset the symptoms may interfere with development of emotion processing, leading to worse functional outcome. This observation is in line with studies suggesting that earlier age of onset is associated with more severe illness.[26] Only the acutely ill individuals did worse on the Emotional Differentiation Task relative to healthy youth, suggesting a state-based deficit, possibly because mania impairs the efficiency of subtle perceptual processes necessary to compare and contrast faces with slight changes in the same emotional expression. Moreover, bipolar disorder youth with ADHD comorbidity performed worse when processing sad expressions only, which is in agreement with studies showing more impaired emotion processing and social perception in bipolar disorder youth with ADHD comorbidity.[27] This study suggests both state- and trait-related emotion processing deficits. However, results are not conclusive because the unmedicated/medicated status was examined in cross-sectional samples of bipolar disorder youth, rather than having the same group of untreated individuals undergo a longitudinal follow-up with treatment.

Importance of Studying the Interface of Affect and Cognition in Bipolar Disorder Youth

Of particular interest for better characterizing the bipolar disorder endophenotype is the study of the dysfunctional interface of cognition and affect. As illustrated in the proposed model affective overreactivity in bipolar disorder may overwhelm cognitive systems, hindering information processing as well as affective and cognitive self-regulation (Fig. 13.1). Indeed, in individuals with bipolar disorder emotional information interferes with cognitive processing on a daily basis—for instance, when a child with bipolar disorder is unable to control his or her anger or frustration after a quarrel with a classmate in order to focus on solving a reading or math problem before the end of the school day. There is growing evidence that emotional interference disrupts attention and working memory processes in bipolar disorder, even when a task does not directly require processing of emotional information. Schenkel and colleagues[28] found that both unmedicated Type I and II bipolar disorder youth performed significantly worse than healthy youth when identifying the intensity of happy and angry expressions on the Chicago-PEAT Task. In addition, during an affective two-back memory task involving happy, angry, and neutral faces, only Type I bipolar disorder youth demonstrated working memory impairments relative to healthy youth, which was worse with negative relative to neutral faces, suggesting more severe social-cognitive impairment and sensitivity to negative emotions in this bipolar disorder subtype.

Furthermore, there is growing evidence that in challenging situations children with bipolar disorder exhibit not only increased emotional reactivity but also reduced attentional performance, such as in tasks with negative contingencies and feedback[29,30] and during semantic processing in the presence of emotional information.[31] Therefore, across different cognitive domains, both children and adults with bipolar disorder might be more sensitive to negative emotions. Of relevance, these deficits may be qualitatively different in bipolar disorder compared to other mood dysregulation illnesses such as severe mood dysregulation (SMD). In fact, Rich et al.[32] provided initial evidence that deficits in attention to emotional stimuli may differ between bipolar disorder and severe mood dysregulation, in that only the bipolar disorder group showed significant emotional modulation of attention. This oversensitivity to emotions in bipolar disorder should be a main target of intervention, since it may be an additional stressor that leads to relapse, that hinders the ability to regulate one's affective reactions, and the ability to develop and maintain coping strategies for familial or social conflict.

Summary and Clinical Considerations

Emotion processing deficits have been extensively documented in bipolar disorder youth. Of clinical relevance, these deficits are detrimental in pediatric bipolar disorder because they deprive the child of normal development of psychosocial skills, such as the ability to interpret facial expressions accurately, to attend and react to social cues in adaptive ways, and to establish and maintain social relations. Moreover, these deficits may contribute to maladaptive cognitive styles, leading to poor self-esteem and social skills, and increasing vulnerability to stress and relapse.[14,30,33] Finally, given the unique pathophysiology and oversensitivity to negative emotions and negative feedback in bipolar disorder youth, it is particularly important to study how interaction of cognitive and affective systems shape the clinical profile of bipolar disorder through development. Early intervention may be beneficial to prevent worsening of emotion processing deficits and dysfunctional interactions between cognitive and affective systems in bipolar disorder.

The Neuropsychological Endophenotype of Bipolar Disorder Youth

One important question that recent studies have tried to address is whether the cognitive deficits in bipolar disorder youth are global across several neuropsychological domains or cluster around specific domains. The main areas of neuropsychological dysfunction that have been reported in meta-analyses of both child and adult bipolar disorder include executive functions, immediate and delayed verbal learning and memory, and attention.[8,34,35] However, it is still a matter of debate whether the neurocognitive deficits are present premorbidly, start at onset, or develop as a consequence of repeated episodes.[36]

Several studies suggest that one of the most impaired neuropsychological domains in bipolar disorder is the verbal memory domain, which may also indicate a disease signature more specific to bipolar disorder than to other mental illnesses (see Horn et al.[37]). Pavuluri et al.[2] examined unmedicated manic and medicated euthymic bipolar disorder youth relative to healthy youth (mean age = 11.7 years, SD = 3.0) using standardized neuropsychological tests assessing attention, executive function, working memory, verbal memory, visual memory, visuospatial perception, and motor skills. Results showed that regardless of medication and illness status, bipolar individuals were impaired in attention, executive functioning, working memory, and verbal learning. ADHD comorbidity in these individuals led to worse performance for tasks related to attention and executive functions. Because medication status did not matter, the authors concluded that these impairments are trait-like characteristics of pediatric bipolar disorder—and suggest dysfunction of prefrontal cortex supporting working memory and mesial temporal lobe systems supporting verbal memory. Moreover, McClure et al.[38] found not only verbal memory and learning problems but also deficits in delayed facial recognition in bipolar disorder youth. These findings hint that deficits in verbal learning and memory, and some aspects of visuospatial memory or memory for faces, may characterize the narrow bipolar disorder phenotype.

Doyle et al.[39] found that bipolar disorder youth, Type I and II, relative to healthy youth exhibited deficits in sustained attention, working memory, and processing speed, when undergoing a comprehensive clinical neuropsychology battery. These deficits were present even after controlling for ADHD comorbidity. Moreover, Rucklidge et al.[40] compared youth with bipolar disorder, youth with ADHD, and the combined bipolar and ADHD type, in 14- to 17-year-old adolescents on tests of processing speed, memory, executive functioning, set shifting, and inhibition. The bipolar disorder–only group differed from healthy youth only in the working memory domain. The ADHD-only group and the combined bipolar and ADHD group were the most impaired, with deficits in processing and naming speed, working memory, and response inhibition. These results highlight the impact of ADHD comorbidity on neurocognitive functioning in bipolar disorder.

Not surprisingly, these cognitive deficits affect IQ measures with important repercussions for academic functioning. Indeed, deficits in attention and working memory, which may persist even in euthymic state and with optimal outcome,[41] prevent youth with bipolar disorder from performing at the level of healthy youth on verbal and visuospatial tasks included in IQ tests. In a recent meta-analysis, Joseph et al.[8] identified deficits in full-scale Intelligence Quotient (FSIQ) and academic functioning. Executive function problems were selectively found for planning, inhibition, and set shifting. Of relevance, the authors noted that the effects tend to disappear in youth bipolar disorder when compared to other pediatric populations. Therefore, to identify neurocognitive phenotypes that are specific to bipolar disorder, it is important to show not only that bipolar disorder youth exhibits deficits relative to healthy youth (i.e., in terms of general psychopathology) but also that these deficits differ from those of other pediatric illnesses, such as ADHD, major depressive disorder, or oppositional defiant disorder, which would imply some differences in the underlying mechanisms of dysfunction.

It is also important to further examine how development of social cognition and social skills may be affected in bipolar disorder.[38,42] Whitney et al.[43] found that children with a parent with bipolar disorder, who had mood dysregulation but not fully syndromal bipolar disorder, exhibited deficits across several neuropsychological domains related to social reciprocity (i.e., social awareness, social cognition, social communication, social motivation, and autistic mannerisms). There were no significant group differences in performance on Theory of Mind or affect recognition tasks. These effects may be due to innate differences in brain development governing socioemotional functioning, or alternatively they may be due to disruptions in normal development caused by mood regulation difficulties.

Effects of Attention-Deficit/Hyperactivity Disorder Comorbidity on Neurocognition in Bipolar Disorder Youth

Because of the high rates of comorbidity between bipolar disorder and ADHD, with prevalence up to 60%,[44] it is important to understand how the ADHD profile influences the clinical manifestations of bipolar disorder. There is growing evidence that bipolar disorder youth with ADHD comorbidity exhibit more severe working memory, attention, and inhibition deficits.[2,39,45] In addition, comorbid individuals have also been found to have a different developmental trajectory relative to bipolar disorder alone, with a profile of earlier onset, greater symptom severity, poorer cognitive functioning, more severe course of illness, and increased number of comorbidities.[46] In line with these findings, during a simple attention task Adler et al.[47] found that, relative to healthy youth, bipolar disorder youth with comorbid ADHD exhibited reduced activation in ventrolateral prefrontal cortex (VLPFC) (a brain region involved in inhibition functions) and increased recruitment of temporo-parietal regions (which are involved in working memory and attention functions).

It is also important to consider that earlier illness onset in the comorbid group may further complicate functional outcome by hindering the development of self-regulation and compensatory strategies that might help manage affective dysregulation in bipolar disorder youth. Taken together, this evidence suggests that the comorbid group may represent a different clinical phenotype, with more severe cognitive and neural deficits. Therefore, future longitudinal studies need to map the cognitive/affective and neural underpinnings of the different developmental trajectory in the comorbid group relative to bipolar disorder alone, which will help inform interventions that can specifically address the increased challenges in the comorbid individuals.

Summary and Clinical Considerations

Youth with bipolar disorder exhibits significant neuropsychological deficits, especially in some aspects of executive functions and in verbal memory, which may persist in euthymic state and may be trait related. Future longitudinal studies may help us better understand whether these deficits precede the onset of illness or are caused by its progression. Bipolar disorder youth with ADHD comorbidity may represent a different clinical phenotype, with more severe deficits and illness outcome. Moreover, the neuropsychological findings agree with reports of structural and functional abnormalities in prefrontal cortex, involved in language and memory functions, and in fronto-limbic systems in bipolar disorder, which seem to underlie the onset of mania and ultimately the course of bipolar disorder illness (see Strakowski et al.[7] for a review).

Executive Functions, Cognitive Flexibility, and Reward-Related Processes in Bipolar Disorder Youth

Clinicians, teachers, and parents alike would easily endorse the view that children and adolescents with bipolar disorder have impaired executive functions. Executive functions are part of a higher order system supervising and monitoring higher order cognitive functions such as attention, working memory, affective and cognitive regulation, planning, and decision making (Fig. 13.1). Executive functions rely heavily on lateral and medial prefrontal cortex and anterior cingulate cortex (ACC).[48] Development of these brain regions through adolescence is accompanied by improvements in cognitive and emotional regulation.[49-53] There is also some consensus that the abnormal development of the interactions between prefrontal cortex and limbic regions is likely responsible for the deficient self-control and affect regulation seen in bipolar disorder.[7,54-56] Moreover, dysfunctional development of executive functions and their interface with reward systems, which are important for motivation and goal-oriented behaviors, may lead to excessive reward-seeking behavior, such as substance abuse, and increased vulnerability to mood swings and impulsivity.[54,57]

One important aspect of executive functions is "cognitive flexibility," that is, the ability to adapt goal-oriented behavior and responses based on changing environmental conditions, such as reward or punishment. Examining this cognitive construct is very useful because it provides insight into the interface between executive functions and the dysfunctional affective system in bipolar disorder. A number of behavioral studies have shown deficits in cognitive flexibility in bipolar disorder. Gorrindo et al.[29] were among the first to document that during a cognitive flexibility task, that is, a probabilistic reversal learning task, 6- to 17-year-old bipolar disorder youth showed worse accuracy than healthy youth both while learning the association between a reward and an object in a pair of stimuli presented repeatedly, and while reversing their learned responses and reidentifying the new reward object after it had been switched without notice. Showing some continuity in the life span of bipolar disorder, these results are in agreement with a study by Pizzagalli et al.[58] in which adult bipolar disorder individuals, relative to healthy youth, showed reduced and delayed reward-related learning, which correlated with self-reported mood symptoms. These results, taken together, suggest a developmental continuity in cognitive flexibility deficits, and that possibly this could be a "trait" marker for early bipolar disorder illness detection.

In another study by Dickstein et al.[59] during a nonprobabilistic intradimensional/extradimensional (ID/ED) shift task of the CANTAB[60] computerized neuropsychological test battery, relative to healthy youth, 6- to 17-year-old narrow phenotype bipolar disorder youth made more errors and required more trials and time to complete a simple reversal. Results were not mediated by mood or ADHD comorbidity. These findings are consistent with those of adult bipolar disorder studies using the ID/ED shift task from the

CANTAB, which found deficits in this task in bipolar disorder relative to healthy youth that were independent of mood.[61,62]

The cognitive rigidity exhibited by bipolar disorder subjects may be a primary deficit, or it may be a consequence of affective overreactivity that interferes with executive functions in lateral prefrontal cortex.[59] In fact, children with bipolar disorder exhibit increased frustration associated with reduced cognitive flexibility in tasks specifically designed to elicit frustration. In an event-related potential (ERP) study by Rich et al.[30] participants underwent an affective Posner Attention Task, with three conditions: a condition with feedback but no contingencies, a condition with contingencies, and a third condition with rigged feedback aimed at causing frustration. Results showed that the bipolar disorder group relative to healthy youth had impaired ability to adapt to contingencies. ERP data showed that on a physiological level the behavioral impairment corresponded to reduced P3 amplitude in parietal regions involved in attention processes, specifically with the rigged task condition. These findings suggest that bipolar disorder youth fail to attend to the task and instead tend to redirect their attention to their own feelings of frustration as elicited during the rigged task.

Poor monitoring functions may also contribute to deficits in cognitive flexibility in bipolar disorder. In a study that used the same affective Posner Task, Rich et al.[32] showed that frustration-inducing negative feedback was accompanied by altered magnetoencephalography (MEG) patterns of activity in right anterior cingulate cortex, a region involved in performance and error monitoring, and in bilateral parietal lobe, involved in visuospatial orienting of attention. These findings indicate that deficient monitoring and control processes in bipolar disorder may lead to failure in assessing one's own performance, in recognizing the need to adjust performance or strategies, and in learning from feedback. Supporting this view, Patino et al.[63] found deficits in conflict monitoring and adaptation in bipolar disorder youth as well as adolescents at familial risk for developing bipolar disorder, during the Eriksen Flanker Task that included neutral, congruent, and incongruent flankers. The results demonstrated that compared with healthy youth they exhibited worse performance on incongruent trials, which are more challenging because they engender more interference, and greater intrasubject response time variability for both incongruent and congruent trials.

An important question is whether bipolar disorder youth exhibit unique cognitive flexibility deficits, or whether these deficits are similar to those exhibited by other pediatric diseases. In this regard, Dickstein et al.[64] examined the specificity of reversal learning impairments in 7- to 17-year-old bipolar disorder youth by comparing these individuals not only to healthy youth but also to youth with severe mood dysregulation, major depressive disorder, anxiety, and healthy youth. The results showed impaired probabilistic reversal learning specifically in bipolar disorder, while the other groups did not differ significantly from healthy subjects. The authors concluded that bipolar disorder youth may fail in using reinforcement expectancy information to guide their behavioral choices, as they are more likely to shift away from a correct response whether they have received either a reward or "spurious" punishment. Reward sensitivity is linked to the motivational drive underlying goal-oriented behavior.[65] Deficits in reward-related processes have been found in both adult and pediatric bipolar disorder, especially in fMRI studies,[58,66,67] suggesting impaired reward systems in bipolar disorder that may affect their ability to learn based on contingencies. These results are in line with fMRI tasks in bipolar disorder population showing disruption of prefrontal cortex and reward circuitries (i.e., fronto-cingulate-parietal and ventral striatal circuits) during reward-related tasks requiring cognitive flexibility.[64,68–70]

Summary and Clinical Considerations

Deficits in executive functions, cognitive flexibility, and self-regulation have been found in bipolar disorder using reversal learning paradigms, and tasks designed to elicit frustration during cognitive performance. The evidence suggests that the impaired cognitive flexibility and self-regulation functions in bipolar disorder may be modulated by emotional overreactivity that interferes with executive functions and possibly reduces performance monitoring. It has also been suggested that altered reward sensitivity in bipolar disorder youth may modulate these deficits. Altogether, the research evidence suggests that interventions that are based on reward contingencies need to keep into account the bipolar disorder youth profile of poor cognitive flexibility, altered responses to contingencies, and problems with learning from contingencies.

Working Memory Deficits in Bipolar Disorder Youth

Working memory is the ability to hold information online and process it for a few seconds, in order to store information in short-term memory. According to the influential model by Baddeley,[71] working memory is a multicomponent system served by distinct subsystems: the "central executive system" (CES) youth functions and directs focused attention, while two "storage buffers" store and manipulate verbal and visuospatial information, and an "episodic buffer" integrates multimodal representations. These working memory functions are performed by an extended network of specialized brain regions, among which the fronto-striatal system underlies the "central executive," while temporo-parietal regions are involved in rehearsal and short-term memory processing.[71–73] Working memory functions develop until late adolescence,[51] and as a consequence, early-onset bipolar disorder may substantially affect their development.

Despite their higher cognitive potential, children and adolescents with bipolar disorder underperform at school, have poor concentration, demonstrate poor planning, become easily frustrated when performing tasks involving multiple steps, and cannot remember more than one or two items at a time. This pattern of poor working memory deficits increases feelings of frustration, and may at least partly contribute to poor affective regulation. Importantly, in terms of academic achievement, complex cognitive skills such as math, reading, or problems solving rely substantially on discrete working memory operations, and working memory deficits result in missing learning milestones and an increasing gap between bipolar disorder youth and healthy peers as schooling progresses and more complex skills need to be learned and mastered.

A burgeoning number of studies have found working memory deficits in adults[74,75] as well as in youth,[1,2,39,41] which persist in time even with optimal clinical outcome.[2,3] These deficits may be intrinsic to bipolar disorder, since they were found to be present regardless of whether the bipolar disorder individuals exhibited ADHD comorbidity.[2,41] Additionally, fronto-striatal-parietal dysfunction has been demonstrated both in bipolar disorder youth[55,76] and in adult bipolar disorder,[77–79] which is suggestive of neural markers in prefrontal cortex and ancillary cognitive regions for working memory deficits in youth with bipolar disorder. Therefore, it is of paramount importance to focus on perfecting paradigms to characterize deficits in specific domains of working memory and, moreover, examine how they may relate to behavior regulation and academic performance.

Importantly, verbal working memory impairment, as assessed by standardized tests, is among the most consistent findings in youth with bipolar disorder when examining different working memory components.[2,8,38,39] Pavuluri et al.[2] examined the impact of neurocognitive function on academic difficulties in pediatric bipolar disorder. They tested 7- to 17-year-old bipolar disorder youth with and without ADHD comorbidity, and healthy youth, using a computerized neurocognitive battery and standardized neuropsychological tests. Moreover, parents completed a structured questionnaire on school and academic functioning. Among the key findings, relative to healthy youth, children with bipolar disorder showed deficits in verbal and visuospatial working memory that were associated with reading difficulties, reduced vigilance, and impaired math ability. Interestingly, a separate logistic regression analysis found that attentional dysfunction predicted math difficulties. ADHD comorbidity worsened deficits in working memory capacity, verbal, visual, and visuospatial memory.

The working memory deficits in bipolar disorder tend to worsen with age. In this regard, a subsequent study by Pavuluri and colleagues found that at a 3-year follow-up, after medication treatment, relative to baseline, bipolar disorder youth had lower verbal memory scores, as assessed by the California Verbal Learning Test (CVLT), and delayed recall, even when they were in euthymic state.[3] This finding suggests that the working memory deficits may be trait specific and separable from the effects of mood dysregulation. It is unclear whether this developmental delay could be a direct effect of the illness, or an indirect disruption of cognitive development due to the illness.

Deficient working memory functions may also affect the ability to regulate one's own behavior, which is often mediated by self-monitoring in the form of internalized language. In fact, it is noteworthy that in the 3 years follow-up study by Pavuluri et al.[3] relative to baseline the bipolar disorder youth group showed an increase in reports of math difficulties from 35% to 62%, and math difficulties were also associated with lower verbal memory scores. McClure et al.[80] examined memory and learning in bipolar disorder youth by using a battery of verbal and visuospatial memory test. They found that bipolar disorder performed worse than healthy youth in verbal learning memory and delayed facial recognition memory, and more so when ADHD comorbidity or acute mood symptoms were involved.

We still do not know whether the working memory problems precede the bipolar disorder illness or are mainly caused by affect dysregulation, although initial evidence suggests that they do not disappear with euthymic state. Therefore, while it is important to study working memory deficits in isolation, it is also crucial to understand how working memory functions are influenced by illness-specific symptoms such as affective dysregulation in bipolar disorder youth (Fig. 13.1). Working memory deficits are exacerbated in bipolar disorder youth when negative valence words[31] or angry faces[28] are presented. Moreover, fMRI studies have shown that emotional content causes a reduction in engagement of executive control systems in prefrontal cortex, accompanied by hyperactivity of the emotional systems that process affect (i.e., amygdala).[3,81–83] These findings have been difficult to replicate using behavioral paradigms. Therefore, there is a need to develop sensitive behavioral paradigms that specifically test these aspects, for example using n-back tasks both with and without emotional content, to examine the way in which working memory and affective systems can work separately or interact in bipolar disorder individuals.

Evidence of Differences in the Severity and Specificity of Cognitive Deficits in Bipolar Disorder Type I and II

There is some evidence that there may be distinct neurocognitive profiles associated with different subtypes of bipolar disorder. It has been found that bipolar disorder Type I exhibits not only more severe manic symptoms but also more severe cognitive dysfunction.[84] While most studies do not distinguish between bipolar disorder type I and II, by differentiating the two neurocognitive phenotypes we can better understand the underlying neural and behavioral pathophysiology that may be related to genes,[85] and we can better differentiate interventions.

Schenkel et al.[84] examined unmedicated and acutely ill Type I and Type II 8- to 18-year-old bipolar disorder individuals, with similar symptom severity, and found that the bipolar disorder Type I group, who had greater incidence of ADHD comorbidity, performed worse than healthy youth in several cognitive domains, including attention, executive functions, working memory, visual memory, and verbal learning and memory. The bipolar disorder Type I group also performed worse than the bipolar disorder Type II group in all domains, with the exception of working memory. The bipolar disorder Type II group performed worse than healthy youth only on verbal learning and memory. Verbal learning and memory deficits were the most significant deficits in both bipolar disorder groups, and they were present regardless of ADHD comorbidity. These results of differential cognitive deficits in bipolar disorder Type I and Type II indicate more severe dysfunction in the Type I group, and they suggest that the neuropathology underlying mania, rather than depression, may be more closely associated with these cognitive deficits. Based on these findings, it will be important to develop differential cognitive interventions based on subtypes of bipolar disorder. Verbally mediated tasks were the most impaired. This finding possibly suggests a reliable endophenotype, which could reflect deficient connectivity between frontotemporal regions in bipolar disorder youth,[86] as also confirmed by diffusion tensor imaging (DTI) data.[87] Similar results regarding Type I and II profile of deficits were obtained with adults with bipolar disorder in a study by Ahn et al.[88] who found that both Type I and II bipolar disorder individuals exhibited worse verbal memory performance compared to healthy youth, while worse visual memory impairment was present only in bipolar disorder Type I. Given the apparent continuity in memory dysfunction between adult and pediatric bipolar disorder,[89] we need to better understand the progression of the underlying cognitive and neural mechanisms. The narrow phenotypes of pediatric and adult bipolar disorder may share some underlying mechanisms with regard to working memory deficits, although the behavioral manifestations may vary in the two groups because of the different levels of cognitive development and the differences in the strategies available to perform cognitive tasks at different ages.

Summary and Clinical Considerations

Working memory deficits are consistently found in bipolar disorder youth and are associated with scholastic underachievement and poor interpersonal functions. These deficits worsen with development and despite optimal clinical outcome.[3] In addition, they tend to be worse in the presence of ADHD comorbidity, and they may differ, both in severity and specificity, in bipolar disorder Type I relative to Type II. An important future direction is that of developing new working memory tasks to study the link between the cognitive deficits and the clinical manifestations in bipolar disorder youth. For example, while it is understandable that working memory capacity is linked to reading problems and math, it is noteworthy that limitations in working memory also predict impulsivity and poor decision making,[90] which underlie the risk-taking and excessive reward-seeking behaviors in bipolar disorder. Along these lines, deficient working memory may also affect the ability to regulate one's own behavior, which is often mediated by self-monitoring in the form of internalized language. Therefore, it seems crucial to invest in developing specific cognitive remediation training programs for this pediatric population that may help reduce the existing cognitive deficits and prevent worsening of cognitive function as the child develops.

Attentional Biases Are Linked to Dysfunctional Interface Between Cognition and Emotion in Bipolar Disorder Youth

Recent studies are focusing on domain-specific information processing biases as potential mediators of the mood dysregulation and poor emotional control typical of bipolar disorder youth. In particular, attention is a fundamental resource for information processing by virtue of directing limited processing resources toward task-relevant stimuli.[91] Attention can be subdivided in three different subdomains: sustained attention, selective attention, and inhibitory attentional control (Fig. 13.1).[91-93] These subdomains are controlled by executive functions and are implemented by distinct yet somewhat overlapping neural circuits, including regions such as the dorsolateral prefrontal cortex, anterior cingulate cortex, striatal, and parieto-temporal regions.[91-93]

Sustained Attention in Bipolar Disorder Youth

Sustained attention is the ability to sustain a certain response during a continuous mental or behavioral activity. Deficits in sustained attention have been reported in children with bipolar disorder using standardized neurocognitive tasks.[2,56,59] Similar deficits in sustained attention were found in adults with bipolar disorder by Bora et al.[94] who found that on the Conners' Continuous Performance Test (CPT)[95] manic bipolar disorder individuals showed increased false responding, perseveration, and vigilance deficits, which were not mediated by medications. Euthymic individuals, on the other hand, showed decreased target sensitivity and response time inconsistency. It remains to be determined whether mood-based effects in sustained attention are stable enough in bipolar disorder youth to be detected and studied during development.

Selective Attention and Attentional Bias to Emotions in Bipolar Disorder Youth

Selective attention is the ability to maintain a behavioral or cognitive set while distracting or interfering stimuli are presented. Of particular interest for bipolar disorder pathophysiology is the interface of selective attention and affect. Studies adopting the affective Stroop task have found that youth with bipolar disorder exhibit more interference in the presence of negative emotional information. One of the first studies to address this issue in euthymic and unmedicated children with bipolar disorder was a study by Pavuluri et al.[55] that used a color matching task to probe affect and attention processes simultaneously. Participants matched the color of words with negative or neutral valence to colored dots presented underneath the words. Findings revealed that relative to healthy youth, youth with bipolar disorder demonstrated greater cognitive interference, as represented by lower accuracy, with emotional valence relative to neutral valence words. These findings suggest that the emotional content of the words, even if it is incidental to the task, affects attention processes during the color matching task. Interestingly the behavioral response patterns were coupled with increased limbic activation and reduced activation in lateral prefrontal regions. Similar results, with increased interference from negative valence stimuli, are obtained in the domain of working memory,[96] suggesting that these effects hold across multiple cognitive domains. We do not know whether this increased interference of emotional information is due to extreme affective overactivity, poor prefrontal/attention function, or a combination of the two processes, with reduced efficiency in coordinating processing strategies.

A very promising candidate for a bipolar disorder endophenotype is the attentional bias construct. A biological mechanism involving subcortical and cortical neural circuits for attentional vigilance[97] ensures an adaptive and automatic attentional bias toward emotionally relevant or potentially harmful stimuli, such as angry faces.[98] However, in anxiety and mood disorders this bias is exaggerated and leads to increased emotional interference and maladaptive functioning.[99] Most studies of attentional bias examined individuals with anxiety disorders, revealing a link between attentional bias to potentially threatening stimuli and clinical anxiety in both adolescents[100] and adults.[101] Brotman et al.[102] found that only bipolar disorder adolescents with lifetime anxiety showed greater attentional bias for angry faces, relative to healthy youth, during a visual-probe paradigm. However it cannot be excluded that this bias was related to the severe anxiety levels, since bipolar disorder adolescents without lifetime anxiety did not differ from healthy youth. Furthermore, a recent adult bipolar disorder study found evidence of an attentional bias away from positive emotional words in mildly depressed bipolar disorder individuals, but not euthymic bipolar disorder individuals, suggesting that the attentional bias may be mood related in bipolar disorder.[103]

A study by Rich et al.[32] that used an "Emotional Interrupt" Task did not find differences between youth with bipolar disorder and healthy youth in the degree of interference caused by emotional images from the International Affective Picture System (IAPS),[104] presented before and after a target (i.e., a circle or square) that the participants needed to respond to. However, it may be easier to ignore emotional information when it is temporally separated from the target stimuli. Some initial evidence of an attentional bias in bipolar disorder youth was provided recently in a linguistic task where both emotional and semantic information were integrated in the experimental stimuli. Passarotti et al.[31] examined emotional interference on attentional processing in 7- to 19-year-old acutely ill youth with bipolar disorder, with and without ADHD, relative to healthy youth, during a synonym matching task where participants decided which of two probe words was a synonym of a target word. On each trial, words could have negative, positive, or neutral valence. Relative to healthy youth, both bipolar disorder groups exhibited worse accuracy for emotional words relative to neutral ones. The attentional bias was greater with negative words and observed regardless of ADHD comorbidity. It is possible that in these individuals selective attention is overly sensitive or biased toward processing emotional content first, which creates interference with the remaining cognitive processes. Alternatively, affective overreactivity in the presence of emotional information may weaken selective attention processes, and leading to greater emotional interference. Either way, by altering attention, memory, and learning, the information processing bias may contribute to compromised self- regulation (Fig. 13.1).[81,105]

Another noteworthy and more recent approach to information processing biases is that of longitudinal studies, since cognitive biases in attention or memory may worsen with age or alter psychosocial development. A recent longitudinal study by Whitney et al.[106] examined "information processing biases" for attention and memory domains in 13- to 18-year-old adolescents with bipolar disorder Type I, shortly after their first manic episode and at 1-year follow-up, after some degree of treatment, in a subset of participants. Specifically, the authors adopted a variation of the dot-probe task using emotional faces (i.e., happy or sad) to test selective attention for neutral relative to emotional faces. Reaction time was expected to be faster for emotional faces if individuals have an intrinsic or automatic bias to orient toward emotional faces. For memory, participants first underwent a Self-referent Encoding Task (SRET), where they decided whether an emotionally valenced word (e.g., "friendly," "angry") described them, and then did an incidental recall task of the SRET adjectives. Results showed no group differences in attentional bias. However, it is possible that bias effects may emerge with other emotions such as anger, which has been found to be effective in eliciting emotional reactivity in youth with bipolar disorder.[81,107,108] For memory bias, while healthy youth endorsed and recalled more positive adjectives both at baseline and follow-up, youth with bipolar disorder recalled more negative words at baseline, and this was independent of mood state. Over time, depression symptoms were associated with impaired memory for positive self-referent adjectives, suggesting that depression symptoms may contribute to negative memory bias in youth with bipolar disorder Type I. The authors conclude that rather early in the illness adolescents may possess a cognitive set reflecting low self-esteem, which may increase vulnerability to future mood episodes. These effects seem to steadily worsen with development. Therefore, early intervention to reduce or eliminate this memory bias would be particularly beneficial at an early age.

Response Inhibition and Impulsivity in Bipolar Disorder Youth

Inhibition function is achieved by age 14 years in healthy children.[51] Poor inhibition functions lead to impulsivity, a key feature of bipolar disorder. Impulsivity has been found to be present both in manic/mixed[109] and euthymic state[110] in adult bipolar disorder. Impulsivity involves several different aspects, including being too quick to act, poor self-control, exhibiting emotional outbursts without considering the consequences, and inability to delay receiving reward in favor of waiting for a better outcome. Because response inhibition skills undergo slow maturation, it is also likely the case that high impulsivity during growth prevents development of appropriate self-regulation skills. Response inhibition in bipolar disorder has been mainly studied using various versions of the Stop Signal Task (SST), which examines the ability to inhibit a prepotent and already on-the-way motor response when a stop cue appears at varying delays from the presentation of a go cue. Performance on this task has been found to strongly correlate with levels of impulsivity in children and adults.[111,112] Moreover, Lombardo et al.[110] found that euthymic adult bipolar disorder Type I had higher scores compared to healthy youth on the Barratt's Impulsivity Scale (BIS-11),[113] which were negatively associated with global functioning.

Most of the inhibition studies in bipolar disorder youth are fMRI studies, which have found altered lateral prefrontal cortex and striatal function during motor inhibition tasks.[83,114,115] However, these studies did not reveal significant group differences other than in the overall accuracy for response inhibition trials, possibly because of reduced power due to the small number of trials in the fMRI task. Moreover, Weathers et al.[116] tried to capture the developmental trajectory of impulsivity in bipolar disorder using an SST. They found age- and diagnosis-related differences in stop trials accuracy as well as differences in anterior cingulate cortex activation, a brain region that monitors performance and errors, during failed inhibition trials, between the child and adult bipolar disorder, and in both groups relative to healthy youth. These results suggest that poor inhibition may be due not only to inhibition processes per se but also to deficient performance monitoring. Inhibition problems have been found in adult bipolar disorder as well. Strakowski et al.[109] examined specific aspects of impulsivity in bipolar disorder Type I manic/mixed adults relative to healthy youth and found that they exhibited independent deficits in sustained attention during a continuous performance test, in response inhibition during an SST and in the ability to delay gratification during a delayed reward task. Moreover, while these deficits did not correlate significantly with severity of symptoms ratings, manic individuals performed significantly worse than mixed individuals, which was expected since mania involves the most severe manifestations of impulsivity. Also Swann et al.[117] found that motor disinhibition in adult bipolar disorder is linked to manic mood, whereas evidence in this regard is less conclusive in children.

Summary and Clinical Considerations

Impulsivity is a fundamental clinical manifestation of bipolar disorder, and as such it deserves a closer examination, including longitudinal studies to capture developmental and illness-specific aspects. While several brain imaging studies have already characterized dysfunctional inhibition circuits in bipolar disorder youth, we still need to further investigate the behavioral manifestations of impulsivity and to implement tasks to study inhibition functions in the presence of emotional challenge in bipolar disorder. It will also be important to disentangle the distinct contributions of affective, reward, and cognitive systems to impulsive behavior. A key question that will drive domain-based research is whether impulsivity is a common dimensional dysfunction across several developmental disorders, with a unified neurobiological mechanism, or whether it is driven by distinct neural mechanisms, with a common behavioral presentation. For instance, there is some evidence that the neural mechanisms of impulsivity may differ between youth with bipolar disorder and ADHD in terms of how affective and cognitive systems influence each other, such that impulsivity may be driven by affective overreactivity in bipolar disorder youth and by poor cognitive control in ADHD youth.[105]

Genes and Cognitive Endophenotypes: Familial Studies in Bipolar Disorder

While bipolar disorder has genetic bases with heritability of approximately 80%,[118] the gene-mapping quest has progressed slowly because of the "complex trait" nature of the illness.[119] Genetic investigation and early intervention may greatly benefit from the identification of *intermediate phenotypes* for youth with bipolar disorder, which are highly heritable biological and behavioral traits prevalent in bipolar disorder,[118] and some unaffected family members. Preliminary evidence suggests that asymptomatic first-degree relatives of bipolar disorder individuals may exhibit intermediate bipolar disorder phenotypes in terms of deficits in verbal memory,[120,121] executive functions,[122] and face emotion processing,[13] as well as anatomical abnormalities in parahippocampal/hippocampal gyri.[123] Nevertheless, at present there are only a small number of family studies on intermediate phenotypes of bipolar disorder.

A few recent studies have examined neurocognitive deficits in healthy siblings and nonbipolar first-degree relatives, because if they do show deficits this evidence would strengthen the idea of a cognitive endophenotype marker linked to genes that may increase vulnerability to bipolar disorder. The main assumption is that the same genes that carry the illness risk should also influence the bipolar disorder endophenotype.[119] Moreover, unaffected first-degree relatives have similar, though less severe, deficits.[124,125] Most of the studies in this area of research were conducted in adults; however, because neurocognitive deficits seem to persist from childhood to adulthood in bipolar disorder, the adult studies suggest important aspects that can be investigated in future studies on pediatric bipolar disorder as well.

Because it is such a prominent area of dysfunction in bipolar disorder, the affective domain may be particularly promising in identifying at-risk relatives. In fact, Gourowitch et al.[120] found impaired memory for face identity in a sample of unaffected cotwins of bipolar disorder individuals. Moreover, Gotlib et al.[120] conducted a cross-sectional study assessing memory biases for emotional self-referent adjectives in healthy offspring of adult bipolar disorder and compared them to age-matched healthy youth. Asymptomatic but high-familial risk children recalled more self-referent negative adjectives than healthy youth on a self-referent encoding task (SRET), suggesting memory biases similar to those found in bipolar disorder youth.[106]

One of the most important candidate domains for a bipolar disorder endophenotype is working memory.[2,8,38,39] Working memory deficits are present in unaffected first-degree relatives who share genetic vulnerability to the disorder,[120,126] which could indicate a trait marker of the illness. Some studies were able to differentiate intermediate phenotypes in bipolar disorder relatively to other closely related illnesses. For instance, Diwadkar et al.[127] assessed parametric working memory and attention performance in 10- to 20-year-old adolescent offspring of bipolar disorder and schizophrenia compared to healthy youth. The tasks used were a delayed spatial memory paradigm with two levels of delay, and a continuous performance test (CPT) for sustained attention. Results showed that although offspring with schizophrenia showed working memory deficits at the longer memory delay, bipolar disorder offspring did not present this pattern. Both groups had deficits in sustained attention, but only bipolar disorder offspring differed significantly from healthy youth in attentional performance. These findings suggest unique but somewhat overlapping vulnerability pathways, for working memory and attention, in adolescent offspring of individuals with bipolar disorder and schizophrenia.

Furthermore, Clark et al.[36] examined whether sustained attention deficits previously found in bipolar disorder could be found in first-degree relatives, using a sustained attention task, namely a rapid visual information processing (RVIP) task, involving monitoring a continuous stream of digits, and looking for prespecified digit strings. Findings indicate that the bipolar disorder individuals showed reduced target sensitivity and slower responses. The deficits were not significant in relatives, but the authors do not exclude that they may have been too small to be detected.

In terms of inhibitory attention functions, in adults, unaffected relatives of individuals with bipolar disorder have been found to exhibit impairment in cognitive tasks that involve aspects of impulsivity, particularly response inhibition.[128] This is also reflected in shared abnormalities between bipolar disorder individuals and their relatives in brain function and functional connectivity within neural networks involved in inhibitory control.[129] Lombardo et al.[110] also found that unaffected siblings of adults with bipolar disorder Type I had higher scores on the total score as well as the motor and nonplanning subscales of the Barratt's impulsivity scale.[113] These findings suggest that impulsivity may be a behavioral marker for familial liability for the illness. In line with these findings, a study by Singh et al.[130] examined different attentional aspects, such as psychomotor inhibition, sustained attention, and inhibitory attentional control, in 12- to 18-year-old adolescents with a nonmanic mood disorder and with a first-degree relative with bipolar disorder Type I disorder, compared to healthy youth. Participants with a nonmanic mood disorder showed abnormal performance in stop signal reaction time and latency during a Stop Signal Task, in sustained attention response bias, and in color naming speed. The results indicate that participants with a nonmanic mood disorder exhibited psychomotor disinhibition, marginal cognitive slowing, and response biases, but no significant deficits in sustained or selective attention.

Finally, Glahn et al.[124] conducted a literature review on neuropsychological deficits in healthy relatives of bipolar disorder and found evidence that executive functions and declarative memory could be neurocognitive endophenotypes for bipolar disorder, although the sample sizes of studies were fairly small, and therefore findings need to be interpreted with caution. Agreeing findings were obtained by Glahn et al.[119] when conducting a large-scale extended pedigree study of cognitive function in bipolar disorder. Participants were 660 Latinos who were members of extended pedigrees, with at least two siblings who had been diagnosed with bipolar disorder, as well as a healthy youth group. In this study, neurocognitive measures found to be heritable were analyzed to identify tests that are impaired in bipolar disorder individuals, that are sensitive to "genetic liability," and that are genetically correlated with affective deficits. The findings suggest that three tests, specifically digit symbol (measuring processing speed), object delayed response (measuring working memory processes) and immediate facial memory (measuring immediate memory for faces), were impaired both in bipolar disorder and nonbipolar first-degree relatives, and additionally were genetically correlated with affective status. These results are remarkable, since this is the first large-scale family-based study to indicate that neurocognitive deficits are linked to genetic liability for the disorder. Glahn et al.[119] propose that the next step for future studies is to examine how these specific cognitive processes are carried out by deficient brain circuits. Additionally, creating working memory tasks specifically for affective disorders, including emotional information that may engender differential interference in individuals relative to healthy youth, may improve task sensitivity to bipolar disorder vulnerability.

Summary and Clinical Considerations

Genetic studies on cognitive phenotypes for bipolar disorder are just starting. While the results are not always agreeing, future studies in this research area will likely contribute to identify behavioral and biological risk markers or intermediate phenotypes for bipolar disorder not only in bipolar disorder individuals but also in siblings at high genetic risk, creating opportunity for early intervention. Future studies will also need to pinpoint protective factors in bipolar disorder and inform interventions accordingly. As Glahn and colleagues[119] point out, molecular genetic studies of bipolar disorder may benefit from using targeted neuropsychological measures as potential endophenotypic markers. Once such markers are identified and well characterized, they may improve power for detecting genes predisposing to bipolar disorder illness and may help improve diagnoses.

Future Directions in Bipolar Disorder Youth Studies

Although much progress has been reached in studying the neurocognitive deficits that characterize youth with bipolar disorder, we still have limited capacity and relatively non-specific paradigms for characterizing the illness-specific neurocognitive deficits that may be potential markers of bipolar disorder. Moreover, we still have an insufficient understanding of how these deficits may affect the outcomes of interventions relying on cognitive function, such as cognitive-behavioral therapy or cognitive remediation.

Moving forward, there is a need to develop explanatory and predictive models on neurocognitive deficits in bipolar disorder youth and to determine whether they are moderated by the mood dysregulation or residual symptoms, or whether intrinsic poor cognitive control may make bipolar disorder individuals more vulnerable to excessive mood swings. It is also possible that cognitive and affective deficits in bipolar disorder influence and exacerbate one another. However, without a systemic and *neuroscience-based information processing model of bipolar disorder dysfunction*, it is difficult to understand and address the complex brain-behavior abnormalities seen in bipolar disorder. Therefore, there is a real need to link cognitive models to neural operations in specialized brain circuits, to provide a better understanding of the correlation between brain pathology and behavioral symptoms, and to better map correlations between neurocognitive deficits and fMRI and other brain imaging findings.[8] Similarly, it is also important to determine whether the cognitive dysfunction comes from a single core deficit, such as poor executive functions (i.e., monitoring) or from multiple and somewhat independent domain impairments, such as working memory, verbal learning, and attention. And, moreover, it is important to know how cognition and affect interact in unique ways to shape the bipolar disorder neuropsychological profile.

Future neurocognitive studies will also need to address some discrepancies present in previous studies, as well as unanswered questions, as suggested by Joseph and colleagues.[8] For instance, there is a lack of consistency in the *diagnostic criteria of bipolar disorder* for study inclusion. Moreover, medication status, mood state, and/or psychiatric comorbidities are not always accounted for in analyses. Additional important questions to be addressed in future studies relate to what deficits or markers precede symptom onset; what causes changes in neuropsychological function with time: Is it development, illness progression, pharmacological treatment, number of episodes, or a combination of the above? Finally, disentangling the possibly different cognitive phenotypes in the bipolar disorder subtypes will likely be very useful in understanding the underlying biological deficits and how they can be best remediated.[131,132]

Furthermore, in order to develop models and interventions that have continuity across the life span, we also need to gain a better understanding of whether the cognitive deficits may be similar or different in children and adults with bipolar disorder. Therefore, we need to better characterize the longitudinal progression of the deficits and examine what cognitive domains become more impaired with time.[8] *Longitudinal studies* will capture the bipolar disorder disease process and will aid the development of tests to assess the range of cognitive/affective dysfunctions and cognitive screenings for neuropsychological interventions at different ages. The findings will ultimately help to answer the question of whether there is phenotypic similarity with development, which will better reinforce the definition of bipolar disorder in youth and inform its treatment.[8]

At present, it is also difficult to develop *cognitive enhancement programs* or teach bipolar disorder children strategies to regulate their behavior if we do not know exactly what specific aspects (e.g., emotional challenge, self-regulation deficits, in information processing bias, deficits in attention and working memory) hinder adaptive functioning the most in bipolar disorder. Disorder-specific treatments must first depend on understanding the underlying cognitive deficits and how they shape clinical symptoms in different developmental illnesses. While there are some initial and informative studies in ADHD on cognitive deficits or remediation, to date there is no evidence that intervention or remediation may have the same outcome in bipolar disorder as in ADHD youth. Previous studies differentiated cognitive deficits in youth with bipolar disorder relative to ADHD, despite some clinical overlap, and showed that negative emotions and mood dysregulation substantially hindered cognitive processes in youth with bipolar disorder in a unique way that was not present in ADHD youth.[82,83,107]

This complex *interconnection between cognitive and affective deficits* is a key aspect in bipolar disorder youth. We need to acknowledge that it results in added complexity and challenges that need to be examined and addressed early in the course of illness. The aim of future studies should be to find out the specific cognitive processes and domains, such as working memory, that are problematic in bipolar disorder in order to inform adaptive training that can lead to substantial improvement, both in terms of performance[133] and at the level of prefrontal cortex function, in the dorsolateral prefrontal cortex and parietal regions that are part of the working memory networks.[134]

A more comprehensive approach will ultimately inform intervention strategies that are more specific to bipolar disorder pathophysiology so that we can improve the quality of life for children and adolescents with bipolar disorder and help develop their full potential at school and home. Cognitive intervention, in turn, may strengthen the same cognitive systems in prefrontal regions that are also involved in affective regulation, thereby helping to improve emotional dysfunction.

Acknowledgments

Many thanks to Mr. Richard C. Whitley for his useful comments and editing on earlier drafts of this chapter.

Author Disclosures

Dr. Passarotti has no conflicts to disclose. She is funded by the National Alliance for Research on Schizophrenia and Depression (NARSAD), the Depressive and Bipolar Disorder Alternative Treatment Foundation (DBDAT), and the National Institute of Drug Abuse (NIDA 1R03DA036656-01A1).

References

1. Dickstein DP, Garvey M, Pradella AG, et al. Neurologic examination abnormalities in children with bipolar disorder or attention deficit/hyperactivity disorder. *Biol Psychiatry*. 2005;58:517–24.
2. Pavuluri MN, Schenkel LS, Aryal S, et al. Neurocognitive function in unmedicated manic and medicated euthymic pediatric bipolar individuals. *Am J Psychiatry*. 2006;163:286–93.
3. Pavuluri MN, West A, Hill S, Jindal K, Sweeney JA. Neurocognitive function in pediatric bipolar disorder: 3-year follow-ups show cognitive development lagging behind health youth. *J Am Acad Child Adolesc Psychiatry*. 2009;48:235–6.
4. Robinson LJ, Ferrier IN. Evolution of cognitive impairment in bipolar disorder: a systematic review of cross-sectional evidence. *Bipolar Disord* 2006;8:103–16. doi:10.1111/j.1399-5618.2006.00277.x
5. Martínez-Arán A, Vieta E, Colom F, et al. Cognitive impairment in euthymic bipolar individuals: implications for clinical and functional outcome. *Bipolar Disord*. 2004;6:224–32. doi:10.1111/j.1399-5618.2004.00111.x
6. Insel T, Cuthbert B, Garvey M, et al. Research domain criteria (RDoC): toward a new classification framework for research on mental disorders. *Am J Psychiatry*. 2010;167:748–51. doi:10.1176/appi.ajp.2010.09091379

7. Strakowski SM, Adler CM, Almeida J, et al. The functional neuroanatomy of bipolar disorder: a consensus model. *Bipolar Disord.* 2012;14:313–25. doi:10.1111/j.1399-5618.2012.01022.x

8. Joseph MF, Frazier TW, Youngstrom EA, Soares JC. A quantitative and qualitative review of neurocognitive performance in pediatric bipolar disorder. *J Child Adolesc Psychopharmacol.* 2008;18:595–605.

9. Dickstein DP, Leibenluft E. Emotion regulation in children and adolescents: boundaries between normalcy and bipolar disorder. *Dev Psychopathol.* 2006;18:1105–31. doi:10.1017/S0954579406060536

10. Geller B, Luby J. Child and adolescent bipolar disorder: a review of the past 10 years. *J Am Acad Child Adolesc Psychiatry.* 1997;36:1168–76. doi:10.1097/00004583-199709000-00008

11. Luby J, Tandon M, Nicol G. Three clinical cases of DSM-IV mania symptoms in preschoolers. *J Child Adolesc Psychopharmacol.* 2007;17:237–43. doi:10.1089/cap.2007.0131

12. Luby JL, Navsaria N. Pediatric bipolar disorder: evidence for prodromal states and early markers. *J Child Psychol Psychiatry.* 2010;51:459–71. doi:10.1111/j.1469-7610.2010.02210.x

13. Brotman MA, Guyer AE, Lawson ES, et al. Facial emotion labeling deficits in children and adolescents at risk for bipolar disorder. *Am J Psychiatry.* 2008;165:385–9. doi:10.1176/appi.ajp.2007.06122050

14. McClure EB, Pope K, Hoberman AJ, Pine DS, Leibenluft E. Facial expression recognition in adolescents with mood and anxiety disorders. *Am J Psychiatry.* 2003;160:1172–4.

15. Seymour KE, Pescosolido MF, Reidy BL, et al. Emotional face identification in youths with primary bipolar disorder or primary attention-deficit/hyperactivity disorder. *J Am Acad Child Adolesc Psychiatry.* 2013;52:537–46.e533. doi:10.1016/j.jaac.2013.03.011

16. Nowicki S Jr, Duke M. Individual differences in the nonverbal communication of affect: the diagnostic analysis of nonverbal accuracy scale. *J Nonverb Behav* 1994;18:9–35. doi:10.1007/BF02169077

17. Kim P, Arizpe J, Rosen BH, et al. Impaired fixation to eyes during facial emotion labelling in children with bipolar disorder or severe mood dysregulation. *J Psychiatry Neurosci.* 2013;38:407–16. doi:10.1503/jpn.120232

18. Rich BA, Vinton DT, Roberson-Nay R, et al. Limbic hyperactivation during processing of neutral facial expressions in children with bipolar disorder. *Proc Natl Acad Sci USA.* 2006;103:8900–5.

19. Shankman SA, Katz AC, Passarotti AM, Pavuluri MN. Deficits in emotion recognition in pediatric bipolar disorder: the mediating effects of irritability. *J Affect Disord.* 2013;144:134–40. doi:10.1016/j.jad.2012.06.021

20. Erwin RJ, Gur RC, Gur RE, Skolnick B, Mawhinney-Hee M, Smailis J. Facial emotion discrimination: I. Task construction and behavioral findings in normal subjects. *Psychiatry Res.* 1992;42:231–40.

21. Wozniak J, Biederman J, Kiely K, et al. Mania-like symptoms suggestive of childhood-onset bipolar disorder in clinically referred children. *J Am Acad Child Adolesc Psychiatry.* 1995;34:867–76. doi:10.1097/00004583-199507000-00010

22. Geller B, Zimerman B, Williams M, Delbello MP, Frazier J, Beringer L. Phenomenology of prepubertal and early adolescent bipolar disorder: examples of elated mood, grandiose behaviors, decreased need for sleep, racing thoughts and hypersexuality. *J Child Adolesc Psychopharmacol.* 2002;12:3–9. doi:10.1089/10445460252943524

23. Silk JS, Steinberg L, Morris AS. Adolescents' emotion regulation in daily life: links to depressive symptoms and problem behavior. *Child Dev.* 2003;74:1869–80.

24. Besel LDS, Yuille JC. Individual differences in empathy: the role of facial expression recognition. *Personality Individ Diff.* 2010;49:107–12. doi:http://dx.doi.org/10.1016/j.paid.2010.03.013

25. Schenkel LS, Pavuluri MN, Herbener ES, Harral EM, Sweeney JA. Facial emotion processing in acutely ill and euthymic individuals with pediatric bipolar disorder. *J Am Acad Child Adolesc Psychiatry.* 2007;46:1070–9. doi:10.1097/chi.0b013e3180600fd6

26. Craney JL, Geller B. A prepubertal and early adolescent bipolar disorder-I phenotype: review of phenomenology and longitudinal course. *Bipolar Disord.* 2003;5:243–56.

27. Friedman SR, Rapport LJ, Lumley M, et al. Aspects of social and emotional competence in adult attention-deficit/hyperactivity disorder. *Neuropsychology.* 2003;17:50–8.

28. Schenkel LS, Passarotti AM, Sweeney JA, Pavuluri MN. Negative emotion impairs working memory in pediatric individuals with bipolar disorder type I. *Psychol Med.* 2012;42:2567–77. doi:10.1017/S0033291712000797

29. Gorrindo T, Blair RJ, Budhani S, Dickstein DP, Pine DS, Leibenluft E. Deficits on a probabilistic response-reversal task in individuals with pediatric bipolar disorder. *Am J Psychiatry*. 2005;162:3.

30. Rich BA, Schmajuk M, Perez-Edgar KE, Pine DS, Fox NA, Leibenluft E. The impact of reward, punishment, and frustration on attention in pediatric bipolar disorder. *Biol Psychiatry*. 2005;58:532–9. doi:10.1016/j.biopsych.2005.01.006

31. Passarotti AM, Fitzgerald JM, Sweeney JA, Pavuluri MN. Negative emotion interference during a synonym matching task in pediatric bipolar disorder with and without attention deficit hyperactivity disorder. *J Intl Neuropsychol Soc*. 2013;19:1–12.

32. Rich BA, Brotman MA, Dickstein DP, Mitchell DG, Blair RJ, Leibenluft E. Deficits in attention to emotional stimuli distinguish youth with severe mood dysregulation from youth with bipolar disorder. *J Abnorm Child Psychol*. 2010;38:695–706. doi:10.1007/s10802-010-9395-0

33. Rich BA, Vinton D, Grillon C, Bhangoo RK, Leibenluft E. An investigation of prepulse inhibition in pediatric bipolar disorder. *Bipolar Disord* 2005;7:198–203. doi:10.1111/j.1399-5618.2005.00183.x

34. Bearden CE, Hoffman KM, Cannon TD. The neuropsychology and neuroanatomy of bipolar affective disorder: a critical review. *Bipolar Disord*. 2001;3:106–50; discussion 151–3.

35. Robinson LJ, Thompson JM, Gallagher P, et al. A meta-analysis of cognitive deficits in euthymic individuals with bipolar disorder. *J Affect Disord*. 2006;93:105–15. doi:10.1016/j.jad.2006.02.016

36. Clark L, Goodwin GM. State- and trait-related deficits in sustained attention in bipolar disorder. *Eur Arch Psychiatry Clin Neurosci*. 2004;254:61–8. doi:10.1007/s00406-004-0460-y

37. Horn K, Roessner V, Holtmann M. Neurocognitive performance in children and adolescents with bipolar disorder: a review. *Eur Child Adolesc Psychiatry*. 2011;20:433–50. doi:10.1007/s00787-011-0209-x

38. McClure EB, Treland JE, Snow J, et al. Memory and learning in pediatric bipolar disorder. *J Am Acad Child Adolesc Psychiatry*. 2005;44:461–9.

39. Doyle AE, Willcutt EG, Seidman LJ, et al. Attention-deficit/hyperactivity disorder endophenotypes. *Biological Psychiatry*. 2005;57:1324–35. doi:10.1016/j.biopsych.2005.03.015

40. Rucklidge JJ. Impact of ADHD on the neurocognitive functioning of adolescents with bipolar disorder. *Biol Psychiatry*. 2006;60:921–8. doi:10.1016/j.biopsych.2006.03.067

41. Pavuluri MN, Passarotti AM, Harral EM, Sweeney JA. An fMRI study of the neural correlates of incidental versus directed emotion processing in pediatric bipolar disorder. *J Am Acad Child Adolesc Psychiatry*. 2009;48:308–19. doi:10.1097/CHI.0b013e3181948fc7

42. Goldstein BI, Levitt AJ. A gender-focused perspective on health service utilization in comorbid bipolar I disorder and alcohol use disorders: results from the national epidemiologic survey on alcohol and related conditions. *J Clin Psychiatry*. 2006;67:925–32.

43. Whitney J, Howe M, Shoemaker V, et al. Socio-emotional processing and functioning of youth at high risk for bipolar disorder. *J Affect Disord* 2013;148:112–7. doi:10.1016/j.jad.2012.08.016

44. DelBello MP, Adler CM, Amicone J, et al. Parametric neurocognitive task design: a pilot study of sustained attention in adolescents with bipolar disorder. *J Affect Disord*. 2004;82(Suppl. 1):S79–88. doi:10.1016/j.jad.2004.05.014

45. Biederman J, Pett CR, Dolan C, et al. A prospective 4-year follow-up study of attention-deficit hyperactivity and related disorders. *Arch Gen Psychiatry*. 1996;53:437–46.

46. Faraone SV, Biederman J, Mick E, et al. A family study of psychiatric comorbidity in girls and boys with attention-deficit/hyperactivity disorder. *Biol Psychiatry*. 2001;50:586–92.

47. Adler CM, Delbello MP, Mills NP, Schmithorst V, Holland S, Strakowski SM. Comorbid ADHD is associated with altered patterns of neuronal activation in adolescents with bipolar disorder performing a simple attention task. *Bipolar Disorders*. 2005;7:577–88. doi:10.1111/j.1399-5618.2005.00257.x

48. Miller EK, Cohen JD. An integrative theory of prefrontal cortex function. *Annu Rev Neurosci*. 2001;24:167–202. doi:10.1146/annurev.neuro.24.1.167

49. Giedd JN, Blumenthal J, Jeffries NO, et al. Brain development during childhood and adolescence: a longitudinal MRI study. *Nat Neurosci* 1999;2:861–3. doi:10.1038/13158

50. Luna B, Thulborn KR, Munoz DP, et al. Maturation of widely distributed brain function subserves cognitive development. *NeuroImage*. 2001;13:786–93.

51. Luna B, Garver KE, Urban TN, Lazar N, Sweeney JA. Maturation of cognitive processes from late child-hood to adulthood. *Cog Dev*. 2004;75:1357–72.

52. Posner MI, Rothbart MK. Developing mechanisms of self-regulation. *Dev Psychopathol*. 2000;12:427–41.

53. Blakemore SJ, Choudhury S. Development of the adolescent brain: implications for executive function and social cognition. *J Child Psychol Psychiatry*. 2006;47:296–312. doi:10.1111/j.1469-7610.2006.01611.x

54. Strakowski SM, Fleck DE, DelBello MP, et al. Impulsivity across the course of bipolar disorder. *Bipolar Disord*. 2010;12:285–97. doi:10.1111/j.1399-5618.2010.00806.x

55. Pavuluri MN, O'Connor MM, Harral EM, Sweeney JA. An fMRI study of the interface between affec-tive and cognitive neural circuitry in pediatric bipolar disorder. *Psychiatry Res*. 2008;162:244–55. doi:10.1016/j.pscychresns.2007.10.003

56. Phillips LK, Ladouceur CD, Drevets WC. A neural model of voluntary and automatic emotion regula-tion: implications for understanding the pathophysiology and neurodevelopment of bipolar disorder. *Mol Psychiatry*. 2008;19:833–57. doi:10.1038/mp.2008.65

57. Cerullo MA, Strakowski SM. The prevalence and significance of substance use disorders in bipolar type I and II disorder. *Subst Abuse Treat Prev Policy*. 2007;2:29. doi:10.1186/1747-597X-2-29

58. Pizzagalli DA, Goetz E, Ostacher M, Losifescu DV, Perlis RH. Euthymic individuals with bipolar dis-order show decreased reward learning in a probabilistic reward task. *Biol Psychiatry*. 2008;64:162–8. doi:10.1016/j.biopsych.2007.12.001

59. Dickstein DP, Treland JE, Snow J, et al. Neuropsychological performance in pediatric bipolar disorder. *Biol Psychiatry*. 2004;55:32–9.

60. *Cambridge Neuropsychological Test Automated Battery (CANTAB)* (Cambridge Cognition Ltd., Cambridge, United Kingdom).

61. Sweeney JA, Kmiec JA, Kupfer DJ. Neuropsychologic impairments in bipolar and unipolar mood dis-orders on the CANTAB neurocognitive battery. *Biol Psychiatry*. 2000;48:674–84.

62. Clark L, Iversen SD, Goodwin GM. Sustained attention deficit in bipolar disorder. *Br J Psychiatry*. 2002;180:313–9.

63. Patino LR, Adler CM, Mills NP, et al. Conflict monitoring and adaptation in individuals at familial risk for developing bipolar disorder. *Bipolar Disord*. 2013;15:264–71. doi:10.1111/bdi.12059

64. Dickstein DP, Gorrostieta C, Ombao H, et al. Fronto-temporal spontaneous resting state func-tional connectivity in pediatric bipolar disorder. *Biol Psychiatry*. 2010;68:839–46. doi:10.1016/j.biopsych.2010.06.029

65. Haber SN, Knutson B. The reward circuit: linking primate anatomy and human imaging. *Neuropsychopharmacology*. 2010;35:4–26. doi:10.1038/npp.2009.129.

66. Ibanez A, Cetkovich M, Petroni A, et al. The neural basis of decision-making and reward processing in adults with euthymic bipolar disorder or attention-deficit/hyperactivity disorder (ADHD). *PLoS One*. 2012;7:e37306. doi:10.1371/journal.pone.0037306

67. Singh MK, Chang KD, Kelley RG, et al. Reward processing in adolescents with bipolar I disorder. *J Am Acad Child Adolesc Psychiatry*. 2013;52:68–83. doi:10.1016/j.jaac.2012.10.004

68. Abler B, Greenhouse I, Ongur D, Walter H, Heckers S. Abnormal reward system activation in mania. *Neuropsychopharmacology*. 2008;33:2217–27.

69. Adleman NE, Kayser R, Dickstein D, Blair RJ, Pine D, Leibenluft E. Neural correlates of reversal learn-ing in severe mood dysregulation and pediatric bipolar disorder. *J Am Acad Child Adolesc Psychiatry*. 2011;50:1173–85.e1172. doi:10.1016/j.jaac.2011.07.011

70. Kim P, Thomas LA, Rosen BH, et al. Differing amygdala responses to facial expressions in children and adults with bipolar disorder. *Am J Psychiatry*. 2012;169:642–9, doi:10.1176/appi.ajp.2012.11081245

71. Baddeley A. Working memory: looking back and looking forward. *Nature Rev*. 2003;4:829–39. doi:10.1038/nrn1201

72. Curtis CE, D'Esposito M. Persistent activity in the prefrontal cortex during working memory. *Trends Cogn Sci*. 2003;7:415–23.

73. Owen AM, McMillan KM, Laird AR, Bullmore E. N-back working memory paradigm: a meta-analysis of normative functional neuroimaging studies. *Hum Brain Mapping*. 2005;25:46–59. doi:10.1002/hbm.20131

74. Ferrier IN, Thompson JM. Cognitive impairment in bipolar affective disorder: implications for the bipolar diathesis. *British Journal of Psychiatry* 2002;180:293–5.

75. Thompson JM, Gallagher P, Hughes JH, et al. Neurocognitive impairment in euthymic individuals with bipolar affective disorder. *Br J Psychiatry*. 2005;186:32–40. doi:10.1192/bjp.186.1.32

76. Passarotti AM, Sweeney JA, Pavuluri MN. Neural correlates of incidental and directed facial emotion processing in adolescents and adults. *Soc Cog Affect Neurosci*. 2009;4:387–96. doi:10.1093/scan/nsp029

77. Adler CM, Holland SK, Schmithorst V, Tuchfarber MJ, Strakowski SM. Changes in neuronal activation in individuals with bipolar disorder during performance of a working memory task. *Bipolar Disord* 2004;6:540–9. doi:10.1111/j.1399-5618.2004.00117.x

78. Haldane M, Cunningham G, Androutsos C, Frangou S. Structural brain correlates of response inhibition in bipolar disorder I. *J Psychopharmacol*. 2008;22:138–43. doi:10.1177/0269881107082955

79. Drapier D, Surguladze S, Marshall N, et al. Genetic liability for bipolar disorder is characterized by excess frontal activation in response to a working memory task. *Biol Psychiatry*. 2008;64:513–20. doi:10.1016/j.biopsych.2008.04.038

80. McClure EB, Monk CS, Nelson EE, et al. A developmental examination of gender differences in brain engagement during evaluation of threat. *Biol Psychiatry*. 2004;55:1047–55. doi:10.1016/j.biopsych.2004.02.013

81. Pavuluri MN, Passarotti AM. Neural bases of emotional processing in pediatric bipolar disorder. *Expert Rev Neurotherap* 2008;8:1381–7. doi:10.1586/14737175.8.9.1381

82. Passarotti AM, Sweeney JA, Pavuluri MN. Differential engagement of cognitive and affective neural systems in pediatric bipolar disorder and attention deficit hyperactivity disorder. *J Intl Neuropsychol Soc* 2010;16:106–17. doi:10.1017/s1355617709991019

83. Passarotti AM, Sweeney JA, Pavuluri MN. Neural correlates of response inhibition deficits in pediatric bipolar disorder and attention deficit hyperactivity disorder. *Psychiatry Res Neuroimaging*. 2010;181:36–43. doi:10.1016/j.pscychresns.2009.07.002

84. Schenkel LS, West AE, Jacobs R, Sweeney JA, Pavuluri MN. Cognitive dysfunction is worse among pediatric individuals with bipolar disorder type I than type II. *J Child Psychol Psychiatry*. 2012;53:775–81. doi:10.1111/j.1469-7610.2011.02519.x

85. Schulze TG. Genetic research into bipolar disorder: the need for a research framework that integrates sophisticated molecular biology and clinically informed phenotype characterization. *Psychiatr Clin North Am*. 2010;33:67–82. doi:10.1016/j.psc.2009.10.005

86. Gogtay N, Ordonez A, Herman DH, et al. Dynamic mapping of cortical development before and after the onset of pediatric bipolar illness. *J Child Psychol Psychiatry*. 2007;48:852–62. doi:10.1111/j.1469-7610.2007.01747.x

87. Pavuluri MN, Yang S, Kamineni K, et al. DTI study of white matter fiber tracts in pediatric bipolar disorder and attention deficit hyperactivity disorder. *Biol Psychiatry*. 2009;65:586–93. doi:10.1016/j.biopsych.2008.10.015

88. Ahn WY, Rass O, Fridberg DJ, et al. Temporal discounting of rewards in patients with bipolar disorder and schizophrenia. *J Abnorm Psychol*. 2011;120:911–21.

89. Geller B, Tillman R, Bolhofner K, Zimerman B. Child bipolar I disorder: prospective continuity with adult bipolar I disorder; characteristics of second and third episodes; predictors of 8-year outcome. *Arch Gen Psychiatry*. 2008;65:1125–33. doi:10.1001/archpsyc.65.10.1125

90. Hinson JM, Jameson TL, Whitney P. Impulsive decision making and working memory. *J Exper Psychol Learning Memory Cog*. 2003;29:298–306. doi:10.1037/0278-7393.29.2.298

91. Kahneman D. *Attention and Effort*. Englewood Cliffs, NJ: Prentice-Hall; 1973.

92. Posner MI, Petersen SE. The attention system of the human brain. *Annu Rev Neurosci*. 1990;13:25–42. doi:10.1146/annurev.ne.13.030190.000325

93. Logan GD, Cowan WB. On the ability to inhibit thought and action: a theory of an act of control. *Psychol Rev*. 1984;91:295–327. doi:10.1037/0033-295x.91.3.295

94. Bora E, Vahip S, Akdeniz F. Sustained attention deficits in manic and euthymic individuals with bipolar disorder. *Prog Neuropsychopharmacol Biol Psychiatry*. 2006;30:1097–102. doi:10.1016/j.pnpbp.2006.04.016

95. Conners CK. *Conners' Continuous Performance Test II: Computer Program for Windows Technical Guide and Software Manual.* Toronto, ON: Multi-Health Systems; 2000.

96. Schenkel LS, Marlow-O'Connor M, Moss M, Sweeney JA, Pavuluri MN. Theory of mind and social inference in children and adolescents with bipolar disorder. *Psychol Med.* 2008;38:791–800. doi:10.1017/S0033291707002541

97. Holmboe K, Nemoda Z, Fearon RM, Csibra G, Sasvari-Szekely M, Johnson MH. Polymorphisms in dopamine system genes are associated with individual differences in attention in infancy. *Dev Psychol.* 2010;46:404–16. doi:10.1037/a0018180

98. Lobue V, DeLoache JS. Detecting the snake in the grass: attention to fear-relevant stimuli by adults and young children. *Psychol Sci.* 2008;19:284–9. doi:10.1111/j.1467-9280.2008.02081.x

99. McClure EB, Monk CS, Nelson EE, et al. Abnormal attention modulation of fear circuit function in pediatric generalized anxiety disorder. *Arch Gen Psychiatry.* 2007;64:97–106. doi:10.1001/archpsyc.64.1.97

100. Pine DS, Mogg K, Bradley BP, et al. Attention bias to threat in maltreated children: implications for vulnerability to stress-related psychopathology. *Am J Psychiatry.* 2005;162:291–6. doi:10.1176/appi.ajp.162.2.291

101. Mogg K, Bradley BP. A cognitive-motivational analysis of anxiety. *Behav Res Ther.* 1998;36:809–48.

102. Brotman MA, Rich BA, Schmajuk M, et al. Attention bias to threat faces in children with bipolar disorder and comorbid lifetime anxiety disorders. *Biol Psychiatry.* 2007;61:819–21. doi:10.1016/j.biopsych.2006.08.021

103. Jabben N, Arts B, Jongen EM, Smulders FT, van Os J, Krabbendam L. Cognitive processes and attitudes in bipolar disorder: a study into personality, dysfunctional attitudes and attention bias in individuals with bipolar disorder and their relatives. *J Affect Disord.* 2012;143:265–8. doi:10.1016/j.jad.2012.04.022

104. Lang PJ. International affective picture system (IAPS): Affective ratings of pictures and instruction manual. Technical Report A-8. Gainesville: University of Florida; 2008.

105. Passarotti AM, Pavuluri MN. Brain functional domains inform therapeutic interventions in attention-deficit/hyperactivity disorder and pediatric bipolar disorder. *Expert Rev Neurotherap* 2011;11:897–914. doi:10.1586/ern.11.71

106. Whitney J, Joormann J, Gotlib IH, et al. Information processing in adolescents with bipolar I disorder. *J Child Psychol Psychiatry.* 2012;53:937–45. doi:10.1111/j.1469-7610.2012.02543.x

107. Passarotti AM, Sweeney JA, Pavuluri MN. Emotion processing influences working memory circuits in pediatric bipolar disorder and attention deficit hyperactivity disorder. *J Am Acad Child Adolesc Psychiatry* 2010;49:1064–80. doi:10.1016/j.jaac.2010.07.009

108. Passarotti AM, Ellis J, Wegbreit E, Stevens MC, Pavuluri MN. Reduced functional connectivity of prefrontal regions and amygdala within affect and working memory networks in pediatric bipolar disorder. *Brain Connect* 2012;2:320–34. doi:10.1089/brain.2012.0089

109. Strakowski SM, Fleck DE, DelBello MP, et al. Characterizing impulsivity in mania. *Bipolar Disord.* 2009;11:41–51.

110. Lombardo LE, Bearden CE, Barrett J, et al. Trait impulsivity as an endophenotype for bipolar I disorder. *Bipolar Disord* 2012;14:565–70, doi:10.1111/j.1399-5618.2012.01035.x

111. Oosterlaan J, Logan GD, Sergeant JA. Response inhibition in AD/HD, CD, comorbid AD/HD+CD, anxious, and control children: a meta-analysis of studies with the stop task. *J Child Psychol Psychiatry.* 1998;39:411–25. doi:10.1111/1469-7610.00336

112. Tillman CM, Thorell LB, Brocki KC, Bohlin G. Motor response inhibition and execution in the stop-signal task: development and relation to ADHD behaviors. *Child Neuropsychol.* 2008;14:42–59. doi:10.1080/09297040701249020

113. Patton JH, Stanford MS, Barratt ES. Factor structure of the Barratt impulsiveness scale. *J Clin Psychol.* 1995;51:768–74.

114. Leibenluft E, Rich BA, Vinton DT, et al. Neural circuitry engaged during unsuccessful motor inhibition in pediatric bipolar disorder. *Am J Psychiatry.* 2007;164:52–60. doi:10.1176/appi.ajp.164.1.52

115. Deveney CM, Connolly ME, Jenkins SE, et al. Neural recruitment during failed motor inhibition differentiates youths with bipolar disorder and severe mood dysregulation. *Biol Psychol.* 2012;89:148–55. doi:10.1016/j.biopsycho.2011.10.003

116. Weathers JD, Stringaris A, Deveney CM, et al. A developmental study of the neural circuitry mediating motor inhibition in bipolar disorder. *Am J Psychiatry*. 2012;169:633–41. doi:10.1176/appi.ajp.2012.11081244

117. Swann AC, Pazzaglia P, Nicholls A, Dougherty DM, Moeller FG. Impulsivity and phase of illness in bipolar disorder. *J Affect Disord*. 2003;73:105–11.

118. MacQueen GM, Hajek T, Alda M. The phenotypes of bipolar disorder: relevance for genetic investigations. *Mol Psychiatry*. 2005;10:811–26. doi:10.1038/sj.mp.4001701

119. Glahn DC, Almasy L, Barquil M, et al. Neurocognitive endophenotypes for bipolar disorder identified in multiplex multigenerational families. *Arch Gen Psychiatry*. 2010;67:168–77. doi:10.1001/archgenpsychiatry.2009.184

120. Gourovitch ML, Torrey EF, Gold JM, Randolph C, Weinberger DR, Goldberg TE. Neuropsychological performance of monozygotic twins discordant for bipolar disorder. *Biol Psychiatry*. 1999;45:639–46.

121. Balanza-Martinez V, Rubio C, Selva-Vera G, et al. Neurocognitive endophenotypes (endophenocognitypes) from studies of relatives of bipolar disorder subjects: a systematic review. *Neurosci Biobehav Rev*. 2008;32:1426–38. doi:10.1016/j.neubiorev.2008.05.019

122. Zalla T, Joyce C, Szöke A, et al. Executive dysfunctions as potential markers of familial vulnerability to bipolar disorder and schizophrenia. *Psychiatry Res*. 2004;121:207–17.

123. Ladouceur CD, Almeida JR, Birmaher B, et al. Subcortical gray matter volume abnormalities in healthy bipolar offspring: potential neuroanatomical risk marker for bipolar disorder? *J Am Acad Child Adolesc Psychiatry*. 2008;47:532–9. doi:10.1097/CHI.0b013e318167656e

124. Glahn DC, Bearden CE, Niendam TA, Escamilla MA. The feasibility of neuropsychological endophenotypes in the search for genes associated with bipolar affective disorder. *Bipolar Disord*. 2004;6:171–82. doi:10.1111/j.1399-5618.2004.00113.x

125. Arts B, Jabben N, Krabbendam L, van Os, J. Meta-analyses of cognitive functioning in euthymic bipolar individuals and their first-degree relatives. *Psychol Med*. 2008;38:771–85. doi:10.1017/s0033291707001675

126. Ferrier IN, Chowdhury R, Thompson JM, Watson S, Young AH. Neurocognitive function in unaffected first-degree relatives of individuals with bipolar disorder: a preliminary report. *Bipolar Disord*. 2004;6:319–22. doi:10.1111/j.1399-5618.2004.00122.x

127. Diwadkar VA, Goradia D, Hosanagar A, et al. Working memory and attention deficits in adolescent offspring of schizophrenia or bipolar individuals: comparing vulnerability markers. *Prog Neuropsychopharmacol Biol Psychiatry*. 2011;35:1349–54. doi:10.1016/j.pnpbp.2011.04.009

128. Christodoulou T, Messinis L, Papathanasopoulos P, Frangou S. Dissociable and common deficits in inhibitory control in schizophrenia and bipolar disorder. *Eur Arch Psychiatry Clin Neurosci*. 2012;262:125–30. doi:10.1007/s00406-011-0213-7

129. Pompei F, Dima D, Rubia K, Kumari V, Frangou S. Dissociable functional connectivity changes during the Stroop task relating to risk, resilience and disease expression in bipolar disorder. *Neuroimage*. 2011;57:576–82. doi:10.1016/j.neuroimage.2011.04.055

130. Singh MK, DelBello MP, Fleck DE, Shear PK, Strakowski SM. Inhibition and attention in adolescents with nonmanic mood disorders and a high risk for developing mania. *J Clin Exp Neuropsychol*. 2009;31:1–7. doi:10.1080/13803390801945038

131. Glahn DC, Bearden CE, Caetano S, et al. Declarative memory impairment in pediatric bipolar disorder. *Bipolar Disord*. 2005;7:546–54. doi:10.1111/j.1399-5618.2005.00267.x

132. Trivedi JK, Goel D, Dhyani M, et al. Neurocognition in first-degree healthy relatives (siblings) of bipolar affective disorder individuals. *Psychiatry Clin Neurosci*. 2008;62:190–6. doi:10.1111/j.1440-1819.2008.01754.x

133. Holmes J, Gathercole SE, Dunning DL. Adaptive training leads to sustained enhancement of poor working memory in children. *Dev Sci* 2009;12:F9–15.

134. Westerberg H, Klingberg T. Changes in cortical activity after training of working memory—a single-subject analysis. *Physiol Behav*. 2007;92:186–92.

The Neural Effects of Intervention in Pediatric Bipolar Disorder

Manpreet K. Singh and Kiki D. Chang

Overview of the Effects of Bipolar Treatment on Brain Structure and Function

Children and adolescents are increasingly being diagnosed with bipolar disorder with approximately 2.5% of youth in the United States ages 13–18 years meeting criteria for a lifetime diagnosis of bipolar I or II disorder with some degree of impairment.[1] An early onset of bipolar disorder in youth has been linked with a more severe course of illness, morbidities such as suicide attempts and substance abuse, and the presence of comorbidities and complications such as poor academic and job performance, interpersonal conflicts, or legal problems.[2-6] Despite vigorous efforts to find effective treatments for bipolar disorder in youths, treatment challenges are frequent[7] and bipolar illness carries high rates of complications, including mortality.[1]

Comprehensive treatment plans are often required for youth with bipolar disorder to address a complex array of symptoms and associated morbidities. In general, a multimodal treatment approach combining pharmacological agents and psychosocial interventions is suggested, with the goal to improve symptoms, provide psychoeducation about the mental illness, and promote treatment adherence for relapse prevention and attenuation of long-term complications from the illness.[7,8] Clinicians are encouraged to advocate for prevention, early intervention, and biopsychosocial treatments that promote the healthy growth and development of all children affected by bipolar disorder, in any cultural context.[8-10] At this point, however, we know relatively little about the mechanisms that underlie treatment and presume that the effects of pharmacological and non-pharmacological interventions on the brain are multifactorial.

An efficient way to elucidate neural mechanisms that underlie the effects of treatment in bipolar disorder is to use magnetic resonance imaging (MRI) technology to assess in vivo brain differences in youth before and after an intervention has occurred. For example, specific differences in brains exposed versus unexposed to medications may suggest intrinsic biological pathways that may clarify the mechanisms by which such treatments are functioning to reduce symptom burden. In some adults with bipolar disorder, medications have been found to have either no effect or a normalizing effect on brain MRI findings in clinical samples compared to healthy subjects.[11] Neuroimaging studies have attempted to examine the effects of medications on brain structural and functional outcomes in post-hoc analyses, and they have not consistently found medication exposure to confound structural, functional, or neurometabolite findings. Specifically, in youth with bipolar disorder, there were no medication effects on reductions in subgenual anterior cingulate gray matter volumes,[12] on increases in dorsolateral prefrontal cortex activations during response inhibition,[13] on reduced thalamic and inferior temporal gyrus activations while anticipating affectively primed rewards,[14] or on intrinsic functional connectivity at rest.[15] Similarly, in youth at risk for bipolar disorder, glutamatergic reductions in the anterior cingulate cortex were not influenced by medication exposure.[16] In other disorders, researchers have tried to avoid the potential confounding effects of medications on brain MRI results altogether by studying only unmedicated or medication-naive youth.[17,18,19,20] While there are some clear advantages to examining unmedicated youth, youth with bipolar disorder who are medication naive are difficult to find and may represent a subset of the population with relatively low symptom severity, thereby limiting generalizability of the results to the overall population.

In this chapter, we will evaluate studies in which medications were not treated as a confound, but rather as a variable of interest on neural outcome. We will review structural, functional, neurochemical, and other neuroimaging modalities employed to study the neurophysiological alterations associated with psychotropic medication exposure in youth with bipolar disorder. In addition, we will review neuroimaging studies examining the effects of psychotherapeutic interventions in an effort to explore potential nonpharmacological treatment effects in bipolar disorder. After reviewing each modality as it applies to youth with bipolar disorder, we will illustrate that pharmacologic interventions during childhood do indeed affect brain structure and function. Finally, we will propose areas of future study that will further explain the biological correlates of treating bipolar disorder.

Methods

A literature search using the National Institutes of Health's PubMed was conducted to identify peer-reviewed neuroimaging studies of children and adolescents with or at risk for bipolar disorder for the period of 1966 to December 2013. The following terms were included in the search: "medication" or "psychotropic" or "psychotherapy" or "treatment" with "bipolar," and "adolescents," "children," "youth," "juvenile," or "pediatric," followed by "neuroimaging," "magnetic resonance imaging (MRI)," "diffusion tensor imaging (DTI)," "functional MRI (fMRI)," or "spectroscopy (MRS)." References from identified articles were also reviewed to ensure that all relevant papers were included.

Results

There are several emerging neuroimaging studies that examined the effect of pharmacological intervention in youth with bipolar disorder. Bipolar symptoms are often severe in youth and create a significant level of impairment such that it is challenging to find youth unmedicated for this disorder when they are enrolled in a neuroimaging study. Some treated youth with bipolar disorder do not show significant departures from healthy development in brain structure and function, possibly due to the normalizing effects of medication. Researchers have used four main methods, either post hoc or a priori, to evaluate the neural effects of medication. First, researchers have examined youth with bipolar disorder who received neuroimaging regardless of treatment exposure and have compared subsamples of youth with and without medication exposure post hoc. Second, researchers have compared neuroimaging outcomes among youth with a variety of different medication exposures. Third, more recent studies have added neural assessments to open-label and randomized controlled clinical trial designs to understand directly the neural effects of medication during a clinical trial. Finally, researchers have compared neural function in treatment responders versus nonresponders and across multiple MRI modalities. Each of these approaches to understanding the neural effects of psychotropic medications has some limitations and strengths. We will provide examples of each of these methods in turn, with the goal of summarizing the current state of the field.

Understanding that medication exposure may influence neural data, several researchers have compared neural data in medicated and unmedicated subgroups. Three structural MRI studies in pediatric bipolar disorder using manual tracing methods characterized volumetric effects on gray matter of medication exposure by comparing youth exposed and unexposed to medication. First, adolescents with bipolar disorder who were exposed to lithium had larger right hippocampal volumes than those who were not exposed to lithium.[21] Second, youth with bipolar disorder who had past mood stabilizer exposure (either lithium or divalproex) had significantly greater posterior subgenual anterior cingulate cortex[22] and amygdala[23] volumes compared to bipolar disorder youth without mood stabilizer exposure and healthy subjects. The effects on white matter microstructure have been less studied, with one post-hoc analysis finding no effects of medication exposure on diffusion tensor imaging (DTI) findings in youth with bipolar disorder.[24] Finally, unmedicated and medicated youth with bipolar disorder showed similar reductions in ventrolateral prefrontal cortex and striatal activations relative to controls during unsuccessful motor inhibition.[25]

Differential neural effects between two medications have also been demonstrated. Pavuluri and colleagues recently investigated the relative effects of risperidone and divalproex on three different cognitive functions in unmedicated manic patients randomized to either treatment and healthy subjects.[26,27,28] In the first task, participants matched the color of a positive, negative, or neutral word with one of two colored circles. They found that after treatment and relative to healthy subjects, the risperidone-treated group showed increased activation in the right pregenual and subgenual anterior cingulate cortex (ACC), and decreased activation in the bilateral middle frontal gyrus, left inferior and medial, and right middle frontal gyri, left inferior parietal lobe, and right striatum. In the divalproex-treated group, relative to healthy subjects, increased activations were found in the right superior temporal gyrus, left medial frontal gyrus, and right precuneus. Second, the differential effects of medication were also evaluated in this sample while they performed a response inhibition task, where a motor response, already "on the way" to execution, had to be voluntarily inhibited on trials where a stop signal was presented.[27] Youth taking risperidone and divalproex differentially engaged an evaluative affective circuit (EAC: bilateral inferior frontal gyrus, middle frontal gyrus, ACC, middle temporal gyrus, insulae, caudate, and putamen) during task performance. Within the EAC, posttreatment and relative to healthy subjects, greater engagement was seen in left insula in the risperidone group and left subgenual ACC in the divalproex group. Finally, during a working memory task under emotional duress, divalproex enhanced activation in a fronto-temporal circuit, whereas risperidone increased activation in the dopamine (D_2) receptor-rich ventral striatum.[28] Thus, risperidone and divalproex yield differential patterns of neural activity during emotion processing, response inhibition, and working memory tasks in youth with bipolar disorder. These studies illustrate that the differential effects of psychotropic medications on the brain may be task dependent and regionally specific. However, these comparative pharmacological functional MRI (fMRI) studies have provided limited knowledge about *how* different medications target different regions while performing various brain functions. Future comparative pharmacological MRI studies must strive to examine the mechanisms that underlie differential neural targets by various psychotropic medications.

Recently, a few researchers have directly examined the effects of pharmacological intervention in fMRI activation in youth with bipolar disorder using prospective studies. The first of such studies was an open-label study by Chang and colleagues,[29] which examined the neural effects of lamotrigine in adolescents with bipolar depression and found that bipolar disorder youth treated with lamotrigine for 8 weeks had less amygdala activation when viewing negative stimuli as depressive symptoms improved; whether the changes in fMRI activation were due to lamotrigine exposure or improvements in depressive symptoms (as a consequence of lamotrigine treatment) could not be determined. Another study examined 17 youth with bipolar disorder after 14 weeks of open-label treatment with a second-generation antipsychotic (SGA) followed by adjunctive lamotrigine monotherapy, and compared fMRI activation to that of healthy subjects while performing an affective color matching task.[30] Researchers observed treatment related decreases in the ventromedial prefrontal cortex (VMPFC) and the dorsolateral prefrontal cortex (DLPFC) in bipolar disorder youth. This same group showed that treatment with an SGA followed by lamotrigine monotherapy enhanced ventrolateral prefrontal cortical (VLPFC) and temporal lobe activity during a response inhibition task, and enhanced VLPFC function was related to clinical treatment response.[31] In this study, behavioral performance was not slowed down in patients on this treatment regimen. This same group also evaluated affective working memory before and after sequential treatment for 8 weeks with an SGA followed by 6 weeks of lamotrigine to previously unmedicated youth with bipolar disorder. This study showed that pharmacotherapy resulted in normalization of symptoms and higher prefrontal cortical and cognitive regional activation in youth with bipolar disorder versus healthy subjects, but it did not normalize amygdala overactivation.[32] Improvement on Young Mania Rating Scale (YMRS) score significantly correlated with decreased activity in the ventromedial prefrontal cortex (VMPFC) within the patient group, suggesting a normalizing effect of treatment on fMRI activation, which may either be due to direct medication effects on the brain or due to symptomatic improvement. A randomized controlled design may be better suited to determine whether neural change that is observed from pre- to postmedication exposure is related to symptomatic improvement.

One randomized controlled trial compared neural activation in a priori regions of interest defined by Brodmann areas (BAs) during a sustained attention task in 23 youth with bipolar disorder randomized to ziprasidone versus placebo and 10 healthy comparison youth at baseline, day 7, and day 28 posttreatment.[33] Compared with placebo, treatment with ziprasidone was associated with greater increases over time in right ventral prefrontal (BA 11 and 47) activation. Interestingly, these effects were not associated with differences in symptom improvement between the treatment groups, suggesting that the observed neural effect of ziprasidone is independent of indices of symptom improvement. However, patients who subsequently responded to ziprasidone showed significantly greater deactivation in the right BA 47 at baseline than those who did not respond to ziprasidone. No significant changes in amygdala activation were detected in association with ziprasidone treatment. Increases in right BA 11 and 47 activation observed during tasks of sustained attention following ziprasidone treatment suggests that ziprasidone may at least partially correct prefrontal dysfunction in currently manic youth. These findings represent the first placebo-controlled evidence for neurofunctional effects of pharmacological treatment in youth with mania.

Other studies have looked more broadly at the effects of pharmacotherapy on neurocognitive systems in pediatric bipolar disorder. Wegbreit and colleagues aimed to determine functional connectivity differences in youth with bipolar disorder who were responders ($n = 22$) versus nonresponders ($n = 12$) to one of three mood-stabilizing medications (divalproex, risperidone, or lamotrigine) and as compared to healthy controls ($n = 14$).[34] Participants performed a color-matching task during fMRI in which they had to match the color of positive, negative, or neutral words with colored dots. A frontolimbic network was identified that showed impaired functional integration in youth with bipolar disorder relative to healthy subjects when participants viewed negatively valenced words. Medication responders in the group with bipolar disorder showed greater connectivity of the amygdala into the network before and after treatment compared with nonresponders, with responders showing a pattern more similar to healthy subjects than to nonresponders. The degree of amygdala functional connectivity predicted medication response as well as the improvement in YMRS scores across responders and nonresponders regardless of medication type. Authors inferred from these results that increased functional integration of the amygdala within the frontolimbic network might be a predictor of broad responsivity to mood stabilizers in bipolar disorder. However, the specific effects of mood stabilizers on task-based or intrinsic functional connectivity patterns associated with pediatric bipolar disorder have yet to be investigated.

In a multimodal neuroimaging study, Chang et al.[35] examined the effects of divalproex on brain structure, chemistry, and function in symptomatic youth at high risk for bipolar disorder. Although there were no detectable effects on brain structure or neurochemistry after 12 weeks of open-label treatment with divalproex, decreases in prefrontal brain activation correlated with decreases in depressive symptom severity.[35] Thus, this change in brain activation may have been due to the intermediate effects of symptom improvement rather than the direct effects of the medication. A placebo-arm may help to differentiate medication effects from those associated with symptomatic change.

Other studies have used magnetic resonance spectroscopy (MRS) in youth with bipolar disorder, primarily employing proton (^{1}H-MRS) acquisitions and focused in key prefrontal cortical regions important for emotion regulation. For example, studies of youth with familial bipolar disorder have shown reduced medial and dorsolateral prefrontal concentrations of N-acetyl aspartate (NAA) and phosphocreatine/creatine (PCr/Cr), healthy nerve cell markers putatively involved in maintaining energy production and myelin formation in the brain.[36] In addition, higher prefrontal myo-inositol (mI) levels, a marker for cellular metabolism and second messenger signaling pathways, have also been found in youth with[37] or at familial risk[38] for bipolar disorder. Both NAA and mI concentrations have been shown to be responsive to lithium treatment in pediatric populations.[39,40] Specifically, Davanzo et al.[39] found that after 1 week of acute lithium treatment, baseline elevated levels of mI/creatine ratios (mI/Cr) in the anterior cingulate cortex in 11 youth with bipolar disorder decreased, and this decrement was higher for lithium responders than lithium nonresponders. However, Patel and colleagues[41] observed that in 12- to 18-year-old youth with bipolar depression, lithium did not have any acute (1 week) or chronic (42 days) effects on mI levels in the medial and lateral prefrontal cortices. In a different study, Patel and colleagues found that after 42 days of lithium administration, 12- to 18-year-old youth with bipolar disorder showed reductions in NAA concentration in the ventromedial prefrontal cortex (VMPFC).[40] In this study, there was a time-by-remission-status interaction of NAA concentrations in the VMPFC, such that youth who remitted developed decreased mean NAA concentration from day 7 to day 42, whereas nonremitters showed an increase in mean NAA concentration during that same time period. The authors speculated that higher lithium levels earlier in the treatment course might have resulted in lithium-induced increases in prefrontal metabolism.[40] However, in adults, chronic lithium exposure has been shown to nonselectively increase NAA concentrations in prefrontal, temporal, parietal, and occipital regions,[42] theoretically increasing neuronal viability and function. Some of these findings suggest that by modulating neurometabolites involved in neuronal cell fluid balance and the second-messenger-related neurometabolite mI, lithium exerts its action either by increasing cellular fluid shifts or by modulating intracellular calcium signaling pathways to deplete membrane inositol lipids.[43,44] These studies provide us clues about the mechanisms by which lithium and other mood stabilizers exert their therapeutic effect[45] and are consistent with the aforementioned neurotrophic effects of lithium on regional brain volumes. Thus, some but not all prior studies have demonstrated that alterations in neurometabolite concentrations may explain the pathophysiology of bipolar disorder[46] and may be sensitive to the effects of psychotropic medications in this population.

Prefrontal neurometabolite levels in youth have also been examined after treatment with divalproex[35] and the atypical antipsychotic olanzapine.[47] In a cohort of youth at high risk for developing bipolar disorder, there were no statistically significant changes in pre- to postdivalproex NAA to Cr (NAA/Cr) ratios, but there was a large effect size ($d = 0.94$) for a decrease in right dorsolateral prefrontal NAA/Cr after treatment with divalproex.[35] This posttreatment *decrease* rather than an expected increase in the NAA/Cr ratio was surprising, given previously proposed neurogenic effects of divalproex leading to increases in NAA.[48] This study may have also been limited by a small sample size, inadequate dose range,[49] short exposure to divalproex, or lack of significant neurobiological impact of divalproex on the neurochemistry of bipolar disorder youth. Hospitalized adolescents with bipolar I disorder who were experiencing a manic or mixed episode achieved remission with olanzapine and demonstrated increases in ventral prefrontal NAA as compared to nonremitting patients, who showed decreases in prefrontal NAA concentrations.[47] Neurogenic effects of these mood-stabilizing agents have been proposed in rat brains[50] and neural stem cells,[51] providing a cellular-level explanation for treatment-related neurometabolite changes. Additional studies examining in vivo metabolite effects of these medications in youth with bipolar disorder would help clarify their role in reversing the pathophysiology of this disorder.

Another prefrontal neurometabolite measurable by ^{1}H-MRS that may be associated with abnormal mood regulation is the excitatory neurotransmitter glutamate, its precursor and storage form glutamine, and a combined contribution of glutamate and glutamine (Glx). Moore and colleagues used ^{1}H-MRS to show decreased levels of glutamine in the ACC in unmedicated youth with bipolar disorder as compared to healthy subjects and medicated youth taking various psychotropics.[52] They also found that unmedicated children with bipolar disorder and significant manic symptoms had lower Glx to creatine (Glx/Cr) ratios in the ACC compared to children with bipolar disorder who were stably treated with risperidone.[53] Mania severity correlated negatively with ACC Glx/Cr levels.

Taken together, these studies suggest that medications appear to have an overall normalizing effect on brain structure, function, and neurometabolites in youth with or at risk for bipolar disorder. Findings from these studies support that medications used to treat bipolar disorder may restore volumetric deficits and improve functional activity in ventrolateral and medial prefrontal regions critical for emotional functioning and regulation. In general, youth with bipolar disorder show decreased activity in amygdala after treatment for mania or depression. In the few instances when increases in amygdala activation relative to healthy subjects were observed regardless of treatment response, authors suggested that residual amygdala hyperactivity may be a trait-like abnormality that may be less responsive to pharmacological intervention.[54] Baseline biochemical abnormalities in magnetic resonance spectroscopic studies compliment abnormalities in fronto-limbic activity in fMRI studies and provide important targets for pharmacological response and outcome (Fig. 14.1).

Overall, these findings are consistent with those reported from studies in adults with bipolar disorder.[55] In adults with bipolar disorder, lithium exposure has been associated with increased volumes in areas important for mood regulation, while antipsychotic agents and anticonvulsants have generally not. Regarding secondary analysis of the medication effects of fMRI and DTI studies, few studies have shown significant effects of medication, although rigorous analyses have not been possible when the majority of subjects were medicated. Medication effects have been more frequently observed in longitudinal studies designed to assess the impact of particular medications on the blood oxygen level–dependent (BOLD) signal. With a few exceptions, the observed effects were normalizing, meaning that the medicated individuals with bipolar disorder were more similar than their

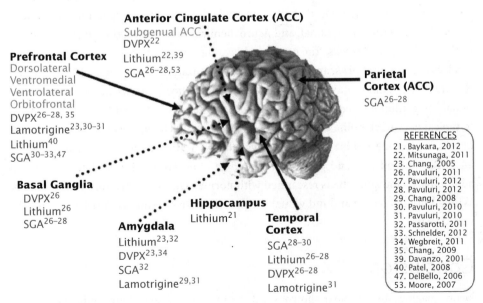

Anterior Cingulate Cortex (ACC)
Subgenual ACC
DVPX[22]
Lithium[22,39]
SGA[26–28,53]

Prefrontal Cortex
Dorsolateral
Ventromedial
Ventrolateral
Orbitofrontal
DVPX[26–28, 35]
Lamotrigine[23,30–31]
Lithium[40]
SGA[30–33,47]

Parietal Cortex (ACC)
SGA[26–28]

Basal Ganglia
DVPX[26]
Lithium[26]
SGA[26–28]

Hippocampus
Lithium[21]

Amygdala
Lithium[23,32]
DVPX[23,34]
SGA[32]
Lamotrigine[29,31]

Temporal Cortex
SGA[28–30]
Lithium[26–28]
DVPX[26–28]
Lamotrigine[31]

REFERENCES
21. Baykara, 2012
22. Mitsunaga, 2011
23. Chang, 2005
26. Pavuluri, 2011
27. Pavuluri, 2012
28. Pavuluri, 2012
29. Chang, 2008
30. Pavuluri, 2010
31. Pavuluri, 2010
32. Passarotti, 2011
33. Schneider, 2012
34. Wegbreit, 2011
35. Chang, 2009
39. Davanzo, 2001
40. Patel, 2008
47. DelBello, 2006
53. Moore, 2007

FIGURE 14.1 Medication effects on selected brain regions in youth with or at risk for bipolar disorder versus healthy subjects. DVPX, divalproex; SGA, second-generation antipsychotic.

unmedicated counterparts to healthy subjects. Larger controlled studies in youth who are initially medication naive would aid in understanding the specific long-term effects of medication exposure on neural structure and function in bipolar disorder.

Clinical Vignette

Although neuroimaging cannot currently be used to diagnose youth with bipolar disorder,[56] we can imagine that this tool will become more accessible and will hopefully lead to more targeted treatments for youth with or at risk for bipolar disorder. In some youth, treatments directed to more specific brain structures such as repetitive transcranial magnetic stimulation have shown some promise for tolerability and efficacy.[57] For the great majority of youth, however, pharmacological and psychosocial interventions will likely remain the mainstay treatments. A hypothetical example follows to illustrate how information from neuroimaging studies might advance our treatments for youth with severe psychiatric illness.

A 16-year-old female presents to the clinic after a week of euphoria, decreased need for sleep, increased goal-directed activities, racing thoughts, grandiosity, distractibility, increased motor activity, and hypersexuality, preceded by a 2-week period of depressed mood, suicidal ideation, irritability, lethargy, and hypersomnia. As these symptoms are clearly impairing function, she meets criteria for bipolar I disorder. Currently unmedicated, she and her family elect to first undergo multimodal neuroimaging. Her structural MRI scan shows that she has reduced volumes in the subgenual ACC, amygdala, and hippocampus. Her fMRI scan shows amygdala overactivation and impaired functional integration of limbic structures with prefrontal areas during emotional and cognitive tasks. Her MRS scan shows increased prefrontal mI, decreased NAA, and decreased glutamine levels. With hope that lithium might treat her acute symptoms as well as restore her structural, functional, and neurochemical aberrancies, the clinician begins a trial of lithium for 12 weeks. The patient achieves remission of her manic symptoms and receives a follow-up MRI scan, which reveals normalization of subgenual ACC, amygdalar, and hippocampal volumes, normalization of activation patterns and improved functional integration between limbic structures and the prefrontal cortex, and restoration to typical neurometabolite concentrations. Three months later, she experiences another depressive episode and is rescanned. Amygdala and VLPFC activations are high during an fMRI emotion task and prefrontal glutamate levels are increased. After 8 weeks of adjunctive lamotrigine she is rescanned with normalization of activation in these areas. With additional family and individual therapy, the patient remains in remission for the next 2 years.

Conclusion

Neuroimaging studies have shown great promise to advance our understanding of potential mechanisms of action of effective treatments for early-onset bipolar disorder.

Reassuringly, in these initial studies, intervention appears to have a normalizing effect on brain structure and function in youth with or at risk for bipolar disorder. The neurotrophic effects of lithium on amygdala and hippocampal volumes are also correlated with symptom improvement, and there appears to be normalization of structure and functional activations while performing a wide array of neurocognitive tasks after treatments with a variety of atypical antipsychotics and mood stabilizers. Additional information is needed to better understand the critical periods of benefit from these interventions and how they compare relative to one another. These kinds of investigations will accelerate the field of child psychiatry and underscore the importance of early identification and prevention of serious mood disorders in youth. Longitudinal studies tracking youth well into adulthood will also provide important supporting evidence for the long-term beneficial effects or deleterious consequences of treatment.

It is also clear from this review that using neuroimaging tools to probe intervention effects in psychiatry may be associated with unique methodological challenges. These include the psychometric effects of repeated scans; how to assess potential relations among the effects of an intervention on symptoms and on specific structural, neurochemical, or brain activation patterns; and how to best make causal inferences about intervention effects on brain function.[58] For example, it is often unclear from the studies described whether neural differences observed after treatment are due to the intervention or due to the symptom improvement that resulted from the intervention (i.e., we do not know whether we are observing a medication effect or a brain improvement effect with symptom change). Future studies should be designed with placebo arms to distinguish these related but separate effects on brain structure and function.

In addition, the study of treatment effects in bipolar spectrum disorders that manifest in childhood presents additional unique challenges due to variance in brain maturation, analysis methods, and the potential for motion artifacts. Methodological advancements to minimize confounds associated with artifact and optimize analytical techniques to enable predictive inferences will be important steps to advance this field. It is also true that the interventions reviewed here were for youth in need of them rather than for typically developing healthy youth experimentally exposed to these interventions, which proves to be ethically challenging. Thus, while it may be the case that lithium restores brain structure and function in youth with bipolar disorder, it is less clear whether it has the same effect in healthy youth. This limits our interpretation of the results as there may be an interaction between certain neural characteristics and medications that produce a unique effect in youth with bipolar disorder that may not be widely generalizable.

There are many justifiable concerns about the adverse effects of psychotropic medication on the developing body and brain of youth. These medications may clearly have adverse peripheral effects on the body, of which the long-term effects are not clear, and may also have central adverse effects, such as extrapyramidal symptoms and sedation. However, we know from prospective observations that the levels of morbidity and mortality from bipolar disorder are very high if left untreated. Therefore, while there are adverse effects that could arise to both the body and the brain, these need to be balanced by the potential *beneficial* effects on the brain, both behaviorally and neurochemically. A comprehensive investigation that evaluates both risks and benefits of intervention is certain to substantiate why behavioral and functional improvements are observed at the clinical level. Moreover, it would be important to determine both predictors of response as well as predictors of adverse effects. For example, is it possible that neuroimaging could help us determine which youth offspring of parents with bipolar disorder being treated for anxiety or depression will respond well to selective serotonin reuptake inhibitors (SSRIs) and which would have a high likelihood of developing antidepressant-induced mania?[59]

When we learn more about the effects of treatment on brain structure and function, and if there is a particular window during development in which they are optimally used (or most problematic), we can begin to develop more targeted and thoughtful approaches to treatment. This knowledge can serve as a guidepost for the next generation of studies and build on emerging treatment biosignatures to personalize interventions for youth with or at risk for bipolar disorder.[54] The possibility remains that acute intervention with proper medications at a critical point in time will allow for shorter duration of treatment needed, and perhaps neuroprotection or neuroplastic change that will then eliminate the need for a lifetime of medications. All practitioners caring for youth with or at risk for bipolar disorder are concerned that these youth achieve full and permanent remission of all symptoms and are able to eventually be on as few medications as possible, if any, prior to reaching adulthood.

Author Disclosures

Dr. Chang serves on the Advisory Board for Sunovion. He is an unpaid consultant to Bristol Myers-Squibb, Otsuka, and GlaxoSmithKline. He receives grant support from GlaxoSmithKline, Merck, and the National Institute of Mental Health.

Dr. Singh has no conflicts to disclose. She receives grant support from the National Institute of Mental Health (K23 MH085919) and Stanford's Child Health Research Institute.

References

1. Merikangas KR, Cui L, Kattan G, Carlson GA, Youngstrom EA, Angst J. Mania with and without depression in a community sample of US adolescents. *Arch Gen Psychiatry.* 2012;69(9):943–51. doi:10.1001/archgenpsychiatry.2012.38

2. Carlson GA, Kotov R, Chang S-W, Ruggero C, Bromet EJ. Early determinants of four-year clinical outcomes in bipolar disorder with psychosis. *Bipolar Disord.* 2012;14(1):19–30. doi:10.1111/j.1399-5618.2012.00982.x

3. Birmaher B, Axelson D, Goldstein B, et al. Four-year longitudinal course of children and adolescents with bipolar spectrum disorders: the Course and Outcome of Bipolar Youth (COBY) study. *Am J Psychiatry.* 2009;166(7):795–804. doi:10.1176/appi.ajp.2009.08101569

4. Pavuluri MN, O'Connor MM, Harral EM, Moss M, Sweeney JA. Impact of neurocognitive function on academic difficulties in pediatric bipolar disorder: a clinical translation. *Biol Psychiatry*. 2006;60(9):951–6. doi:10.1016/j.biopsych.2006.03.027

5. Wilens TE, Martelon M, Anderson JP, Shelley-Abrahamson R, Biederman J. Difficulties in emotional regulation and substance use disorders: a controlled family study of bipolar adolescents. *Drug Alcohol Depend*. 2013;132(1–2):114–21. doi:10.1016/j.drugalcdep.2013.01.015

6. Goldstein TR, Ha W, Axelson DA, et al. Predictors of prospectively examined suicide attempts among youth with bipolar disorder. *Arch Gen Psychiatry*. 2012;69(11):1113–22. doi:10.1001/archgenpsychiatry.2012.650

7. Chang K. Challenges in the diagnosis and treatment of pediatric bipolar depression. *Dialogues Clin Neurosci*. 2009;11(1):73–80.

8. McClellan J, Kowatch R, Findling RL. Practice parameter for the assessment and treatment of children and adolescents with bipolar disorder. *J Am Acad Child Adolesc Psychiatry*. 2007;46(1):107–25. doi:10.1097/01.chi.0000242240.69678.c4

9. Chang K, Howe M, Gallelli K, Miklowitz D. Prevention of pediatric bipolar disorder: integration of neurobiological and psychosocial processes. *Ann NY Acad Sci*. 2006;1094:235–47. doi:10.1196/annals.1376.026

10. Miklowitz DJ, Chang KD. Prevention of bipolar disorder in at-risk children: theoretical assumptions and empirical foundations. *Dev Psychopathol*. 2008;20(3):881–97. doi:10.1017/S0954579408000424

11. Phillips ML, Travis MJ, Fagiolini A, Kupfer DJ. Medication effects in neuroimaging studies of bipolar disorder. *Am J Psychiatry*. 2008;165(3):313–20. doi:10.1176/appi.ajp.2007.07071066

12. Singh MK, Chang KD, Chen MC, et al. Volumetric reductions in the subgenual anterior cingulate cortex in adolescents with bipolar I disorder. *Bipolar Disord*. 2012;14(6):585–96. doi:10.1111/j.1399-5618.2012.01043.x

13. Singh MK, Chang KD, Mazaika P, et al. Neural correlates of response inhibition in pediatric bipolar disorder. *J Child Adolesc Psychopharmacol*. 2010;20(1):15–24. doi:10.1089/cap.2009.0004

14. Singh MK, Chang KD, Kelley RG, et al. Reward processing in adolescents with bipolar I disorder. *J Am Acad Child Adolesc Psychiatry*. 2013;52(1):68–83. doi:10.1016/j.jaac.2012.10.004

15. Dickstein DP, Gorrostieta C, Ombao H, et al. Fronto-temporal spontaneous resting state functional connectivity in pediatric bipolar disorder. *Biol Psychiatry*. 2010;68(9):839–46. doi:10.1016/j.biopsych.2010.06.029

16. Singh M, Spielman D, Adleman N, et al. Brain glutamatergic characteristics of pediatric offspring of parents with bipolar disorder. *Psychiatry Res*. 2010;182(2):165–71. doi:10.1016/j.pscychresns.2010.01.003

17. Guyer AE, Choate VR, Detloff A, et al. Striatal functional alteration during incentive anticipation in pediatric anxiety disorders. *Am J Psychiatry*. 2012;169(2):205–12.

18. Chantiluke K, Halari R, Simic M, et al. Fronto-striato-cerebellar dysregulation in adolescents with depression during motivated attention. *Biol Psychiatry*. 2012;71(1):59–67. doi:10.1016/j.biopsych.2011.09.005

19. Freitag CM, Luders E, Hulst HE, et al. Total brain volume and corpus callosum size in medication-naïve adolescents and young adults with autism spectrum disorder. *Biol Psychiatry*. 2009;66(4):316–9. doi:10.1016/j.biopsych.2009.03.011

20. Dickstein DP, van der Veen JW, Knopf L, Towbin KE, Pine DS, Leibenluft E. Proton magnetic resonance spectroscopy in youth with severe mood dysregulation. *Psychiatry Res*. 2008;163(1):30–9. doi:10.1016/j.pscychresns.2007.11.006

21. Baykara B, Inal-Emiroglu N, Karabay N, et al. Increased hippocampal volumes in lithium treated adolescents with bipolar disorders: a structural MRI study. *J Affect Disord*. 2012;138(3):433–9. doi:10.1016/j.jad.2011.12.047

22. Mitsunaga MM, Garrett A, Howe M, Karchemskiy A, Reiss A, Chang K. Increased subgenual cingulate cortex volume in pediatric bipolar disorder associated with mood stabilizer exposure. *J Child Adolesc Psychopharmacol*. 2011;21(2):149–55. doi:10.1089/cap.2010.0094

23. Chang K, Karchemskiy A, Barnea-Goraly N, Garrett A, Simeonova DI, Reiss A. Reduced amygdalar gray matter volume in familial pediatric bipolar disorder. *J Am Acad Child Adolesc Psychiatry*. 2005;44(6):565–73. doi:10.1097/01.chi.0000159948.75136.0d

24. Barnea-Goraly N, Chang KD, Karchemskiy A, Howe ME, Reiss AL. Limbic and corpus callosum aberrations in adolescents with bipolar disorder: a tract-based spatial statistics analysis. *Biol Psychiatry*. 2009;66(3):238–44. doi:10.1016/j.biopsych.2009.02.025

25. Leibenluft E, Rich BA, Vinton DT, et al. Neural circuitry engaged during unsuccessful motor inhibition in pediatric bipolar disorder. *Am J Psychiatry*. 2007;164(1):52–60. doi:10.1176/appi.ajp.164.1.52

26. Pavuluri MN, Passarotti AM, Lu LH, Carbray JA, Sweeney JA. Double-blind randomized trial of risperidone versus divalproex in pediatric bipolar disorder: fMRI outcomes. *Psychiatry Res*. 2011;193(1):28–37. doi:10.1016/j.pscychresns.2011.01.005

27. Pavuluri MN, Ellis JA, Wegbreit E, Passarotti AM, Stevens MC. Pharmacotherapy impacts functional connectivity among affective circuits during response inhibition in pediatric mania. *Behav Brain Res*. 2012;226(2):493–503. doi:10.1016/j.bbr.2011.10.003

28. Pavuluri MN, Passarotti AM, Fitzgerald JM, Wegbreit E, Sweeney JA. Risperidone and divalproex differentially engage the fronto-striato-temporal circuitry in pediatric mania: a pharmacological functional magnetic resonance imaging study. *J Am Acad Child Adolesc Psychiatry*. 2012;51(2):157–70.e5. doi:10.1016/j.jaac.2011.10.019

29. Chang KD, Wagner C, Garrett A, Howe M, Reiss A. A preliminary functional magnetic resonance imaging study of prefrontal-amygdalar activation changes in adolescents with bipolar depression treated with lamotrigine. *Bipolar Disord*. 2008;10(3):426–31. doi:10.1111/j.1399-5618.2007.00576.x

30. Pavuluri MN, Passarotti AM, Parnes SA, Fitzgerald JM, Sweeney JA. A pharmacological functional magnetic resonance imaging study probing the interface of cognitive and emotional brain systems in pediatric bipolar disorder. *J Child Adolesc Psychopharmacol*. 2010;20(5):395–406. doi:10.1089/cap.2009.0105

31. Pavuluri MN, Passarotti AM, Harral EM, Sweeney JA. Enhanced prefrontal function with pharmacotherapy on a response inhibition task in adolescent bipolar disorder. *J Clin Psychiatry*. 2010;71(11):1526–34. doi:10.4088/JCP.09m05504yel

32. Passarotti AM, Sweeney JA, Pavuluri MN. Fronto-limbic dysfunction in mania pre-treatment and persistent amygdala over-activity post-treatment in pediatric bipolar disorder. *Psychopharmacology (Berl)*. 2011;216(4):485–99. doi:10.1007/s00213-011-2243-2

33. Schneider MR, Adler CM, Whitsel R, et al. The effects of ziprasidone on prefrontal and amygdalar activation in manic youth with bipolar disorder. *Isr J Psychiatry Relat Sci*. 2012;49(2):112–20.

34. Wegbreit E, Ellis JA, Nandam A, et al. Amygdala functional connectivity predicts pharmacotherapy outcome in pediatric bipolar disorder. *Brain Connect*. 2011;1(5):411–22. doi:10.1089/brain.2011.0035

35. Chang K, Karchemskiy A, Kelley R, et al. Effect of divalproex on brain morphometry, chemistry, and function in youth at high-risk for bipolar disorder: a pilot study. *J Child Adolesc Psychopharmacol*. 2009;19(1):51–9. doi:10.1089/cap.2008.060

36. Chang K, Adleman N, Dienes K, Barnea-Goraly N, Reiss A, Ketter T. Decreased N-acetylaspartate in children with familial bipolar disorder. *Biol Psychiatry*. 2003;53(11):1059–65.

37. Patel NC, Cecil KM, Strakowski SM, Adler CM, DelBello MP. Neurochemical alterations in adolescent bipolar depression: a proton magnetic resonance spectroscopy pilot study of the prefrontal cortex. *J Child Adolesc Psychopharmacol*. 2008;18(6):623–7. doi:10.1089/cap.2007.151

38. Cecil KM, DelBello MP, Sellars MC, Strakowski SM. Proton magnetic resonance spectroscopy of the frontal lobe and cerebellar vermis in children with a mood disorder and a familial risk for bipolar disorders. *J Child Adolesc Psychopharmacol*. 2003;13(4):545–55. doi:10.1089/104454603322724931

39. Davanzo P, Thomas MA, Yue K, et al. Decreased anterior cingulate myo-inositol/creatine spectroscopy resonance with lithium treatment in children with bipolar disorder. *Neuropsychopharmacology*. 2001;24(4):359–69. doi:10.1016/S0893-133X(00)00207-4

40. Patel NC, DelBello MP, Cecil KM, Stanford KE, Adler CM, Strakowski SM. Temporal change in N-acetyl-aspartate concentrations in adolescents with bipolar depression treated with lithium. *J Child Adolesc Psychopharmacol*. 2008;18(2):132–9. doi:10.1089/cap.2007.0088

41. Patel NC, DelBello MP, Cecil KM, et al. Lithium treatment effects on Myo-inositol in adolescents with bipolar depression. *Biol Psychiatry*. 2006;60(9):998–1004. doi:10.1016/j.biopsych.2006.07.029

42. Moore GJ, Bebchuk JM, Hasanat K, et al. Lithium increases N-acetyl-aspartate in the human brain: in vivo evidence in support of bcl-2's neurotrophic effects? *Biol Psychiatry*. 2000;48(1):1–8.

43. Soeiro-de-Souza MG, Dias VV, Figueira ML, et al. Translating neurotrophic and cellular plasticity: from pathophysiology to improved therapeutics for bipolar disorder. *Acta Psychiatr Scand*. 2012;126(5):332–41. doi:10.1111/j.1600-0447.2012.01889.x

44. Demuro A, Parker I. Cytotoxicity of intracellular aβ42 amyloid oligomers involves Ca2+ release from the endoplasmic reticulum by stimulated production of inositol trisphosphate. *J Neurosci*. 2013;33(9):3824–33. doi:10.1523/JNEUROSCI.4367-12.2013

45. Glitz DA, Manji HK, Moore GJ. Mood disorders: treatment-induced changes in brain neurochemistry and structure. *Semin Clin Neuropsychiatry*. 2002;7(4):269–80.

46. Yildiz-Yesiloglu A, Ankerst DP. Neurochemical alterations of the brain in bipolar disorder and their implications for pathophysiology: a systematic review of the in vivo proton magnetic resonance spectroscopy findings. *Prog Neuropsychopharmacol Biol Psychiatry*. 2006;30(6):969–95. doi:10.1016/j.pnpbp.2006.03.012

47. DelBello MP, Cecil KM, Adler CM, Daniels JP, Strakowski SM. Neurochemical effects of olanzapine in first-hospitalization manic adolescents: a proton magnetic resonance spectroscopy study. *Neuropsychopharmacology*. 2006;31(6):1264–73. doi:10.1038/sj.npp.1300950

48. Manji HK, Moore GJ, Chen G. Clinical and preclinical evidence for the neurotrophic effects of mood stabilizers: implications for the pathophysiology and treatment of manic-depressive illness. *Biol Psychiatry*. 2000;48(8):740–54.

49. Kowatch RA, Fristad M, Birmaher B, et al. Treatment guidelines for children and adolescents with bipolar disorder. *J Am Acad Child Adolesc Psychiatry*. 2005;44(3):213–35.

50. Hashimoto R, Fujimaki K, Jeong MR, et al. [Neuroprotective actions of lithium]. *Seishin Shinkeigaku Zasshi*. 2003;105(1):81–6.

51. Laeng P, Pitts RL, Lemire AL, et al. The mood stabilizer valproic acid stimulates GABA neurogenesis from rat forebrain stem cells. *J Neurochem*. 2004;91(1):238–51. doi:10.1111/j.1471-4159.2004.02725.x

52. Moore CM, Frazier JA, Glod CA, et al. Glutamine and glutamate levels in children and adolescents with bipolar disorder: a 4.0-T proton magnetic resonance spectroscopy study of the anterior cingulate cortex. *J Am Acad Child Adolesc Psychiatry*. 2007;46(4):524–34. doi:10.1097/chi.0b013e31802f5f2c

53. Moore CM, Biederman J, Wozniak J, et al. Mania, glutamate/glutamine and risperidone in pediatric bipolar disorder: a proton magnetic resonance spectroscopy study of the anterior cingulate cortex. *J Affect Disord*. 2007;99(1–3):19–25. doi:10.1016/j.jad.2006.08.023

54. Mayanil T, Wegbreit E, Fitzgerald J, Pavuluri M. Emerging biosignature of brain function and intervention in pediatric bipolar disorder. *Minerva Pediatr*. 2011;63(3):183–200.

55. Hafeman DM, Chang KD, Garrett AS, Sanders EM, Phillips ML. Effects of medication on neuroimaging findings in bipolar disorder: an updated review. *Bipolar Disord*. 2012;14(4):375–410. doi:10.1111/j.1399-5618.2012.01023.x

56. Chang K, Adleman N, Wagner C, Barnea-Goraly N, Garrett A. Will neuroimaging ever be used to diagnose pediatric bipolar disorder? *Dev Psychopathol*. 2006;18(4):1133–46. doi:10.1017/S0954579406060548

57. Mattai A, Miller R, Weisinger B, et al. Tolerability of transcranial direct current stimulation in childhood-onset schizophrenia. *Brain Stimul*. 2011;4(4):275–80. doi:10.1016/j.brs.2011.01.001

58. Dichter GS, Sikich L, Song A, Voyvodic J, Bodfish JW. Functional neuroimaging of treatment effects in psychiatry: methodological challenges and recommendations. *Intl J Neurosci*. 2012;122(9):483–93. doi:10.3109/00207454.2012.678446

59. Goldsmith M, Singh M, Chang K. Antidepressants and psychostimulants in pediatric populations: is there an association with mania? *Paediatr Drugs*. 2011;13(4):225–43. doi:10.2165/11591660-000000000-00000

Integration and Future Direction

Toward Improving Outcomes for Youth With Bipolar Disorder

Luis Rodrigo Patino Duran, Peirce Johnston,
Caleb M. Adler, Melissa P. DelBello,
and Stephen M. Strakowski

Phenomenology and Diagnosis

Looking toward a future of better managing bipolar disorder in youth, certainly one of the greatest challenges facing both researchers and clinicians is accurate and timely diagnosis; this challenge is especially acute when attempting to identify the illness at the earliest presentation, as discussed in Chapters 2 and 3. Several lines of evidence suggest that the early course of bipolar disorder exhibits progressive shortening of euthymic periods between affective episodes, so any ability to intervene in this period of illness might interrupt this progression and perhaps the lifelong risk of recurrent mania and depression that characterizes bipolar disorder.[1] In fact, it would be ideal to identify individuals at imminent risk for developing bipolar disorder prior to the onset of a full manic episode in order to prevent the illness altogether. Indeed, several investigators are beginning to clarify prodromal features that precede the defining mania or hypomania; as described in Chapter 1, these features can be present sometimes years before the full episode. Studies of interventions in the prodromal period might lead to prevention strategies and ultimately improve long-term outcomes. Consequently, a better understanding of these prodromal features could affect diagnosis and thus treatment through all stages of life in people with bipolar disorder. Toward this end, in Chapter 1 Dr. Duffy describes a staging system for bipolar disorder that classifies young people with known familial risk from Stage 0 to Stage 4, taking into consideration many factors, including the subject's trajectory of development, course of illness, family history, and other risk factors.[2] A staging process such as this one might lead to a targeted treatment approach that could delay or diminish the impact of the illness.

To achieve this goal of preventing illness onset or progression, the future of pediatric bipolar disorder will need to move past a simple focus on irritability toward an increasingly robust understanding of the variety of prodromal presentations, which includes premorbid anxiety syndromes, such as panic disorder, generalized anxiety, and obsessive-compulsive disorder, as described in Chapter 4. How these prodromal syndromes intersect between the onset of bipolar illness *per se* and actual co-occurrence of separate illnesses require careful longitudinal and treatment studies to best interpret symptom combinations. Clarifying illness co-occurrence and comorbidity in these young people, both prior to and after the onset of the first manic episode, will undoubtedly be necessary in order to disentangle any overlap of truly different diagnoses (i.e., diseases) or else to further refine our definition of bipolar disorder at its very onset to better understanding its variable symptomatic presentation.

One common problem discussed in previous chapters of this book is that imprecise history-taking significantly contributes to struggling with establishing a diagnosis of bipolar disorder in youth. Up to 90% of individuals with pediatric bipolar are diagnosed with at least one comorbidity so that there is potential for various interpretations of symptoms and syndromes as well as a tremendous need for clarity of how these interact to impact treatment response and course of illness.[3] Moreover, it can take many years for bipolar individuals to receive a correct diagnosis. In addition, a precise understanding of an individual's baseline behaviors versus manifestations of early bipolar symptoms is paramount to differentiate temperamental components from incipient affective illness. In other words, clinicians must keep in mind that acquiring this information requires many assessments and a longitudinal observation over an extended period of time before an accurate diagnosis or diagnoses can be made. A thorough review of diagnoses in youth, particularly when treatment is not working, is necessary for clinicians to identify the most appropriate therapy. The benefits of such exactitude are not only a clearer picture of each bipolar individual but also purer data for future researchers; moreover, comparative effectiveness studies are then needed to demonstrate how this precision impacts treatment and course of illness. Although advances in technology, such as imaging, promise objective diagnostic markers, these do not yet exist and the technology is typically limited by the quality and interpretation of clinical data; consequently, large prospective longitudinal clinical studies integrated with new technologies are needed to better define pediatric bipolar illness, its onset, and its early course.

Neurobiological investigation will undoubtedly play a major role in future discoveries of bipolar disorder etiology, clinical presentation, and diagnosis. For example, the finding from proton magnetic response spectroscopy (HMRS) that a higher ratio of glutamate and glutamine to myo-inositol-containing compounds appears in the anterior cingulate cortex of children with only attention-deficit/hyperactivity disorder (ADHD) versus those with comorbid bipolar disorder and ADHD suggests this technology might help in diagnostic assessments.[4] In other words, this type of research suggests that as neuroimaging techniques improve, at some point they likely will guide diagnostic decision making in pediatric bipolar disorder (as well as other psychiatric conditions). Most studies looking at the genetic or neurobiological underpinnings of pediatric bipolar disorder as potential sources of diagnostic biomarkers have compared bipolar and healthy youth; given the diagnostic complexity of the condition, however, additional work in bipolar youth with common comorbidities, such as oppositional defiant disorder, conduct disorder, and substance use disorders, as well as compared to other diagnostic groups (e.g., youth with anxiety disorders), are sorely needed.

Hopefully, in the future establishing a diagnosis of pediatric bipolar disorder will incorporate a battery of information, including clinical assessment, neuroimaging, genetics, developmental course, environmental events, and other factors as suggested in the staging model previously reviewed. As evidenced in many chapters throughout this book, as the field begins to integrate across the various approaches, the study of pediatric bipolar disorder and ultimately its diagnosis is in the midst of a possible paradigm shift from an approach that is driven purely by clinical assessment and then trial-and-error pharmacological management of illness episodes or secondary prevention toward a model that centers on primary prevention. To achieve this shift, integrating detailed clinical assessments with neuroimaging, genetic and other approaches over time (i.e., longitudinally) across diverse cohorts of individuals will be needed to better elucidate a process to correctly identify pediatric bipolar disorder prior to or early on after illness onset.

Treatment

Beyond establishing an accurate diagnosis and describing the phenomenology of bipolar disorder, well-recognized developmental differences between youth and adults make the treatment of early-onset bipolar disorder, to say the least, complex. For example, adults typically exhibit distinct episodes of depression and mania, whereas the pattern of illness observed in young people is often characterized by mixed or dysphoric mood states accompanied by irritability and other behavioral symptoms that may be persistent over time.[5] Moreover, children and adolescents seem to experience more symptomatic periods and may be more susceptible to rapid cycling than adults.[6] As previously reviewed, most individuals with pediatric bipolar disorder also experience co-occurring conditions, most commonly attention-deficit/hyperactivity and anxiety disorders. These differences in presentation could be related to differences in brain development between adults and youth, differences in the stages of neuroprogression of bipolar disorder, or may constitute a subset of bipolar disorder related to age at onset that has a different course of illness. Regardless, it is notable that these types of complex presentations when they occur in adults with bipolar disorder often herald treatment nonresponse.[6]

In the midst of the challenges of recognizing and managing bipolar disorder in children and adolescents, it is also clear that children and adolescents with bipolar disorder require prompt treatment to ameliorate symptoms and to prevent (or at least reduce) the psychosocial morbidity that accompanies the illness. In fact, early detection and treatment seem paramount since earlier onset and longer duration of illness are associated with poor rates of recovery.[7] Again, early intervention might prevent illness progression, improving long-term outcome. Delays in treatment early in the course of illness risk potentially worsening outcomes many years later.

Because of its complexity, treatment of pediatric bipolar disorder requires a multimodal approach that includes pharmacologic and psychosocial interventions as reviewed in detail in Section 2 of this book. Although medication is the cornerstone of any treatment approach, adjunctive psychosocial interventions and complementary-medicine approaches are often necessary for maximal outcomes. As reviewed in Section 2, several effective treatments have been identified for pediatric bipolar disorder in manic/mixed and depressed phases of illness. These data support several conclusions regarding treatment options for pediatric bipolar disorder. Second-generation antipsychotics are highly efficacious for treatment of acute manic/mixed episodes, although tolerability remains a major concern and their efficacy across other phases of illness are much less established. The evidence regarding traditional mood stabilizers (e.g., lithium, valproate) suggests that these may be less efficacious than antipsychotics among youth; however, this conclusion remains tentative pending additional placebo-controlled trials.[8] Also, evidence emerging from psychosocial interventions in both youth at risk for bipolar disorder and individuals with bipolar disorder highlight the advantages of a multimodal approach in the treatment and hopefully one day prevention of early-onset bipolar disorder.[9] However, the number of studies of treatment interventions in youth with or at risk for bipolar disorder remains relatively low, so that many treatment decisions in routine clinical practice likely arise by extrapolating from experiences in adults. Unfortunately, given differences in brain development and illness course between youth and adults, the validity of this approach is questionable. Obviously, more research is desperately needed, particularly across illness phases and over time.

In addition, because it is highly unlikely that any given medication will be proven universally effective in youth with bipolar disorder (or in any age group for that matter), more studies searching for adequate personalized predictors of treatment response are of vital importance to achieve individualized treatment strategies. These predictors can range from demographic characteristics, symptomatic clusters, family history, pharmacogenetic markers, cognitive deficits, to neuroimaging traits. Moreover, given that it will be unlikely that any single study will be sufficiently powered to detect predictors of treatment response to all available treatment options, efforts must be taken to have an available pool of data to collectively search for those predictors. Systematic data collection, similar data designs, and uniform rater reliability in efficacy measurements that are shared across research groups would be one initial step in this endeavor. Vigorous and concerted efforts to address these and other questions will ensure that the momentum of progress in the treatment of pediatric bipolar disorder is sustained over the coming years.

Beyond our scientific and academic understanding of bipolar disorder and its treatment, we must consider that health (and more so mental health) is an individual experience. Notions of an effective treatment may differ between health providers and people struggling with illness. At the community level, on the other hand, cost-effectiveness and feasibility are quintessential, but often times are overlooked in clinical trials. Bridging this gap is one of the future challenges that the field of therapeutics in early-onset bipolar disorder will need to tackle. One recent approach is found in the Patient-Centered Outcomes Research Institute (PCORI). PCORI's mission extends beyond efficacy measurements of treatments toward "real-world" effectiveness. By doing so, PCORI should help people make informed health care decisions and improve health care delivery and outcomes, by producing and promoting high-integrity, evidence-based information that comes from research guided by people with bipolar disorder, their caregivers, and the broader health care community.[10]

Neurobiology of Bipolar Disorder

As reviewed earlier, our understanding of the neurobiological underpinnings of bipolar disorder have greatly advanced in the past decades, thanks in part to progress made in neuroimaging techniques (i.e., PET, MRI, fMRI, DTI, sMRI) that have allowed us to peek into the developing brain of both youth with bipolar disorder and healthy individuals. Through these techniques investigators have been able to identify and track cortico-limbic abnormalities that are implicated in the development of bipolar disorder. Studies suggest abnormalities in the structure, function, and connectivity among brain networks, including prefrontal cortex, amygdala, and ventral striatum. Evidence from studies using these imaging modalities also supports the notion that trajectories of cortico-limbic development during adolescence and young adulthood differ between bipolar disorder and healthy subjects and may represent underlying illness risk.[11] By studying and comparing individuals from different stages of disease progression, we are starting to understand the processes behind developing bipolar disorder.

As noted in Chapters 12 and 13, the most consistent findings in youth with bipolar disorder have been located in the amygdala. There is also evidence supporting amygdala abnormalities in adolescents at familial risk for bipolar disorder, suggesting these are early abnormalities in the progression of bipolar disorder that are potential targets for early detection, treatment, and possibly prevention strategies.[12] On the other hand, the ventral striatum is also highly implicated in bipolar disorder.[13] However, despite reports of both structural and functional findings in the striatum in adult and adolescent bipolar disorder and at-risk individuals in general, there are fewer studies of the ventral striatum specifically, and results have varied.[14] There have been few direct comparisons of the amygdala and ventral striatum among individuals with bipolar disorder and those with other psychiatric conditions (e.g., major depressive disorder), so illness specificity of these findings remains unclear; however, there is preliminary evidence suggesting that some features of abnormalities in these structures may differ among psychiatric disorders, such as in the type of functional abnormalities that are elicited by stimuli of particular valences and cognitive types.[15]

Among the cortical structures involved in pediatric bipolar disorder, the ventral prefrontal cortex, known for its role in regulating emotionally appropriate behavior and modulating responses of the amygdala and ventral striatum, is of paramount importance.[16] Decreases in ventral prefrontal cortex volume and dysregulated responses have been found in adults with bipolar disorder across mood states and in at-risk individuals, suggesting that they are associated with risk for the illness. Also, consistent with the continued maturation of the ventral prefrontal cortex during adolescence and young adulthood, ventral prefrontal cortex abnormalities seen in youth with bipolar disorder progress during this time period.[17] This observation suggests that adolescence and young adulthood may be periods during which reduction in factors that are detrimental to ventral prefrontal cortex development, such as stress and substance abuse, may help reduce the impact of such abnormalities and potentially delay onset or decrease illness progression.

With respect to white matter findings, diffusion tensor imaging (DTI) studies have found frontotemporal abnormalities in intra- and interhemispheric white matter in bipolar adults, adolescents, and at-risk individuals. These findings may represent a neurobiological trait of bipolar disorder, so they could be considered as a candidate endophenotype to target in identification, treatment, and prevention strategies.[18]

Of course, structural and functional abnormalities found in youth with bipolar disorder are phenotypically expressed in the form of cognitive and other behavioral deficits. Cognitive impairments in individuals with bipolar disorder had been traditionally thought to be mild and limited to acute mood episodes; however, a growing body of evidence challenges this assumption. This suggestion is even more evident in youth with bipolar disorder. Studies across disease stages have consistently revealed the presence of cognitive and information processing deficits in this population, particularly in the domains of emotion processing, working memory, cognitive flexibility, executive function, and attention.[19] These deficits persist during interepisodic asymptomatic periods; they interfere with the course of healthy cognitive and emotional development and with progression of illness. They may also lead to poor psychosocial adjustment and functioning. Cognitive deficits could potentially be markers of neuropathology, disease vulnerability, and treatment response in youth with bipolar disorder.

Although considerable advances have been made elucidating the neurobiology of bipolar disorder in youth, this task is far from complete. Future studies into the neurobiology and neuroprogression of bipolar disorder will have to tackle obstacles that have plagued the study of neurobiology of mental disorders. As suggested previously, a better integration across illness course, treatment trials, and developmental stages is necessary. Moreover, study designs must become more specific and better powered. For example, sample sizes in neuroimaging studies tend to be low; hence, the average statistical power of neuroimaging studies is also low. Low-powered studies undermine the reliability of neurobiological findings.[20] In general, three main problems contribute to producing unreliable findings in studies with low power, even when all other research practices are ideal. They are as follows: the low probability of finding true effects; the low positive predictive value when an effect is claimed; and an exaggerated estimate of the magnitude of the effect when a true effect is discovered (e.g., "the winner's curse"). There is also frequently a tendency for publications to significantly overestimate the relative importance of findings. Future endeavors may seek to increase sample sizes and reliability of the neurobiological findings in youths with bipolar disorder while bringing increased intellectual modesty toward understanding the human brain and its function. One possible option to this end is the adoption of large-scale collaborative consortia. Through collaborations, researchers can perform one or many replications to increase total sample size (and therefore statistical power) while minimizing labor and resource impact on any one contributor.

On the other hand, overreliance on magnetic resonance imaging (MRI) to understand and define neurobiological abnormalities found in bipolar disorder is worth discussing. Despite the exceptional topographic resolution that MRI techniques offer, tracking the function of brain structures involved in bipolar disorder has been challenging, in part because such techniques offer poor temporal resolution. Switching from block designs to event-related designs in fMRI help to link temporal relationships between brain activity and task, but this does not completely resolve the problem. Alternatives such as electroencephalography and magnetoencephalography measure functional brain activity by detecting the variations in electrical and magnetic fields across the scalp, respectively, which reflect neuronal activity in the brain. While these techniques offer superb temporal resolution, topographic resolution (particularly subcortical) is far from ideal. In the future, investigating human brain function could potentially be improved by employing a multimodal neuroimaging approach. The integration of different noninvasive electrophysiological and hemodynamic (fMRI and functional near-infrared spectroscopy) neuroimaging modalities during motor and cognitive tasks can potentially complement each technique's limitations.

Neuroimaging studies have facilitated our understanding of potential mechanisms of action of effective treatments for early-onset bipolar disorder. Reassuringly, at least in these initial studies, intervention appears to have a normalizing effect on brain structure and function in youth with or at risk for bipolar disorder. For example, the neurotrophic effects of lithium on amygdala and hippocampal volumes are correlated with symptom improvement, and there appears to be normalization of structure and functional activations while performing a wide array of neurocognitive tasks after treatment.[21] Additional information is needed to better understand the critical periods of benefit from these interventions, and how they compare relative to one another. These kinds of investigations will accelerate the field of child psychiatry and underscore the importance of early identification and prevention of serious mood disorders in youth. Longitudinal studies tracking youth well into adulthood would provide important supporting evidence for the long-term beneficial effects or deleterious consequences of specific treatments.

It is also clear from Section 3 that using neuroimaging tools to probe intervention effects in psychiatry may be associated with unique methodological challenges. These include the psychometric effects of repeated scans; how to assess potential relations among the effects of an intervention on symptoms and on specific structural, neurochemical, or brain activation patterns; and how to best make causal inferences about intervention effects on brain function. For example, it is often unclear from the studies described whether neural differences observed after treatment are due to the intervention or due to the symptom improvement that resulted from the intervention (i.e., we do not know whether we are observing a medication effect or a brain improvement effect with symptom change). Future studies should be designed with placebo arms to distinguish these related, but separate effects on brain structure and function.

In addition, the study of treatment effects in bipolar disorder that manifest in childhood presents additional unique challenges due to variance in brain maturation, analysis methods, and the potential for motion artifacts. Methodological advancements to minimize confounds associated with artifact and to optimize analytic approaches to enable predictive inferences will be important steps to advance this field. It is also true that interventions reviewed in this book were for youth in need of them rather than for typically developing healthy youth experimentally exposed to these interventions; although this approach has scientific merit, it proves to be ethically challenging, so innovative methods to manage these problems of interpretation are needed. For example, while it may be the case that lithium restores brain structure and function in youth with bipolar disorder, it is unknown whether it has the same effect in healthy youth. This limitation clouds our interpretation of results, as there may be interactions between certain neural characteristics and medications that produce unique effects in youth with bipolar disorder that may not be widely generalizable to youth with other psychiatric disorders or in health.

There are justifiable concerns about the adverse effects of psychotropic medication on the developing body and brain of youth. Psychotropic medications clearly have adverse peripheral effects on the body, from which the long-term impact is not clear, and may also have central adverse effects. However, we know from prospective observations that morbidity and mortality from bipolar disorder are very high if it is left untreated. Therefore, while there are adverse effects that could arise in both the body and the brain, these effects need to be balanced by the potential beneficial effects on the brain and the potential negative effects of neuroprogression when bipolar disorder is left untreated. A challenge to the field is to therefore acquire enough risk/benefit information for both treatments and the absence of treatments to better guide people with bipolar disorder, their families, and their clinicians to make the best long-term choices. Learning about the precise mechanisms and effects that treatment has on brain structure and function, and also whether there is a particular window during development in which they are optimally used (or most problematic), we could begin to develop more targeted and thoughtful approaches to illness management. This knowledge could serve as a guide for the next generation of studies and build on emerging treatment biological markers to personalize interventions for youth with or at risk for bipolar disorder. The possibility remains that acute interventions with proper medications at a critical point in time will allow for shorter duration of treatment needed, and perhaps neuroprotection or neuro-plastic change that will then eliminate the need for a lifetime of medications (i.e., prevent illness progression and recurrence). For now, practitioners caring for youth with or at risk for bipolar disorder must commit to striving for these youth to achieve maximal remission of symptoms and restoration of function using as few medications as possible.

In addition to neuroimaging, genetic studies offer considerable promises to bet-ter understand the etiology of bipolar disorder, identify treatment markers to personal-ize therapy, and aid in assessing risk and assigning diagnosis. These studies use variable approaches, including familial risk analyses, candidate gene analyses, linkage analyses, and genome-wide association studies (GWASs), as described in Chapter 5. Using single-nucleotide polymorphisms (SNPs) technology, several promising genes have been identi-fied that may contribute to the expression of pediatric bipolar disorder. Although well reviewed in Chapter 5, several of these warrant comment.

As noted in Chapter 5, the gene that encodes the alpha subunit of the L-type cal-cium channel, CACNA1C, has now been identified in two large bipolar GWASs, suggest-ing its likely association with bipolar illness.[22] There is a long history of calcium metabolic abnormalities identified with bipolar illness, although the specific meaning of these find-ings has been elusive. Another example is the discovery that TRANK3 has been found to be more highly expressed after valproic acid is given. Findings like these might indicate changes in the underlying neuropathology or markers of changing neurophysiology in the face of effective treatment. Additional work in this regard might not only clarify the etiology of treatment response but might also identify early response markers to improve treatment efficacy. These two examples suggest the promise of genetic analyses in pediat-ric bipolar disorder. Current and future studies should continue to better define bipolar disorder's polygenic nature. There is no doubt that further—and very large—sequencing studies are warranted.

Another potential benefit from the study of SNPs will be further clarification of diagnosis. For instance, in the largest GWAS of neuropsychiatric disorders to date, indi-viduals with ADHD, autism spectrum disorders, bipolar and major depressive disorders, and schizophrenia were found to have three SNPs significantly linked with respect to shared effects across all five conditions, with one of those SNPs (rs1024582) found mainly associated with bipolar disorder and schizophrenia. Clearly, there are conflicting data over the last decade about whether bipolar disorder and schizophrenia are on a spectrum or are discrete disorders. Although the symptoms appear to cover a spectrum, treatment response to lithium suggests discrete conditions. Cross-disorder findings such as these challenge current diagnostics. Consequently, a component of the future of the study of bipolar disorder is to clarify what, genetically, distinguishes bipolar disorder from other illnesses and also what may be common among them.

Given the inability of genetics to identify a specific link to bipolar illness, an alternative approach has been to attempt to find endophenotypes for bipolar disorder that may more directly map onto genetic variations. Several endophenotypes have been proposed, including measures of circadian rhythm disruption, neurocognitive impairment, and temperament. As discussed in Chapter 5, the expression of bipolar disorder may be tied to genes known to be associated with circadian rhythm functions (CLOCK, PERIOD, VIP). SNPs linked to temperament have been recently uncovered, including several specific SNPs associated with hyperthymic, dysthymic, or irritable temperaments. There are ongoing investigations of SNPs suspected to be linked to delusionality and suicidality. Needed most in this research is replication and verification via much larger samples or alternative endophenotypes that are more predictably linked to specific genetic allelic patterns.

The role of the environment will necessarily be another focus, as there is compelling evidence that environmental risk factors, including early childhood maternal loss, early sexual and/or physical abuse, *T. gondii* infection, and head injury and seizures, contribute to the onset of bipolar disorder. The precise role of these and other (yet unelaborated) environmental stressors is not clear, but the expression of bipolar disorder, although highly heritable (at 80%–85%) is not completely under genetic control. Furthermore, the interaction between genetic susceptibilities and environmental risk factors has not been fully explored in pediatric bipolar disorder. Consequently, understanding environmental factors could provide strategies to interrupt illness onset and progression. In addition, there is promising research with respect to protective environmental interventions: the potential role of LCn-3, an omega fatty acid that may be associated with decreased lifetime prevalence of not only bipolar disorder but also unipolar depression, and the seeming promise of lithium's role in correcting dysregulation in immune-inflammatory signaling homeostasis. These findings are described in Chapter 6.

Conclusions

Ultimately, like other branches of psychiatry, the next advances in understanding the neurobiological basis of pediatric bipolar disorder will involve sophisticated integrative studies across technologies. Continued refinement of the expression of brain processes as they are linked to genetic variability and clinical behaviors in pediatric bipolar disorder require relatively large (probably multisite and multi-investigator) studies that combine technologies to isolate neural and genetic processes underlying specific symptomatic domains. Studies across developmental stages are relatively rare, but they are a critical next step to provide the healthy brain developmental context to interpret findings in bipolar disorder. These longitudinal studies are difficult and expensive, but they offer the best approach to an illness that is lifelong and progressive. As prodromal periods are better defined, preonset treatments can be applied and integrated with these discovery technologies to refine understanding of how the first manic episode (and onset of illness) occurs in order to prevent it. Increasing emphasis on treatment effectiveness across populations and age groups will also play an important next step in the evolution of treatments designed specifically for youth with bipolar illness, not simply extrapolated incompletely from adults with bipolar disorder. Although the challenges facing the field remain significant, progress has been steady. A move into longer term, multitechnology approaches to understanding illness offers the promise of a potential paradigm shift into how we think about pediatric bipolar disorder (and other psychiatric conditions). The future is bright for our people suffering from these conditions; we will undoubtedly continue to make progress.

Author Disclosures

Dr. Johnston has no conflicts to report.

Dr. Adler has received research support from Astra Zeneca, Amylin, Eli Lilly, GlaxoSmithKline, Lundbeck, Martek, Merck, Novartis, Otsuka, Pfizer, Takeda, and Shire. He has been on the lecture bureau for Merck and Sunovion, for which he has received honoraria.

Drs. DelBello and Patino Duran have received research support from each of the following: AstraZeneca, Eli Lilly, Johnson and Johnson, Janssen, Pfizer, Otsuka, Sumitomo, Depression and Bipolar Alternative Treatment Foundation, NIDA, NIMH, NIAAA, NARSAD, GlaxoSmithKline, Merck, Novartis, Sunovion, Lundbeck, Purdue, Somerset, and Shire.

Dr. DelBello has served on the lecture bureau for Bristol-Myers Squibb, Otsuka, and Merck, and as a consultant for Pfizer, Eli Lilly, Dey, Lundbeck, and Sunovion.

Dr. Strakowski serves as data-safety and monitoring board chair for Sunovion, Inc. and Novartis, Inc. He is an EAP consultant to Procter & Gamble and has performed grant reviews for the NIH. He has previously published with Oxford University Press.

References

1. Duffy A. The early natural history of bipolar disorder: what we have learned from longitudinal high-risk research. *Can J Psychiat.* 2010;55(8):477–85.
2. Berk M, Hallam KT, McGorry PD. The potential utility of a staging model as a course specifier: a bipolar disorder perspective. *J Affect Disord.* 2007;100(1–3):279–81.
3. Joshi G, Wilens T. Comorbidity in pediatric bipolar disorder. *Child Adolesc Psychiatr Clin N Am.* 2009;18(2):291–319, vii–viii.
4. Moore CM, Biederman J, Wozniak J, et al. Differences in brain chemistry in children and adolescents with attention deficit hyperactivity disorder with and without comorbid bipolar disorder: a proton magnetic resonance spectroscopy study. *Am J Psychiatry.* 2006;163(2):316–8.
5. Chang K. Adult bipolar disorder is continuous with pediatric bipolar disorder. *Can J Psychiatry.* 2007;52:418–25.

6. Ketter TA, Wang PW. Predictors of treatment response in bipolar disorders: evidence from clinical and brain imaging studies. *J Clin Psychiatry*. 2002;63(Suppl. 3):21–5.

7. Birmaher B, Axelson D, Strober M, et al. Clinical course of children and adolescents with bipolar spectrum disorders. *Arch Gen Psychiatry*. 2006;63:175–83.

8. Fraguas D, Correll CU, Merchán-Naranjo J, et al. Efficacy and safety of second-generation antipsychotics in children and adolescents with psychotic and bipolar spectrum disorders: comprehensive review of prospective head-to-head and placebo-controlled comparisons. *Eur Neuropsychopharmacol*. 2011;21(8):621–45.

9. Miklowitz DJ. A review of evidence-based psychosocial interventions for bipolar disorder. *J Clin Psychiatry*. 2006;67(Suppl. 11):28–33.

10. Clancy C, Collins FS. Patient-Centered Outcomes Research Institute: the intersection of science and health care. *Sci Transl Med*. 2010;2(37):37.

11. Cousins DA, Grunze H. Interpreting magnetic resonance imaging findings in bipolar disorder. *CNS Neurosci Ther*. 2012;18(3):201–7.

12. DelBello MP, Adler CM, Strakowski SM. The neurophysiology of childhood and adolescent bipolar disorder. *CNS Spectr*. 2006;11(4):298–311.

13. Cerullo MA, Adler CM, Delbello MP, Strakowski SM. The functional neuroanatomy of bipolar disorder. *Int Rev Psychiatry*. 2009;21(4):314–22.

14. Deveney CM, Connolly ME, Jenkins SE, et al. Striatal dysfunction during failed motor inhibition in children at risk for bipolar disorder. *Prog Neuropsychopharmacol Biol Psychiatry*. 2012;38(2):127–33.

15. Pavuluri MN, Passarotti A. Neural bases of emotional processing in pediatric bipolar disorder. *Expert Rev Neurother*. 2008;8(9):1381–7.

16. Strakowski SM, Adler CM, Almeida J, et al. The functional neuroanatomy of bipolar disorder: a consensus model. *Bipolar Disord*. 2012;14(4):313–25.

17. Schneider MR, DelBello MP, McNamara RK, Strakowski SM, Adler CM. Neuroprogression in bipolar disorder. *Bipolar Disord*. 2012;14(4):356–74.

18. Vederine FE, Wessa M, Leboyer M, Houenou J. A meta-analysis of whole-brain diffusion tensor imaging studies in bipolar disorder. *J Prog Neuropsychopharmacol Biol Psychiatry*. 2011;35(8):1820–6.

19. Nieto RG, Castellanos FX. A meta-analysis of neuropsychological functioning in patients with early onset schizophrenia and pediatric bipolar disorder. *J Clin Child Adolesc Psychol*. 2011;40(2):266–80.

20. Button KS, Ioannidis JP, Mokrysz C, et al. Power failure: why small sample size undermines the reliability of neuroscience. *Nat Rev Neurosci*. 2013;14(5):365–76.

21. Baykara B, Inal-Emiroglu N, Karabay N, et al. Increased hippocampal volumes in lithium treated adolescents with bipolar disorders: a structural MRI study. *J Affect Disord*. 2012;138(3):433–9. doi:10.1016/j.jad.2011.12.047

22. Craddock N, Sklar P. Genetics of bipolar disorder. Lancet. 2013 May 11;381(9878):1654–62.

Index

choline, 208*t*, 221–22
chromium, 208*t*, 218
chromosomes, 299
cingulate regions
   ACC. *See* anterior cingulate cortex
   in Affective Priming Task, 288
   executive functions and, 295
   fractional anisotropy values in, 265
   HMRS profiles of, 57–58
   mental flexibility and, 294
   mood stabilizers and, 252
   posterior cortex, 283*f*, 284, 286, 294
   reward-related processes in, 315
   working memory and, 292
cingulum bundle, 264–65
circadian rhythm, 7, 100, 101, 190, 357
Clinical Global Impression - Improvement (CGI-I)
   scale, 74*f*, 161, 164
clinical management, 197
clinical staging model, 6–10, 136–140, 348–49
CLOCK gene, 101, 357
clonazepam, 217
clozapine, 167
Cluster A traits, 138
coenzyme Q10 (CoQ10), 207*t*, 214–15
cognition
   academic functioning and, 316
   ACC and, 288, 291
   in ADHD, 326
   affective dysfunction and, 305, 326–27
   in attention, 319
   in BP-1 vs. BP-2, profiles for, 317
   brain pathophysiology and, 288, 291, 297
   early intervention and, 142
   emotion processing and, 282, 284, 295–96, 300, 309, 326
   as endophenotype, 100, 323, 357
   executive functions and, 295–96
   exercise and, 228
   future research on, 325–27
   genetics and, 101, 323–25
   Kraepelin on, 4
   mood dysregulation and, 326
   phenotypes for, 311
   phenotypic heterogeneity in, 94
   research on, 353
   response inhibition and, 289–291
   in reversal learning task, 294
   working memory and, 292–93
cognitive switching, 294–95
cognitive-behavioral therapy (CBT)
   for anxiety and bipolar disorders, 72
   assumptions of, 192, 196
   for CD with bipolar disorder, 66–67
   child and family-focused, 196

   for depression, 199
   in early interventions, 135, 137
   on goal-directed behavior, 190
   for OCD with bipolar disorder, 75
   for ODD, 61
   psychoeducation group based on, 198
   QALY for, 148
   RCTs of, 196–97
   STEP-BD study on, 194, 196
combination drug therapy, 58, 70, 159, 174–79
communication enhancement training (CET), 193–94
community mental health centers (CMHCs), 200
complementary and alternative medicine (CAM), 205–31
complementary treatment, 205
COMT gene, 101, 219, 299
conduct disorder (CD)
   abuse and, 120–21
   with bipolar disorder, 17, 18*t*, 20*t*, 29, 39, 56, 62–68
   criteria for, 51
   genetics in, 65
   MAOA and, 120–21
   MDD and, 63
   pharmacotherapy for, 61, 66
   prevalence of, 17
   prospective studies on, 139
   SUD and, 17, 63–64
   sugary beverages and, 116
Continuous Performance Test (CPT), 290, 319, 323
copy number variations (CNVs), 99–100
corona radiata, 266, 298
corpus callosum, 262–63, 267–68, 298
corticolimbic regions, 244–45, 251, 263, 268–69, 352
cost utility analyses (CUAs), 148
Course and Outcome of Bipolar Youth (COBY) study, 17–19, 44–45
creatine, 215, 297, 339–340
creatine kinase, 215
creatine monohydrate, 207*t*, 214, 215
creatinine, 160*t*
crime, violent, 120–21
cucurmin, 216–17
C vitamin, 214, 220
cycle length
   in adult onset, 5
   amygdala and, 248
   in ASD with bipolar disorder, 80
   chromium and, 218
   definition of, 5
   delay in treatment and, 142
   early vs. late onset and, 20–21*t*

genetics and, 299
light therapy and, 227
in pediatric onset, 22, 82
trauma and, 112
cyclothymia, 9, 45–46, 101, 138–39, 171
cyclothymic temperament, 139
cysteine, 213
cytochrome P450 enzyme, 165
cytokines, 119, 120*f*, 207*t*, 209*t*, 210,
   216–17, 229

Declaration of Helsinki, 141, 149–150
declarative memory, 101, 324
delusions, 19, 20*t*, 101, 182, 357. *See also*
   hallucinations
demyelination, 263
Denmark, 110–11, 115
deoxyribonucleic acid (DNA), 110, 215, 219
Deplin, 220
depression
   acupuncture and, 229–230
   affective temperaments and, 101
   antidepressants for, 113
   CBT for, 199
   CD and, 63
   concentration in, 48
   CUAs for, 148
   DALY for, 148
   diet and, 226
   DMDD and, 49–50
   exercise and, 227–28
   family-focused therapy for, 140
   family studies of, 102, 138
   fatty acids and, 116–17, 140, 210, 357
   genetic studies on, 102, 104, 121
   irritability and, 35
   lithium for, 140
   major. *See* major depressive disorder
   minerals and, 217–18
   multinutrient supplement and, 116
   with multiple sclerosis, 115
   prospective studies on, 139
   psychosis and, 51
   RAINBOW program and, 196
   SAM-e and, 213
   smoking and, 209*t*
   stress and, 112
   sugary beverages and, 116
   vitamins and, 116, 218–224
depressive episodes
   acupuncture and, 229
   ADHD and, 59
   age at onset of, 138
   agitation in, 48
   antidepressants for, 174–76

antipsychotics for, 175
biomarkers of, 244
in clinical staging model, 137–38
diet and, 226
DSM on, 44–45
duration of, 5, 34
"extreme attributions" in, 196
fMRI studies in, 258
gender and, 5
genetic studies on, 104
initial, 6, 46
irritability in, 34–35, 47
lamotrigine for, 175–76
light therapy for, 227
lithium for, 175–76
in OCD with bipolar disorder, 73
OFC for, 174–76
offset of, 15, 46
in OSBP, 42, 44–45
psychosis with, 46–47, 50
psychotherapy in, 196
quetiapine for, 175
SSRIs for, 174
stress and, 112, 190
substance abuse during, 46
SUD and, 7, 9
suicide during, 9, 46
temporal sequence of, 119, 137–38
triggers for, 193, 209*t*, 228–29
developmental disorders, 40, 58
dextroamphetamines, 212–13
DGKH gene, 97*t*, 98
DHH gene, 97*t*, 98
diagnosis
   accurate and timely, 348–350
   "clinically meaningful," 57
   controversy on, 13
   Kraepelin's approach to, 4
Diagnostic Analysis of Nonverbal
   Accuracy (DANVA), 307
*Diagnostic and Statistical Manual of
   Mental Disorders* (*DSM*), xv, 13–16,
   35–44, 137
Diagnostic Interview for Children and
   Adolescents - Revised (DICA-R), 18*t*
Diagnostic Interview for Genetic Studies
   (DIGS), 20*t*
dialectical behavior therapy (DBT), 196–97
diet
   epidemiological studies on, 210, 226
   gluten in, 117, 119, 120*f*
   ketogenic, 209*t*, 226–27
   probiotic, 209*t*, 227
   research on, 115–16, 206, 225–26, 228
   Western, 225–26

puberty and, 5
studies on, 18*t*
of SUD with bipolar disorder, 58, 67–68, 81
Penn Computerized Neuropsychological Battery,
    308
Penn Emotional Acuity Task (PEAT), 308
PERIOD gene, 357
peripheral blood mononuclear cells (PBMCs), 119,
    120*f*
pharmacotherapy. *See also specific drugs*
    brain pathophysiology and, 335, 341–42
    effectivity of, 189
    for maintenance treatment, 176–78
    management strategies for, 156–57, 182–83
    research on, 355–56
phenobarbital, 163
phenytoin, 163
phosphate, 215
phosphatidyl choline, 208*t*, 221
phosphocreatine, 215, 339
phospholipids, 208*t*, 213, 221
phosphorus magnetic resonance spectroscopy
    (PMRS), 214
physical abuse, 76, 112, 136, 191
polycystic ovary syndrome (PCOS), 161, 163
positron emission tomography (PET), 257
posterior association cortex, 264
posterior cingulate cortex, 283*f*, 284, 286, 294
posterior parieto-temporal activity, 290
posttraumatic stress disorder (PTSD)
    ADHD and, 76
    with bipolar disorder, 39, 58, 75–76, 77*f*, 78
    carbamazepine for, 72, 78
    DMDD and, 50
    explosive behavior in, 51
    irritability in, 51
    pharmacotherapy for, 72, 78
    prevalence of, 75
    psychosis and, 40
    psychotherapies for, 78
    SUD and, 75
prefrontal cortices
    ACC and, 286
    ADHD and, 290–92, 295–96
    ADHD with bipolar disorder and, 290, 312
    amygdala and, 245, 251, 256, 264, 269,
        285–87
    antipsychotics and, 337–38, 341*f*
    attention and, 319
    cingulum bundle and, 264
    connections between, 262
    creatine and, 339–340
    development of, 244–46, 252–54
    DHA and, 211
    divalproex and, 261, 339–340, 341*f*

emotion processing and, 259–262, 269, 284–291,
    295–96, 300, 317, 319
executive functions and, 290–91, 295–96,
    313–14
family studies of, 253
fMRI studies of, 259–262
gender and, 252
hippocampus and, 264
illustration of, 283*f*, 341*f*
lamotrigine and, 337–38, 341*f*
lesions of, 251, 259
limbic system and, 245, 305, 313
lithium and, 252, 339–340, 341*f*
MDD and, 254, 261–62
mental flexibility and, 294
mesial temporal structures and, 263–64, 311
mood stabilizers and, 252, 254
motor inhibition and, 321, 336
motor skills and, 291
myo-inositol and, 339
NAA and, 339–340
olanzapine and, 340
pharmacotherapy and, 298, 341
phosphocreatine and, 339
research on, 244, 251–52, 353
response inhibition and, 335
resting-state connectivity in, 296
in reversal learning task, 294
SMD and, 294
sMRI studies of, 251–54
stress and, 269, 353
striatum and, 245, 251, 269
structural integrity of, 299
substance abuse and, 269
uncinate fasciculus and, 264
volume of, 251–54, 269, 298
white matter connecting tracts with, 267
working memory and, 291–93, 311, 316–17
YMRS scores and, 338
ziprasidone and, 338
pregnancy
    divalproex and, 163
    fetal asphyxia during, 120
    fetal neural tube defects during, 163, 219
    lithium and, 159
    maternal health during, 110–11
    pharmacotherapy during, 179–180
    stress during, 110–11
    vitamins during, 219, 222
pregnenolone, 217
premotor cortex, 292
preschoolers, 41, 65–66
probiotic diet, 209*t*, 227
processing speed, 311, 324
pro-inflammatory agents, 120*t*, 140